Physiotherapy
a psychosocial approac

Second Edition

D1129017

Physiotherapy
a psychosocial approach

Second Edition

Edited by

Sally French BSc, MSc(psych), MSc(Soc), MSCP, Dip TP

Senior lecturer, Department of Health Studies, Brunel University College, Isleworth, UK
Freelance lecturer, writer, researcher and physiotherapist

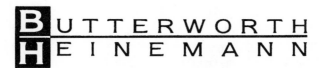

Butterworth-Heinemann
Linacre House, Jordan Hill, Oxford OX2 8DP
A division of Reed Educational and Professional Publishing Ltd

℞ A member of the Reed Elsevier plc group

OXFORD   BOSTON   JOHANNESBURG
MELBOURNE   NEW DELHI   SINGAPORE

First published 1992
Second Edition 1997

© Reed Educational and Professional Publishing Ltd 1997

British Library Cataloguing in Publication Data
A catalogue record for this book is available from the British Library

Library of Congress Cataloguing in Publication Data
A catalogue record for this book is available from the Library of Congress

ISBN 0 7506 2608 9

Typeset by David Gregson Associates, Beccles, Suffolk
Printed and bound in Great Britain by Martins the Printers, Berwick upon Tweed

Contents

Contributors

Richard J. Butler BSc, MSc, PhD
Consultant Clinical Psychologist, Leeds Community and Mental Health Services NHS Trust. Honorary Lecturer in Sports Psychology, University of Leeds, Leeds, UK. Visiting Research Fellow in Sports Psychology, Chichester Institute, Chichester, UK

Michael Calnan BSc, MSc, PhD
Professor of Sociology of Health Studies, Director of the Centre for Health Service Studies, University of Kent, Canterbury, UK

Tina Everett Grad Dip Phys, MCSP, SRP, FETC
Head of Physiotherapy Services, Oxfordshire Mental Healthcare NHS Trust, Warneford Hospital, Oxford, UK

Sally French BSc, MSc (Psych), MSc (Soc), MCSP, Dip TP
Senior Lecturer, Department of Health Studies, Brunel University College, Isleworth, UK. Freelance lecturer, writer, researcher and physiotherapist

Stephanie Kitchener BSc, MSc, MCSP
Senior Physiotherapist, Royal Free Hospital, London, UK

Paul Lawrence BEd, MPhil
Senior Lecturer of Students with Learning Difficulties, North Tyneside College of Further Education, North Tyneside, UK

Mary F. McAteer PhD, MEd, MCSP, MICSP, Dip TP
Lecturer, School of Physiotherapy, University College Dublin, Dublin, Ireland

Susan Neville MA, MCSP, Dip TP
Principal Lecturer, Department of Health Studies, University of East London, London, UK

Jane S. Owen Hutchinson BA, MA, MA (Ed), Grad Dip Phys, Cert Ed., Cert Health Ed., Dip TP, Dip Rehab Couns
Manager, Physiotherapy Support Services, Royal National Institute for the Blind, London, UK

M. Jane Riddoch PhD, CPsychol, MCSP
Senior Lecturer, School of Psychology, University of Birmingham, Birmingham, UK

Helen Roberts BA, Maîtrise, DPhil
Head of Childcare Research and Development, Barnardo's, Barkingside, UK. Honorary Senior Fellow, Social Statistics Research Unit, City University, London, UK

Julius Sim BA, MSc, PhD, MCSP
Principal Lecturer, School of Health and Social Sciences, Coventry University, Coventry, UK

Janet M. Simpson PhD, MSc, CPsychol, AFBPsS
Senior Lecturer in the Rehabilitation of Elderly People, St George's Hospital Medical School, London, UK

John Swain BSc, PGCE, MSc, PhD
Reader in Disability Studies, Faculty of Health, Social Work and Education, University of Northumbria, Newcastle-upon-Tyne, UK

Ayesha Vernon BA, Cert Ed, PhD
Researcher in Disability Studies and Multiple Oppression, Peterborough, UK

Jan Walmsley BA, PGCE, MSc, PhD
Senior Lecturer, School of Health and Social Welfare, Open University, UK

Christopher A. Whittaker MEd, DAES, ACP, TCert
Senior Lecturer, Faculty of Health, Social Work and Education, University of Northumbria, Newcastle-upon-Tyne, UK

Preface

This new edition of *Physiotherapy: a psychosocial approach* has been completely revised and updated to meet the continuing needs of physiotherapy students and practitioners. Like its predecessor it draws together a wide range of topics, mostly in the fields of psychology and sociology, and applies them to physiotherapy practice. Many of the authors are physiotherapists themselves and are, therefore, in a unique position to apply their theoretical expertise to physiotherapy. Although the book is written for physiotherapists, most of the topics are relevant to other health workers. The book aims to be informative, analytical and stimulating; it is well referenced for those readers who wish to pursue individual topics in greater depth.

The book is divided into four sections. In the first section psychosocial issues which impinge upon health care are examined. These include broad topics, such as inequalities in health, and specific topics such as ageism and health care for people from ethnic minorities. The second section focuses on the experience of illness and disability including, stress, pain, lay beliefs about health and illness and death, dying and bereavement. Section three explores communication in physiotherapy practice and includes chapters on clinical interviewing, counselling and interpersonal communication. Section four examines various psychosocial aspects of physiotherapy practice including health education, child development, ethical decision-making and psychological treatment in physiotherapy practice.

Several new authors, all of whom are experts in their fields, have contributed to this edition. Some new topics have also been included to reflect changing ideas and practice; Chapter 7 considers the attitudes of health professionals to disabled people, Chapter 24 considers the changing roles of physiotherapists who work with clients with learning difficulties and Chapter 27 poses challenging questions about disabled people and sexuality.

I would like to thank all the authors for contributing chapters to this book. Thanks are also extended to Caroline Makepeace from Butterworth-Heinemann for her constant encouragement, and to all the physiotherapists, physiotherapy lecturers and students who have given me useful and positive feedback on the first edition. I would also like to thank my sister, Jo Laing, whose expertise as an English teacher was invaluable when editing the text and Jill Whitehouse for allowing me to use an expanded version of the following article: French, S. (1994) Attitudes of Health Professionals towards Disabled People: a review of the literature. *Physiotherapy*. **80**(10), 687–693.

Most of all I would like to thank the many physiotherapy students I have taught over the years who have enabled me to gain the expertise and confidence I needed to write and edit this book.

Sally French

Psychosocial Influences on Health Care Practice

1

Society and the changing nature of illness and disease

Sally French

Before approximately 10 000 BC people lived as hunter-gatherers, moving around in small groups without any settled agriculture. Although there are few reliable records from this period, it is believed that the infectious diseases were not a common cause of death. Life expectancy was, nonetheless, short, due to starvation, hunting accidents and exposure. The first agricultural revolution occurred around 8000 BC resulting in large, more settled communities where crops were cultivated and animals domesticated. This increased the density of the population, creating favourable conditions for the spread of infectious diseases which were to remain the main health hazard of human beings until recent times (Gray, 1993). There were frequent episodes of plague, cholera, dysentery and typhoid, but although these epidemics and pandemics were very dramatic, giving rise to enormous loss of life in an extremely short space of time, they probably had less effect on overall mortality than endemic diseases such as tuberculosis.

Starvation was also a major cause of death, though according to Sharpe (1987), it did not occur on a large scale in England after 1625, as by then agricultural practice had resulted in the production of greater supplies of food for the population. Malnutrition, however, was extremely common creating great susceptibility to infection. In addition the low resistance of infected individuals meant that diseases took a longer time to subside resulting in large scale spread.

Malnutrition, poverty and disease are intimately related. Xerophthalmus, which is a common cause of blindness among children in developing countries, is associated with malnutrition and infectious disease. Sanders (1985) explains that when recovering from such diseases as chickenpox and measles, the body needs greater quantities of vitamin A and if this is not available visual impairment results. Similarly diarrhoea, which is the most common cause of childhood death in many parts of the developing world, is more likely to affect malnourished children and in turn leads to further malnutrition through anorexia and loss of nutrients. Malnutrition and poverty are also 'transmitted'; a malnourished mother will tend to have small sickly babies who will be susceptible to infection. There may also be difficulty with breast feeding. This early deprivation, both before and after birth, can affect the health status of the individual throughout life. In addition, if large numbers of people are ill or seriously malnourished there may be an insufficient workforce to provide enough food to meet the needs of the community.

Infections pass from one person to another most easily and rapidly in overcrowded conditions. This explains why many diseases in modern industrial societies are not widely prevalent until children go to school, as their first years are spent mainly within the confines of the small nuclear family. In earlier times and in many developing countries today, diseases such as measles and whooping cough occur in younger children who live in poor and overcrowded conditions. Their immaturity, together with malnourishment, lowers their resistance, leading the disease to run a more severe course, frequently resulting in death.

Until the latter part of the seventeenth century in Britain, any tendency for the population to increase was kept in check by malnutrition and the infectious diseases. The birth rate was high but, when in a situation of poverty, this can lead to an increase in mortality; it puts pressure on the mother's health and predisposes to small sickly babies who will only be breast fed until the next one arrives, leading to malnutrition (Gray, 1993). Tuberculosis was very common and there were frequent 'mortality crises' brought about by pandemics and epidemics. After about 1680 the population started to increase, at first modestly, but later very rapidly. Between approximately 1750 and 1850, for example, the population of England rose from 6 to 15 million. The rise in population was due to increased fertility and reduced mortality. Increased fertility was the main factor until 1870 but after that decreased mortality became more important (Royle, 1987).

There has been much speculation regarding the factors responsible for the rise in fertility at this time, including more marriage, earlier marriage, better nutrition and healthier mothers (Daunton, 1995). Various theories have also been put forward to account for the decline of infectious diseases, including more education, improved personal hygiene and medical intervention, but it is commonly believed that improved nutrition and public hygiene were most important. Chinn (1995) comments on the bad housing, overflowing sewers, polluted air and unhealthy burial places which existed during the nineteenth century. In addition large numbers of people used the same toilet and well and the water was frequently contaminated. It is interesting to note that at the time of the sanitary reforms of the mid-nineteenth century it was believed that disease was spread by foul smells and gases, illustrating that theory does not necessarily have to precede effective practice (Chinn, 1995).

Sanders (1985) lists various factors which improved health in Britain after 1850 including purification of water, efficient disposal of sewage, provision of safe milk, improved hygiene, better nutrition, improved living and working conditions and, to a lesser extent, preventative and curative medical measures. Diseases such as typhus and cholera declined (Chinn, 1995) and other diseases, such as syphilis and scarlet fever, became less severe. There is also no doubt that increased political awareness and greater opportunity for a larger section of society to become politically active were very important. Despite these improvements the average life expectancy at birth in England in the decade 1881–1890 was only 43.6 years and it was far lower than this in some parts of the country (Chinn, 1995). This was a slight improvement on the 1820s when life expectancy at birth in Britain was 39 years (Daunton, 1995).

Despite the overall increase in fertility and reduction in mortality, the health status of different sections of society was very uneven, a situation which persists today (Jacobson *et al.*, 1991). Thus health depends not only on wealth but on how that wealth is distributed, who has the power and how society is ordered. Various social changes which eventually reduced poverty and increased wealth caused great hardship to certain sections of society for an extended period of time. The enclosure of common land in the nineteenth century, for example, resulted in greater production of food but also forced poor people off the land which had been their only livelihood. Similarly, the industrial revolution eventually created wealth, part of which was used to improve social conditions, but the centralization of work forced people from cottage industries in the countryside to factories in the cities where they worked long, hard hours for little reward and where overcrowding at home and inhumane work practices created ideal conditions for the development of illness and the spread of infection.

Although reforms were gradually made this did not occur without substantial opposition, and foremost in the minds of employers was the need to maintain a healthy workforce to increase production, rather than any humanitarian concerns. Similarly war in recent British history facilitated the development of medical services in order to ensure that present and future generations would be fit enough to fight. The Emergency Medical Service of the Second World War had a strong influence on the ideology and structure of the National Health Service.

From 1870 there was a rapid decline in mortality from the infectious diseases in Britain and the Western World. This marked the start of the slow move away from infectious disease towards chronic disease which comprise the main health problems faced in industrial countries today (Gray, 1993). The infections did, however, remain a considerable health hazard until recent times and even now they are by no means eliminated. Many air-borne diseases, such as influenza and measles, still have a high incidence though they rarely give rise to large scale mortality or serious morbidity. Rapid international travel makes the spread of infections easier, however, and new infections still arise as the development of AIDS so clearly illustrates.

In Britain and other wealthy countries, the fall in the mortality rate from 1870 coincided with a fall in the birth rate resulting in a gradual slowing of population growth. Since the Second World War it has remained virtually static though subject to fluctuation. The reasons for the decline in fertility remain controversial. It is likely that as child mortality fell parents became more confident that their children would survive, and it has been suggested by Sanders (1985) and Sagan (1987) that various economic and political changes, including compulsory education, restriction of child employment and the development of state benefit, made children less of an economic asset to their parents. How far children were an economic advantage is, however, a matter for debate. The high incidence of infanticide in Europe until the last quarter of the nineteenth century, which Turshen (1989) suggests was a way of keeping the population in check, throws doubt on these ideas, as do the large numbers of children abandoned at this time. Education, improved self-esteem, choice and a range of opportunities to pursue in life have all been found to reduce the desire for early and prolonged motherhood (The Child Mothers, *Horizon*, BBC, 1990).

Health and illness in Britain today

In Britain today heart disease, respiratory disease and cancer account for about 70% of all deaths. A similar pattern exists in other industrial countries, although there are many interesting differences in the incidence of specific diseases. Most of the increase in the incidence of these diseases can be attributed to the altered age structure of the population as they are all basically diseases of old age. This is not to imply that they are inevitable and that nothing can be done to reduce their incidence as they appear to be related to behavioural and social factors such as eating habits, pollution, cigarette smoking, alcohol consumption, lack of exercise and the maldistribution of wealth, which in principle can all be changed (Jacobson *et al.*, 1991). The various factors causing disease, illness and impairment in contemporary Britain, as well as their uneven distribution among groups within society, will be discussed in detail in Chapter 2.

A quarter of all deaths in Britain are the result of cancer and cancer of the lung is by far the most common cancer, claiming 24 671 lives in England and Wales in 1988 (Jacobson *et al.*, 1991). It is known to be closely associated with cigarette smoking. The other major cancers are those of the large intestine, breast and stomach. Pneumonia is the most common fatal respiratory disease. This is not surprising as frail, elderly people with underlying respiratory pathology are particularly susceptible.

There are about 550 deaths per year resulting from industrial accidents in Britain, and at least 500 000 industrial injuries (Jacobson *et al.*, 1991). Industry is also fully or partially responsible for many diseases such as asbestosis and bronchitis, though this is notoriously difficult to prove. Turshen (1989) believes that industry resists public health regulations and that it welcomes the germ theory of disease, which became dominant at the end of the nineteenth century, as it conceptualizes disease as biological and arising randomly rather than being the product of social and political processes.

Although accidents account for relatively few deaths, loss in terms of years of life is very great, far exceeding deaths from cancer. Years of life lost is calculated by subtracting the age at which the individual dies from the mean age of death for that society (Gray, 1993). Motor cycle accidents, in particular, account for a large number of years lost in the Western World although in developing countries the infectious diseases are much more important. 'Accident' is, perhaps, the wrong word to use because such deaths are not randomly distributed throughout the community and can usually be explained.

So far this discussion has focused on mortality. Measuring morbidity and tracing changes over time is far more difficult. Unlike mortality, illness is subjective, meaning different things to different individuals. People vary widely in whether or not they use the health service, how much they use it and how they deal with their symptoms from day to day. Lack of historical data makes any coherent discussion of past morbidity patterns difficult and is complicated by the way in which disease has been classified at different times. For example, much is written about 'sweating sickness' which is not a category used or understood today (Gray, 1993). Scarlet fever and diphtheria were classified as one disease until 1855 and the category 'old age' was in use until the beginning of the twentieth century, but it is no longer considered to be a cause of death.

The diseases which are now in evidence are largely chronic and are associated with old age, although there is much evidence to suggest that the cause is partly social and behavioural. These diseases include heart disease, respiratory disease, cancer, stroke, circulatory diseases, neurological diseases and arthritis. They are not all life threatening. Most physical impairment is associated with these diseases with only a tiny minority of disabled people having hereditary or congenital conditions. The latter tend to be emphasized, however, giving the false impression that disabled people comprise a small minority within society. The number of disabled people does, of course, depend on how disability is defined. Reports by Bone and Meltzer (1989) and Martin *et al.* (1989) estimate the number to be approximately 6 million, though many believe this to be an under-estimation. It is clear from the report by Martin *et al.* (1989) that most impairment is acquired in later life.

People with mental illness comprise a large percentage of the patient population today. Mental disorder is the second most common reason for visiting the general practitioner (Jacobson *et al.*, 1991). Whether there has been an increase in mental illness, or what the incidence of mental illness was in the past is, however, impossible to say. Psychiatry is a young science and there is still enormous difficulty regarding classification and categorization of the various symptoms and syndromes. Although the classification system has steadily improved, reliability is still far from perfect (Davison and Neale, 1990). Rosenhan (1980), in his famous study, demonstrated that psychiatric workers could not distinguish mentally ill from 'normal' people.

Mental illness can be viewed in biological, psychological and social terms (Tyrer and Steinberg, 1987; Pilgrim and Rogers, 1993; Donaghy, 1995). Szasz (1961) believes that mental illness is nothing more nor less than a myth, Laing (1967) that it is a type of super-sanity, Braginsky *et al.*(1969) that it is a form of malingering and Goffman (1961) that it is a convenient way of removing from society those whom powerful people regard as undesirable. Pilgrim and Rogers (1993) state that people from certain ethnic minorities and women are more likely to be labelled mentally ill than others, and Davison and Neale (1990) note that a diagnosis of schizophrenia is more often given to working class people living in cities than to others.

Confinement in stark impoverished institutions and the stigma attached to the label of mental illness are, in themselves, recognized as being sufficient to produce or worsen disturbed behaviour, thought or feeling. The stigma will also determine people's willingness to acknowledge psychiatric symptoms within themselves as well as their readiness to seek help. Distinguishing 'normal' from 'abnormal' behaviour and mental processes is, however, fraught with problems and varies from time to time and from place to place. Homosexuality, for example, has been defined as an illness, as a criminal activity and, more recently, as normal behaviour. People in severe poverty may not have the luxury of attending to their psychological needs and may be part of a culture which considers such 'symptoms' as tiredness, depression and anxiety a normal part of life.

Before 1850 it was common for those classified as 'mad' to live either with their families or in workhouses with others considered deviant such as criminals and beggars (Jones, 1993). However, some private madhouses for the rich were established as early as the fifteenth century. There were many scandals centred around these madhouses where it was possible for people to have their relatives admitted and confined (Jones, 1993). By the mid-eighteenth century asylums specifically for the insane were opened with public funds, as well as with money from religious philanthropists. The inmates were frequently chained and treatments included beating, purging, semi-starvation, and confinement. Gradually a more humanitarian approach, termed 'moral treatment' was practised. In the York Retreat opened in 1796, for example, the treatment consisted of good food, fresh air, occupation and exercise (Jones, 1993). It is described by Davison and Neale (1990):

> 'York Retreat was established on a country estate. It provided the mentally ill with a quiet religious atmosphere in which to live, work and relax. They discussed their difficulties with attendants, worked in the garden and took walks in the countryside'.

This situation was not to continue. In the second half of the nineteenth century a large number of public mental asylums were erected and mental disturbance was 'medicalized'; the asylums were termed 'mental hospitals' and the people in them 'patients'. The number of people confined to these institutions rapidly increased and, as they did, the philosophy and treatment practices, which were initially humanitarian, were gradually eroded resulting in stark institutions of confinement and harsh treatment. The situation became progressively worse, for as the numbers rose the asylums became more expensive to run leading to cost cutting measures rendering conditions even worse. In 1850 the total number of people in England and Wales confined to mental asylums was 7140, by 1930 this figure had risen to 119 659 and by 1961 to over 130 000. The number of people in each institution also rose from a few hundred in 1850 to one or two thousand by the mid-twentieth century. Although the number of institutions rose, for example from 24 in 1850 to 98 in 1930, this was insufficient to accommodate the many people classified as insane (Jones, 1993).

The rate of insanity rose from 12.66 per 10 000 to 19.12 per 10 000 between 1844 and 1960 (U205 Course Team, Open University 1985a). This huge expansion probably had more to do with industrialization, which created an unwillingness or inability to tolerate unusual or deviant behaviour, than a real increase in mental disturbance. The growing influence and power of the medical profession at this time may also have been influential. Wide-scale concern for people incarcerated in mental handicap and psychiatric hospitals did not occur until the second half of the twentieth century. These hospitals are now being closed and, to some extent, intellectual disability and mental illness are undergoing 'demedicalization' although many criticize the way in which this is taking place and are sceptical about the motives behind it. (For more detail on institutions and community care, the reader is referred to Chapter 3.)

Health and illness in developing countries today

In many developing countries today, birth, death and morbidity are poorly documented making accurate statistics impossible. Nevertheless, it is clear that their health status is similar to that of industrial countries, such as Britain, 200 years ago, with high infant mortality, low life expectancy, malnutrition and a high incidence of infectious diseases such as tuberculosis and measles. It is also interesting to note that because of the large size of the population in developing countries, they also experience more deaths from 'Western' diseases such as cancer and stroke than in the West. Although some improvement in the health status of developing countries has occurred it has been much slower than that of developed countries, thus the gap between them has widened.

In this chapter individual developing countries will not be discussed, although in reality they show considerable variation. In Sri Lanka, for example, the gross national product (the total output of a national economy expressed in monetary terms) is low but the health of the population is relatively good due to equitable distribution of resources. In some richer countries the health of certain sections of society are far worse than that experienced in Sri Lanka (U502 Course Team, Open University, 1985b).

At the present time the population of the developing countries is growing much faster than that of the developed world. In 1990 approximately three-quarters of the world's population lived in the developing countries and this figure is expected to rise considerably by the turn of the century (Gray, 1993). As noted above, the population of Britain went through a similar period of growth in the nineteenth century. This pattern of low to high growth, eventually returning to low levels again, has been termed the 'demographic transition' (Gray, 1993). The industrial countries have reached the end of this transition and are now experiencing low mortality and low fertility rates resulting in an ageing population. The developing countries, on the other hand, are at the earlier stage of population growth which, together with high mortality rates, has given rise to a population with a large number of young people and relatively few old people.

Much 'victim blaming' occurs in discussion of developing countries. On the surface it seems only common sense for people in poverty to restrict the size of their families, the reasons for not doing so are often put down to ignorance, lack of education and irresponsibility. Having a large family may, however, be an advantage when in a situation of poverty, children can help with everyday chores and even earn money or goods from a young age. They may be the parents' only insurance against destitution when old due to lack of pensions and other state provisions. People with larger families may be entitled to more land and there is always the possibility of one child obtaining a good job which will raise the living standards of the whole family. Thus population growth can be viewed as a symptom of poverty rather than the cause of it. Sanders (1985) points out that poor families in India must have 6.5 children to be 95% sure that one son will survive. He believes that a decline in mortality is almost a necessity for a decline in fertility. According to Sagan (1987) economic growth also leads to better educated women who tend to become pregnant later and who have ambitions other than motherhood.

Much attention is given to developing countries at times of acute food shortages. These episodes are usually interpreted in terms of drought, poor agricultural practice, war, ignorance and religious ideologies which prohibit or restrict contraception and encourage population growth. Although some of these factors may be important, what is often forgotten is that people in the developing countries are already seriously malnourished or ill and it therefore takes little to reduce them to starvation. Maldistribution, rather than the lack of resources, is often the root cause of famine, many people simply do not have sufficient money to buy available food. Such inequality lies within developing countries as well as between them and developed countries. There may be discrimination on the grounds of class, gender and religious affiliation, with most of the wealth, including the best land, being owned by foreign capitalists and elite groups within society.

Turshen (1989) points out that the large, powerful food industries of the developed world have contributed to the food shortages and malnutrition of developing countries by using available land for non-arable crops; tea and coffee, animal feed and luxury goods for export. Some developing countries export more food than they import, or exchange it for commodities which only the elite can afford. The development of a world market has meant that foreign industries have destroyed or undermined those of developing countries. It is worth remembering that:

> 'The gulf in wealth between rich and poor countries is so great that the 10% or so of population growth attributable to the industrial countries will consume approximately the same volume of the world's natural resources as the 90% of increase located in the Third World countries'. (U205 Course Team, Open University, 1985b)

Despite the similarity of poverty and disease in many developing countries to that of industrial countries 200 years ago, many have argued that the origins of the problem are dissimilar. As the industrial revolution grew and industrial trade increased, so too did colonization. The colonies served the interests of the colonial powers, not the indigenous populations, which led to the stripping of their wealth and the use of fertile land to grow crops for export (Gray, 1993).

The colonists evicted many people from the land, working the new plantations with slave labour. They also introduced many new viruses and bacteria into these countries. Although there is much controversy, many believe that the rich industrial countries continue to create and maintain poverty in the developing countries. As Sanders (1985) puts it '... the over-development of the one depends on and creates the under-development of the other'.

The medical contribution

The view that medicine made a major contribution to improvements in health of the British population, by controlling infectious diseases, has been disputed. The reason for this scepticism is that much of the decline in mortality had occurred before any effective treatment was available and was due to improved diet and social conditions. McKeown (1979) and Sagan (1987) provide a great deal of evidence to illustrate this point. Mortality from tuberculosis, for example, declined sharply before the introduction of antibiotics or the BCG inoculation.

McKeown (1979) illustrates a similar pattern of decline for many other infectious diseases including poliomyelitis, measles, whooping cough and diphtheria. In the case of some of these diseases, in particular poliomyelitis, diphtheria and tuberculosis, medicine does appear to have had some effect as mortality rates dropped more sharply after medical measures were introduced. Royle (1987) notes that the incidence of smallpox declined dramatically after the introduction of compulsory inoculation in 1871 although Sagan (1987) remains sceptical as the disease was already declining rapidly. For other diseases, for example measles and whooping cough, the decline in mortality has been no greater since the introduction of inoculation than it was before, making an assessment of the medical contribution difficult.

McKeown (1995) notes that with regard to diarrhoea, cholera and dysentery, 95% of the decline in incidence had occurred before intravenous therapy was introduced in the 1930s and that medical treatment had no influence on the decline of typhus and typhoid. Sagan (1987) believes that 'much of public health practice is instituted after the problem has already been solved' and Turshen (1989) states that 'medical efficiency was discovered when it was already largely irrelevant'. However, earlier medical intervention may not have helped very much as it is relatively ineffective if nutrition and environmental conditions are seriously inadequate. Turshen (1989) believes that it is wasteful to concentrate on a particular disease rather than on the underlying social, political and economic organization of that society. He refers to vaccines as 'a quick fix' and suggests that improvement in living standards and nutrition would help to eliminate many diseases.

It must also be said that some of the infectious diseases which medicine has, in a small way, helped to reduce, were always rare. McKeown (1979) points out that before the First World War tetanus was only responsible for seven deaths per million and both poliomyelitis and smallpox were relatively uncommon diseases. Thus the reduction or eradication of such diseases, though important, had little effect on overall mortality or morbidity rates.

McKeown has been criticized for focusing exclusively on the infectious diseases and the biomedical role of medicine rather than medicine's role in prevention and the alleviation of symptoms. He also says little about the development of anaesthetics and aseptic procedures in the nineteenth century. Despite these omissions his ideas have not been seriously undermined.

How far medical intervention helps to prevent, control and reduce suffering from illness, disease and impairment today is an issue of much dispute. Sagan (1987) points out that there is no relationship between expenditure on health care and health, and Sanders (1985) considers that the training of health professionals is unnecessarily long and that they have too much power.

Sagan (1987) states that most medical procedures have never been adequately evaluated and that there is little evidence that expensive provision, such as coronary care units, make any difference to survival or recovery rates. He complains of the over use of antibiotics and surgical procedures, such as Caesarian section and hysterectomy, and believes that widespread screening does more harm than good by creating stress and labelling people as ill, thereby actually creating illness. Turshen (1989) makes the point that screening, when used to uncover stigmatizing conditions, such as AIDS, can be used unfairly to discriminate against people. Disabled people have also voiced their concerns about the damaging and irrelevant treatment they have received (Swain et al., 1993; French, 1994). McKeown (1979) believes that, with the exception of dentistry, '... there is no wholly effective treatment for the non-fatal diseases which trouble people from day to day', though he acknowledges advances in many areas of medicine including obstetric practice, replacement surgery and genetics. There has also been success with some of the rare forms of cancer, and the drugs used in psychiatric practice have enabled many mentally ill people to lead independent and productive lives.

There has also been much criticism of medical care in developing countries (Coleridge, 1993). Medical services have been patterned on those of industrial countries with an orientation towards cure rather than prevention. Although medical technology has had some success in alleviating disease, the underlying causes remain unchallenged. Large sums of money have been spent on sophisticated teaching hospitals where indigenous health workers tend to congregate. Sanders (1985) states that the cost of construction of one teaching hospital in Zambia could have been used to build 250 health centres in the countryside where most people live. He concludes that their own traditional practices and practitioners have been discredited and believes that for health care to be successful in developing countries it must be demystified and democratic and carried out by ordinary local people.

Developing countries lose far more doctors and nurses than they gain through emigration and frequently cannot afford to pay such highly trained people. In parts of India children as young as nine are taught to recognize the signs and symptoms of the common diseases and are given the responsibility for educating people in their community and making sure they are immunized (All Our Children, BBC1, 1990).

Various suggestions have been put forward regarding how medicine should change in order to address the political, social and behavioural origins of illness, disease and impairment. McKeown (1979) believes that there should be specialist doctors of environmental health to investigate and control the many health hazards that are present in all aspects of daily life. He is convinced that far more weight should be given to the social origins of ill-health in medical education and that patients' needs outside hospital should be addressed more fully. Similarly Finkelstein (1993) advocates the transfer of disability issues from The Department of Health to The Department of the Environment.

Tudar Hart (1984) agrees that doctors should abandon their traditional role, of merely attempting to cure disease once it has occurred, but rather should strive to conserve the health of the entire population. To illustrate doctors' passivity he points out that even though diphtheria toxoid was available from 1913, doctors still concentrated their efforts on treating the disease which cost the lives of thousands of children. Similarly, although it is known that cigarette smoking is one of the major health hazards of our time, this knowledge has not been reflected in clinical practice. Tudar Hart describes the role of doctors as one of 'shopkeepers passively responding to sick customers' and urges them to become 'active guardians' of their registered populations. He advocates a large medical team, including people with social knowledge and skills, and an expansion of preventative medicine and health education which, he contends, should be a central component of the medical curriculum. He believes that we need '… a new kind of doctor, with new functions within a new structure'.

Turshen (1989) believes that the split between clinical medicine and public health is a great obstacle and that the education of health professionals and others should be integrated. He thinks all health professionals should be educated in the social sciences, advocates integrated research which includes a social perspective, and urges health workers to be sceptical of science.

Others are more critical of medicine. Illich (1995), one of the main critics, views the medical profession, not as an altruistic body orientated to the needs of sick and disabled people, but as a self-interested monopoly which creates illness and dependency giving rise to 'the medicalization of everyday life'. He believes that medical rhetoric and impressive technology have fostered the false impression that medicine is highly effective.

Illich believes that medicine has done more harm than good by creating a large amount of iatrogenic disease – disease which is caused by medicine. He view iatrogenesis in physical terms, for example addiction to barbiturates, surgical accident, unnecessary treatment and infection contracted while in hospital, and in social and psychological terms, for example dependence on medical professionals, the de-skilling of people with regard to the management of illness and the 'medicalization' of everyday aspects of life, such as birth and death, which he believes reduces people's ability to cope and fosters unhealthy responses. His views are echoed by many disabled people including Oliver (1993) and Davis (1993). In addition it is now queried whether mental illness and learning disability should ever have been described in medical terms. McKeown (1979) believes that, 'doctors have always tended to over-estimate the effectiveness of their intervention and to under-estimate the risks'.

In contrast to this, Navarro (1995) puts no blame on medical professionals with regard to medical practice, but rather views them as pawns in a capitalist system which values profit more than health. He believes that if there is a conflict of interest between health and capital accumulation, then health will always come last. Ideas and ideologies which conflict with capitalism are likewise suppressed and neglected in education and research, and decision-making is heavily weighted in favour of powerful groups within society. Thus dangerous industrial processes may be allowed to continue in order to ensure high profits, regardless of the health consequences for people carrying them out. Cigarette smoking, which is known to cause thousands of premature deaths every year, is still promoted, people are encouraged to eat starchy food, which leads to obesity, and poor housing, low incomes, unemployment and stressful environments persist regardless of the effect they have on health.

Attempts to improve health are invariably focused on the individual and his or her behaviour, a process which Ryan refers to as 'victim blaming'. Navarro (1995) and others such as Doyal (1983, 1995) believe that medicine is an agent of the state treating illness, disease and impairment as it arises rather than confronting the underlying causes thus maintaining the status quo. To take a political and social, rather than a medical approach to the problems of illness, disease and impairment would obviously be more expensive than the provision of a health service and would disrupt power relationships within society on which capitalism is based.

Turshen (1989) agrees that clinical medicine does not threaten vested interests as a public health approach would and believes that the germ theory of disease maintains the political and social status quo. He believes that immunization campaigns are, 'only as good as the analysis of the political situation in which they are mounted'. Turshen views access to health as access to education, employment and decision-making, not merely admission to medical care. Clearly health, illness, impairment and disease are tied as much to sociology, politics and history as they are to biology. Yet introducing sociology and politics into medical and paramedical education is problematic, for as well as broadening professionals' views it also challenges fundamental assumptions about medicine on which practice is based.

McKeown (1979) thinks that to tell students at the start of their medical education that most patients are not cured by medicine and that health does not primarily depend on medical intervention is like a 'slap in the face', and Sanders (1985) believes that, 'it is not in the interests of the medical profession to examine, and still less to confront, the fundamental social roots of illness'. The introduction of a social perspective into medical and paramedical education has been slow to develop, though May and Clarke (1980) believe that its inclusion is one of the most striking developments in medical education in recent times.

Despite this, sociology is still a Cinderella subject in medical and para-medical education, with few hours being allocated to it when compared with disciplines like anatomy and physiology. Its integration with other subject areas also tends to be poor, emphasizing its peripheral status. Sociology in medicine is usually perceived in terms of providing a context in which to consider 'real' biological medicine rather than being a central component of medicine, and because of the breadth of sociology when applied to health, illness, disease and impairment, the more contro-versial issues can easily be avoided. This is especially so if it is merged with psychology under the title of 'behavioural sciences'. Sociological concepts are complex and if taught superficially they can easily reinforce prejudices and stereotypes rather than dispel them.

It is interesting to speculate on why sociology has found its place in medical and paramedical education at all. It may be an attempt to give these professions a more human face, in the light of growing criticism from patients regarding the interpersonal behaviour of professionals, though it has been suggested that this more humanistic style may merely be a tactic for getting patients to comply and conform now that the old authoritarian approach is unacceptable (Norell, 1987). The growing popularity of alternative medicine, whose practitioners have tended to take a more 'holistic' approach, is also posing a threat to orthodox medi-cine in the competition for patients.

Conclusion

Where does all this leave the physiotherapist? Turshen (1989) believes that both practice and education need to be radically transformed if health is to be improved substantially. He states:

> '… we need a radical transformation of public health work and the epidemiology that supports it so that it is no longer orientated to the control of single diseases. Concepts of complex social prevention, the integration of social science in medicine, concepts of social class, knowledge of political economy, and the goals of equity and access must inform public health work and education in the health professions'.

References

All Our Children (1990) BBC1. 3rd June.

Braginsky B. M., Braginsky D. D. and Ring K. (1969) *Methods of Madness: The Mental Hospital as a Last Resort*. London: Holt, Rinehart and Winston.

Bone M., Meltzer H. (1989) *The Prevalence of Disability Among Children. Report 3*. Office of Population Censuses and Surveys. London: HMSO.

The Child Mothers (1990) *Horizon* BBC2. 4th June.

Chinn C. (1995) *Poverty Amidst Prosperity: The Urban Poor in England 1834–1914*. Manchester: Manchester University Press.

Coleridge P. (1993) *Disability, Liberation and Empowerment*. Oxford: Oxfam.

Daunton M. J. (1995) *Progress and Poverty: An Economic and Social History of Britain 1700–1850*. Oxford: Oxford University Press.

Davis K. (1993) The crafting of good clients. In *Disabling Barriers – Enabling Environments* (Swain J., Finkelstein V., French S., Oliver M., eds). London: Sage.

Davison G. C., Neale J. M. (1990) *Abnormal Psychology*, 5th ed. New York: John Wiley.

Donaghy M. (1995) Models of mental disorder. In *Physiotherapy in Mental Health* (Everett T., Dennis M., Ricketts E., eds). Oxford: Butterworth-Heinemann.

Doyal L. (1983) *The Political Economy of Health*. London: Pluto Books.

Doyal L. (1995) *What Makes Women Sick: Gender and the Political Economy of Health*. London: Macmillan.

Finkelstein V. (1993) Disability: a social challenge or an administrative responsibility? In *Disabling Barriers – Enabling Environments* (Swain J., Finkelstein V., French S., Oliver M., eds). London: Sage.

French S. (ed.) (1994) *On Equal Terms: Working with Disabled People*. Oxford: Butterworth-Heinemann.

Goffman E. (1961) *Asylums*. Harmondsworth: Penguin Books.

Gray A. (ed.) (1993) *World Health and Disease*. Buckingham: Open University Press.

Illich I. (1995) The epidemics of modern medicine. In *Health and Disease: A Reader* (2nd edn). (Davey B., Gray A., Seale C., eds). Buckingham: Open University Press.

Jacobson B., Smith A., Whitehead M. (eds) (1991) *The Nation's Health: A Strategy for the 1990s*. King Edward's Hospital Fund for London.

Jones K. (1993) *Asylums and After*. London: The Athlone Press.

Laing R. D. (1967) *The Politics of Experience*. New York: Pantheon Books.

McKeown T. (1979) *The Role of Medicine*. Oxford: Basil Blackwell.

McKeown T. (1995) The medical contribution. In *Health and Disease: A Reader*, (2nd edn) (Davey B., Gray A., Seale C., eds). Buckingham: Open University Press.

Martin J., Meltzer H., Elliot D. (1989) *The Prevalence of Disability Among Adults. Report 1*. Office of Population Censuses and Surveys. London: HMSO.

May D., Clarke I. (1980) Cuckoo in the nest: some comments on the role of sociology in the undergraduate medical curriculum. *Journal of Medical Education*, **14**, 105–112.

Navarro V. (1995) The mode of state intervention in the health sector. In *Health and Disease: A Reader* (2nd edn). (Davey B., Gray A., Seale C., eds). Buckingham: Open University Press.

Norell J. (1987) Uses and abuses of the consultation. In *While I'm Here Doctor* (Elder A., Samual O., eds). London: Tavistock Publications.

Oliver M. (1993) Disability and dependency: a creation of industrial societies? In *Disabling Barriers – Enabling Environments* (Swain J., Finkelstein V., French S., Oliver M., eds). London: Sage.

Pilgrim D., Rogers A. (1993) *A Sociology of Mental Health and Illness*. Buckingham: Open University Press.

Rosenhan D. L. (1980) On being sane in insane places. In *Readings in Medical Sociology* (Mechanic D., ed.). New York: The Free Press.

Royle E. (1987) *Modern Britain: A Social History 1750–1985*. London: Edward Arnold.

Sagan A. (1987) *The Health of Nations*. New York: Basic Books.

Sanders D. (1985) *The Struggle for Health*. London: Macmillan.

Sharpe J. A. (1987) *Early Modern England. A Social History*. London: Edward Arnold.

Swain J., Finkelstein V., French S., Oliver M. (eds) (1993) *Disabling Barriers – Enabling Environments*. London: Sage.

Szasz T. S. (1961) *The Myth of Mental Illness*. New York: Harper and Row.

Tudar Hart J. (1984) A new kind of doctor. In *Health and Disease: A Reader* (Black N. et al., eds). Milton Keynes: Open University Press.

Turshen M. (1989) *The Politics of Public Health*. London: Zed Books.

Tyrer P., Steinberg D. (1987) *Models of Mental Disorder*. Chichester: John Wiley.

U205 Course Team (1985a) *Caring for Health: History and Diversity*. Milton Keynes: Open University Press.

U205 Course Team (1985b) *The Health of Nations*. Milton Keynes: Open University Press.

2

Inequalities in health
Sally French

'It is one of the greatest of social injustices that people who live in the most disadvantaged circumstances have more illness, more disability and shorter lives than those who are more affluent.' (Benzeval *et al.*, 1995a)

In 1980 a research working group, chaired by Sir Douglas Black, produced *The Black Report* which documented inequalities in health in Britain since the Second World War. This report is summarized by Townsend and Davidson (1982). The Health Education Council commissioned an update of the evidence leading to a second report, *The Health Divide* in 1987. This report is summarized by Whitehead (1988). Both reports clearly demonstrate that health is closely associated with social class, favouring those in the higher social classes, and that the National Health Service has been unsuccessful in bringing about health equality. All of these issues are reiterated by Whitehead and Dahlgren (1995).

The overall standard of health has improved for the entire British population over the course of this century (Jacobson *et al.*, 1991). The standardized mortality rate for babies under one year, for example, was 10% in 1900 and is now approximately 1%. Life expectancy has also increased, with more people living into middle and old age. Whitehead (1989) reports that life expectancy increased by 2 years in the short period between 1973 and 1983 and Hendricks and Hendricks (1978) state that people born in 1960 can expect to live 20 years longer than those who were born in 1900. Despite this major overall improvement there is little evidence that the gap in health status between the social classes has reduced, in fact Whitehead (1988) believes it has widened in most respects, though she cites post-neonatal deaths (deaths between one month and one year of age) as an area where the gap between the social classes has narrowed.

Social class

Social class is a complex concept and no totally adequate way of measuring it exists. Some measures which have been used are educational level, housing tenure, car ownership, income, crowding, neighbourhood and occupation. They are all crude measurements but nevertheless tend to produce similar results which greatly increases their validity. Whitehead (1988) believes that, 'There can be no doubt that these inequalities exist however imperfect the measuring tool'. Furthermore Jacobson *et al.* (1991) point out that if two or more systems of classification are used simultaneously even larger social class differences can be seen.

The Registrar General's classification of social class, based on occupation, is the most frequently used measure. Knowledge of occupation provides some indication of living standards, life style and income. Using this measure the social class of single people is classified according to their own occupation and the social class of families is derived from the husband's occupation, though the occupation of his wife is now recorded in the Census. The Registrar General's classification divides occupations into six social classes (Table 2.1).

Table 2.1   Registrar General's classification of social class based on occupation

Social class		Occupation
1.	Professional	Doctor, lawyer
2.	Managerial and lower professional	Physiotherapist, teacher
3N.	Skilled non-manual	Clerk, secretary
3M.	Skilled manual	Plumber, electrician
4.	Semi-skilled	Bus driver, postman
5.	Unskilled	Labourer, road sweeper

A serious short-coming of this system is that it fails to classify unemployed people who tend to be the poorest members of society.

Measuring health

Measuring health is fraught with problems, not least because it is so difficult to define and encompasses social and psychological well-being which are very subjective and individualistic. The mortality rate is frequently used to judge the health status of a population because it is by far the most objective measure and is a fairly sensitive indicator of health. It is not an entirely adequate measure, however, because many diseases and impairments do not lead to an early death, thus mortality rates do not give an adequate picture of morbidity rates. Morbidity is defined in different ways according to time, culture and individual beliefs. Furthermore, not everyone reports disease, illness or impairment to medical authorities, thus its true extent remains obscure.

Social class differences in health

Mortality rates and morbidity rates rise as socioeconomic class falls (Jacobson *et al.*, 1991; Fox and Benzeval, 1995; Morris, 1995). The most striking contrasts are seen when social classes one and five are compared. The mortality rate of social class five is approximately twice that of social class one, dropping to a 50% increase in old age (Fox and Benzeval, 1995). Jacobson *et al.* (1991) state that the life expectancy of a child born to a family in social class five is 8 years shorter than that of a child born to a family in social class one, and that the excess avoidable deaths of manual workers aged 16 to 74 years, between 1979 and 1983, was 42 000. They state '... the total excess mortality associated with manual work social classes amounts to the equivalent of a major air crash or shipwreck every day'. Jacobson *et al.* (1991) found that the mortality rate for men in social classes four and five was higher than that for men in social classes one and two for 62 of 66 diseases, and of the 70 major causes of death among women 64 gave rise to greater mortality in social classes four and five than in social classes one and two.

The Black Report and *The Health Divide* show that people from the higher social classes have the lowest infant mortality rate, the lowest suicide and parasuicide rate and the lowest rate of mental illness. They also experience less stillbirths, prematurity, illness and impairment. Chronic illness and impairment are more prevalent in manual workers who also experienced poor psychological well-being and physical fitness when compared with professional workers (Jacobson *et al.*, 1991).

People from social classes one and two have larger babies than people in social classes four and five. Mothers in social class five are three times more likely than mothers in social class one to give birth to babies weighing less than 2.5 kg. Such babies are more likely to be both physically and intellectually impaired. Cerebral palsy increases in prevalence as social class falls. Impairments of a purely genetic origin tend not to show class differences but those where the cause is thought to be partly or wholly environmental, such as spina bifida and certain types of deafness, are more common in social classes four and five.

There are also differences in physical attributes among the social classes. Knight (1984) found that people in social classes one and two are considerably taller than those in social classes four and five. Such differences also reflect family size and birth position, regardless of class, with children from large families and those born latest, having the shortest stature.

Similar differences in health status can be found when measures of social class, other than the Registrar General's classification are used. Lynch and Delman (1981) found that in the British Army coronary heart disease varied according to rank with those in the lowest rank being six times more likely to have the disease than those in the highest rank. People who are unemployed have worse health records than those who are employed (Jacobson *et al.*, 1991; Benzeval *et al.*, 1995b); the mortality rate of unemployed men and their wives is 20% higher than those who are employed and suicide rates are double those of employed people. However, unemployment alone may not necessarily cause this increase in illness as unemployed people are disadvantaged in so many ways and may experience low self-esteem and social isolation. Income is closely associated with health especially at the lower levels and the health of people who own their own homes is better than those who rent them either privately or as council tenants (Fox *et al.*, 1986; Fogelman *et al.*, 1987; Jacobson *et al.*, 1991; Best, 1995). People from ethnic minority groups are over-represented in social classes four and five and are also more likely to be unemployed. This, together with communication problems and racism, means that their access to health care services is severely restricted. (For further information on health care and people from ethnic minority groups, the reader is referred to Chapter 5.)

Gender differences in health

In the developed world women live considerably longer than men. According to Whitehead (1988) women could expect to live 5 years longer than men in 1950 and over 6 years longer than men in 1981. Hart (1985) states that, with the exception of social class one, death rates for males are higher than those for females regardless of class. There is evidence, however, that this gap is narrowing because women are now more prone to some of the major causes of death such as lung cancer and accidents (Jacobson *et al.*, 1991). At the present time life expectancy for males at birth in Britain is approximately 72 years and that for females approximately 78 years. Three-quarters of people over the age of 85 in Britain are women.

The ratio of male to female deaths is roughly two to one in childhood with many more boys dying in accidents. In under-developed countries males tend to live longer than females, though for both sexes overall life expectancy is short due to large numbers of people dying in childhood and early adult life. The low life expectancy of women is due to high mortality associated with childbirth and sometimes gender discrimination in terms of the distribution of resources. In British society the gap between the sexes regarding mortality was very much less at the turn of the century. Waldron (1980) believes that about half the difference in mortality rates between the sexes is due to behavioural factors, such as higher levels of cigarette smoking, alcohol consumption and accidents among men. Leviatan and Cohen (1985) focus on the environment, believing it to be generally more hazardous for men. They note that in the kibbutz, where the environment is similar for both sexes, the difference in mortality rate between them is smaller. There may also be a genetic basis for the difference. It is likely that a combination of factors operates.

In contrast to this, women show greater morbidity than men, though this is mainly confined to old age (Jacobson *et al.*, 1991). Boys and young adult males are more prone to illness and impairment than females in this age group but there is little difference in overall morbidity between the sexes in middle life. The type of morbidity is, however, different, for example women are more likely than men to experience rheumatoid arthritis. Women are also more prone to mental illness, especially young women in social class five. The reasons for this are uncertain. Cochrane (1983) and Pilgrim and Rogers (1993) suggest that doctors are more prone to label women as mentally ill and women may be more inclined than men to define themselves in this way. The social disadvantages and stress women experience, in terms of low paid, low status employment and their additional responsibilities of child care and housework may also help to explain their high incidence of mental illness. (For further information on sex, gender and health care, the reader is referred to Chapter 4 and to Morris (1994).)

Regional inequalities in health

Townsend and Davidson (1982) found that Scotland, Wales and northern England have greater mortality and morbidity rates than southern England and East Anglia. A very similar pattern has emerged in *The Health Divide* (Whitehead, 1988). There are clear differences in health status between these regions for men and married women though the pattern is less marked for single women. These differences cannot be accounted for in terms of social class. The typical class differences are present in every region, though they are larger in the regions of highest mortality and morbidity. In south-east England people in every social class have better health than their counterparts elsewhere in the country. When the mortality rate of social classes four and five are combined for women in East Anglia, it is less than that of women in social classes one and two in Scotland. The concept of a north/south divide is, however, too simplistic as there are enormous differences within regions (Aggleton, 1990).

There are marked regional variations in the incidence of disease, for example neural tube defects are more common in Scotland, Wales and Northern Ireland than elsewhere in Britain. A fuller explanation of these regional differences in health remains obscure. There are climatic and cultural differences between the regions as well as dissimilarities in environmental conditions such as the composition of the water. It is probable, however, that the greater material disadvantage in Scotland, Wales and the north of England, when compared with the south, is the main factor creating inequalities in health.

Distribution of resources in the National Health Service have been grossly unequal, favouring southern England despite its low mortality and morbidity rates. The London teaching hospitals, in particular, have absorbed a large proportion of available resources. In 1976 the Government implemented the recommendations of the Resource Allocation Working Party (The RAWP Report), which recommended geographical reallocation of resources. Unfortunately, the recommendations were implemented by cutting the resources of the richer regions rather than increasing the overall budget, however, since the RAWP report inequalities in NHS resource allocation have been reduced.

Jones *et al.* (1983) point out that equality in NHS and other resources has the potential to increase inequalities in health rather than reduce them. Equality means 'equal shares' whereas equity means 'fair shares'. Given the existing inequalities in health and advantage, a fair distribution of resources rather than an equal distribution is required.

There is, however, little correlation between the distribution of NHS resources and mortality or morbidity rates (Benzeval *et al.*, 1995b). East Anglia is the healthiest area of Britain yet has always been under-resourced when compared with many other regions. It should also be appreciated that the RAWP report did not address inequalities in resources among medical specialities which remain marked, favouring the acute services. In addition there are vast differences in the quantity and quality of services provided by local authorities and many believe that much more money should be channelled into community care, indeed this was one of the recommendations of *The Black Report*.

The role of medicine in reducing inequalities in health should not be over-estimated. Jacobson *et al.* (1991) believe that the percentage of deaths which are potentially preventable through medical treatment is about 5% and that medical intervention has had little impact on death rates from common diseases such as cancer. (For further discussion of the role of medicine in health, the reader is referred to Chapter 1.)

International comparisons of health

Accurately measuring the health status of different nations, particularly morbidity rates, is extremely difficult and unreliable due to the different ways in which the information is collected, classified and defined (Aggleton, 1990). When compared with 14 other north-western European countries, England and Wales had the seventh lowest infant mortality rate in 1966 but its position dropped to ninth by 1984 (Whitehead, 1988). Infant mortality in Britain is high when compared with Nordic countries such as Sweden and Denmark, but, in contrast the mortality rate of young adults in Britain is lower than almost anywhere else in the world because of a low rate of accidents. Suicide rates are also very low in Britain though suicide is still the third most common cause of death among young people (Ridley, 1993).

By middle age, mortality rates are again very high in Britain when compared with Nordic countries, Scotland being particularly high. Jacobson et al. (1991) state that Britain has the highest mortality rate for coronary heart disease and lung cancer in the world and the highest rate for breast cancer in western Europe. Despite these differences every country appears to experience inequalities in health with poor health being concentrated among the disadvantaged groups in society. The amount a country spends on its health service is not closely related to the health status of its people (Benzeval et al., 1995b).

Recent improvements in health

Despite the rather dismal picture regarding inequalities in health, there have been several important improvements in the health of the British population in recent years which should not be ignored. Jacobson et al. (1991) note that there was an unexplained 30% reduction of deaths from stroke between 1973 and 1983 with a similar decrease in many other developed countries. There has also been a small decrease in coronary heart disease, although death rates in Britain remain worse than anywhere else in the world. Dental health has improved among children and death rates on the roads in 1985 were lower than those for the previous three decades, despite a tremendous increase in the volume of traffic. Teenage pregnancies have reduced, as the use of contraception has increased, more women are now breast feeding and there has been a sharp, unexplained reduction in parasuicide among women since the mid 1970s. There has also been a sharp reduction in babies born with abnormalities of the central nervous system; for example between 1976 and 1985 there was a decrease of 63% of babies born with spina bifida, only about one-third of which can be explained in terms of screening and abortion (it is, however, a debatable point whether screening and abortion of impaired fetuses is ethical or desirable and for further discussion of this the reader is referred to Morris (1991) and Chapter 25 in this book).

Other health statistics show a mixed picture. For example, suicide rates have decreased among women but have increased among young men and lung cancer has declined in men but has increased in younger women reflecting smoking habits (Jacobson et al., 1991).

Explaining inequalities in health

The artefact explanation

The artefact explanation of health inequalities suggests that the concepts of 'health' and 'class' are too complex to be measured reliably and that any relationship between them is artificial and of little causal significance.

Making comparisons between health status and class over time is methodologically problematic. The Registrar General's classification of social class has undergone various changes over the years and the occupational structure of British society has also altered. Social class five has reduced in size since the Second World War and the professional classes have expanded. It is argued that the poor health status of those in social class five is due to the relocation of young people to other occupational groups, leaving a disproportionate number of older workers who are more prone to ill-health. However, Hart (1985) and Blane (1991) point out that the differences which exist are far more pronounced among younger people.

The failure to reduce the gap between the health status of the social classes is also believed to be counter-balanced by the shrinkage of social class five. Comparing the health status of the previously small professional classes with those of today is also problematic for it is likely that their status and life style have little in common. There is a great deal of variability both within and between occupational classes but when disease is measured according to particular occupations the gap between social classes tends to increase.

It has also been argued that people may be assigned a different social class when they die from that which they receive on the Census (Blane, 1991). However, a longitudinal study by Goldblatt (1989) found that when individuals are assigned the same social class, both in the census and when they die, inequalities in health remain, though they are smaller.

An argument against the artefact explanation is that social class differences still exist when measures other than occupation are used, for example income, housing or education. Whitehead (1988) points out that some studies imply that measuring social class by occupation tends to decrease rather than exaggerate the differences. Many studies have controlled for effects such as age of individuals and size of social class yet the results do not alter to any great extent.

Inequalities in health apply to much larger sections of society, not just those who are unskilled, for example the mortality rate of people in social class three is higher at every age than that of people in social classes one and two. Hart (1985) believes that inequality in mortality risk is not an artefact but a real phenomenon of advantage and disadvantage and Whitehead (1988) states, 'Whether social position is measured by income, housing tenure, household possessions or education, a similar pattern emerges on inequalities of health between the top and the bottom of the social scale, consistent with that found by using occupational status'. Blane (1991), Jacobson *et al.* (1991) and Fox and Benzeval (1995) believe that the artefact explanation can be largely discounted.

Natural and social selection

This theory proposes that the fittest members of society will be upwardly mobile whereas those who are unfit will drift down to the lower social classes. Thus inequalities in health are explained by a 'survival of the fittest' principle.

Illsley (1986) studied social class mobility on marriage. He demonstrated an upward social trend for tall, healthy women and a downward trend for short, less healthy women. Those who moved up the social scale had less perinatal mortality than those who moved down. This demonstrates a process of selective mating. There is also a tendency for people suffering from alcoholism to be downwardly mobile. However, this downward path is not inevitable, Fogelman *et al.* (1987), using data from the National Child Development Study which has followed a cohort of children since 1958, found that the health of those people who had remained in the same social class differed more than those who had been upwardly or downwardly mobile.

Class gradients for mortality and morbidity are generally steeper in early adulthood, if the theory of natural and social selection were correct one would expect to see the most marked differences in later adult life. Whitehead (1988), Jacobson *et al.* (1991) and Fox and Benzeval (1995) all conclude that the selection effect accounts for only a small proportion of the difference in health status between the social classes.

The behavioural/cultural explanation

There is considerable evidence that people from social classes four and five indulge in behaviours such as cigarette smoking and alcohol consumption more than their counterparts in social classes one and two. The decline in cigarette smoking has been much more marked in the non-manual than the manual classes. Most people accept that this type of behaviour can lead to a high incidence of diseases such as lung cancer, coronary heart disease and chronic bronchitis (Townsend, 1995). The distribution of cigarette smoking according to social class is very similar to that of lung cancer and coronary heart disease and is estimated to cause 100 000 premature deaths in Britain each year (Jacobson *et al.*, 1991).

People from the manual classes tend to report illness less often than others and use the preventative services less. They make less use of dental services and are under-represented in preventative programmes such as cervical screening and antenatal care (Jacobson *et al.*, 1991). Middle class people are able to make more use of consultation time, they ask more questions and more information is communicated to them (Ley, 1988). The level of use of the health service among people from social classes four and five certainly does not match their high incidence of illness.

The behavioural/cultural explanation of inequality in health status among the social classes focuses on the individual and his or her culture as the main determinants of health; thus excessive consumption of refined food and alcohol, cigarette smoking, lack of exercise, and under use of preventative services and contraception are believed to lie at the root of ill health. People in the lower social classes are thought to know little about their own health requirements or that of their families and to lack the motivation to change their habits. Ryan (1976) regards this explanation as a form of 'victim blaming' which is politically convenient because it maintains the status quo.

Lewis (1967), an anthropologist, put forward 'the culture of poverty' theory which states that human existence in any environment gives rise to elaborate systems of norms, ideas and patterns of behaviour which, though initially socially and biologically adaptive, tend to persist when the factors which gave rise to them have changed or no longer exist. Thus a diet which at one time was the best available may persist despite an abundance of alternative, more nutritious foodstuffs. Similarly dangerous work practices, which in the past could not be avoided, may persist and lead to accidents even though safer techniques are available. Hart (1985) believes that '… the behaviour in question is not a series of random individual acts. It is a group phenomenon, a cultural norm rather than a personal habit'.

Smoking, for example, may be a symbol of adulthood rather than simply an addictive habit. Hart (1985) argues that it is easier to redefine the meaning of smoking, from something desirable to something undesirable, if there are substitutes for it. Alternative symbols and sources of enjoyment are more likely to be available to those in the professional classes, where people are more mobile and where group solidarity and group sanctions are less evident. The 'culture of poverty' thesis has been widely criticized by sociologists who cite instances where change has been rapid, for example in the use of contraception. Blaxter and Paterson (1982) found that problems of disadvantaged mothers stemmed from lack of skill in dealing with the system rather than with their cultural beliefs. (For further information on social class and the use of health care, the reader is referred to Chapter 8)

The materialist explanation

'The association between social class and health shows that death and disease are socially constructed, as opposed to being randomly distributed throughout the population.' (Blane, 1991)

The materialist explanation regards inequalities in health as being primarily due to inequalities in the distribution of wealth in our society. It is the explanation favoured in both *The Black Report* (1980) and *The Health Divide* (1988). In Britain a very small proportion of the population own most of the wealth with a large minority owning very little. Benzeval *et al.* (1995a) believe that income inequality is greater in Britain than in most other developed countries. Thus health and illness cannot be divorced from politics.

The extent of poverty in Britain is considerable though the number of people living in poverty does depend on how it is defined. A frequent definition of poverty is an income of no more than 40% above the level of supplementary benefits (Jacobson *et al.*, 1991). Using this definition, in 1985 one in three people in Britain lived in poverty including 85% of unemployed people, two-thirds of single parents and about 50% of families with three or more children. Diet, housing and facilities such as cars, telephones and household appliances all correlate with income.

Durward (1984) calculated that it is not possible for pregnant women on low incomes to follow dietary advice and Graham (1986) found that families on low incomes had difficulty providing their children with a healthy diet. Poor people spend proportionately twice as much of their income on food as people on higher incomes (Jacobson *et al.*, 1991). Even among high income groups, the quality of diet diminishes as family size increases. Baird (1975) suggests that the nutritional state of females before they are born affects their later reproductive capacity and the health of their own children. In this way deprivation can be said to be 'transmitted' with health being determined by the individual's life history.

Jacobson *et al.* (1991) and Best (1995) note that homelessness and poor housing are associated with respiratory illness, accidents and mental illness. High illness and accident rates among children from social class five can sometimes be explained in terms of living in damp, high-rise accommodation which so often leads to physical disease and stress. This type of accommodation is also unsuitable for play so children are less likely to be supervised. The high proportion of single parents on low incomes in social class five make it more necessary for them to take paid employment, and as child-minders cannot be afforded children may be left alone. In addition, inner-city areas, where such families are often located, tend to offer less amenities in terms of medical services, sporting facilities and safe play areas. They also predispose children to behavioural and emotional problems (Jacobson *et al.* 1991). The fact that people from social class five visit their doctors less than other people (when the amount of illness they experience is taken into account) and make less use of preventative services may be viewed as entirely rational when their social situation, including poor public transport and lack of car ownership, is taken into account.

Although occupational accidents and diseases only account for a small proportion of morbidity, manual workers are subject to more risk than non-manual workers. They are more likely to be in contact with hazardous substances, such as asbestos and coal dust which are known to cause serious disease, accidents occur more frequently and noise is more often a problem. Manual workers tend to have less job security, fewer fringe benefits, less favourable pensions, shorter holidays and poorer sick leave arrangements than skilled and professional workers (Jacobson *et al.*, 1991).

Occupational risk is, however, difficult to define, for example, there is an ongoing debate concerning the health risks of working with video display units and sedentary work. Stress, shift work and access to drugs may all be instrumental in causing disease. It is usually the case, however, that the work environment is just one of many factors giving rise to disease, this makes it possible for employers and government to focus on aspects other than those directly associated with the work place, such as personal habits.

People in social classes four and five tend to be disadvantaged in medical consultations. Consultation time between general practitioners and working class patients tends to be shorter than that between general practitioners and middle class patients. Middle class patients tend to ask more questions and receive more information (Morgan, 1991). White males also participate in the consultation more than women or people from ethnic minorities (Morgan, 1991). Whitehead (1988) states that general practitioners make more home visits to people in the professional classes and Blaxter (1984) found that they are more likely to refer professional patients to a specialist. Thus the working class patient tends to get less benefit from medical encounters and may be less likely to return for treatment or to comply with advice. This can be viewed as due, not to ignorance or lack of motivation on the part of the patient, but to poor communication resulting from a difference of status and culture.

People in social classes four and five are likely to have multiple stresses in their lives, a situation which has been found to predispose people to illness. A supportive social network of relatives and friends protects people from the ill effects of stress, depression and anxiety. There is a romantic notion that poor people are more likely than others to be part of a large supportive social network, but in reality this is not so, especially since the clearance of the slums. Poor people are usually more isolated than those with higher incomes as they are less able to run a car, afford to go out or use the telephone regularly. Whitehead (1988) points out that even when behavioural factors like smoking, drinking, diet and lack of exercise are controlled in research, the social class differences in morbidity are still present.

Jacobson *et al.* (1991) point out that in human society the interests of some groups of people are achieved by manipulating or suppressing other groups and putting them at risk. For example the tobacco, alcohol and confectionery industries spend billions of pounds each year promoting their products while government benefits by the receipt of large sums in taxation. The organization ASH UK reported in 1993 that the government spends £100 million in advertising and promoting tobacco products. Government has the power to reduce health risks and inequalities. Seat belt legislation, for example, has had a large effect on accident rates. Road safety could be further improved for pedestrians and cyclists by providing more zebra crossings and cycle tracks. Legislation can protect people from harmful agents such as drugs and pollution and from inadequate incomes by the redistribution of wealth. Government also has the power to increase inequalities in health by failing to respond to dangers such as pollution, by creating unemployment or declaring war.

The interaction between behavioural factors and material disadvantage

'The notion that inequalities in health result from a cultural preference among working class people for a life that is 'short and sweet' is not supported by the evidence.' (Jacobson, 1991)

People have a variety of ways of dealing with their situation in the short term, and although their behaviour may go against professional advice, it is usually entirely rational given the social circumstances they are in, even if they fully understand the risks. Smoking, for example, may ease tension and help someone cope with a difficult family or work situation, eating the 'wrong' foods may be one of the few sources of pleasure available, giving up breast feeding early may enable a mother to go back to work and provide for other members of her family, and giving children sweets may help to keep them quiet and happy in a crowded flat or bed-and-breakfast accommodation. Campkin (1987) points out that trying to change a person's behaviour may only serve to cause him or her more stress and guilt, perhaps leading to an increase in the behaviour, furthermore if behaviour change does occur there is the potential for other more serious problems to surface as the coping strategy keeping them at bay has been removed. The role of social factors in determining health has been less thoroughly investigated than biological or psychological factors (Fox and Benzeval, 1995).

Jacobson *et al.* (1991) believe that material and behavioural factors relating to health and illness are totally interrelated. They emphasize the importance of social, economic and political factors in shaping a person's behaviour and believe that:

'... there is a limit to the extent to which risk factors such as smoking, poor diet and physical inactivity can be changed without altering the circumstances in which they arise'.

Blane (1991) agrees that behaviour and environment cannot be separated. Stillbirth and low birth weight, for example, are positively correlated with poverty, young maternal age, smoking, short stature and large families. Low intelligence can be compensated for by an enriching environment and a person's level of education will greatly influence his or her choice of occupation and ability to comprehend information. Ley (1988) found that much health education literature could only be understood by people who had had a college education. A person's behaviour, attitudes, beliefs and state of mind are greatly influenced by the present situation, his or her culture and past experience. The apparent apathy of disadvantaged people towards their health may reflect feelings of powerlessness and low self-esteem (Sagan, 1987). Jacobson *et al.* (1991) believe that health education would be more successful among working class people if their material disadvantages were reduced.

The cause of disease is often multifactorial with biological, social and behavioural components. Jacobson *et al.* (1991), for example, point out that cigarette smoking increases the risk of lung disease from asbestos tenfold and that lower levels of sugar consumption and the adding of fluoride to toothpaste have both caused a reduction in tooth decay. In addition one adverse circumstance can so easily lead to another, for example childhood accidents are positively correlated with parental illness, and disability often leads to poverty. How a person behaves can also affect his or her social situation, for example a depressed or anxious person may lose friends and have difficulty finding work.

Implications for physiotherapists

The Black Report and *The Health Divide* make many recommendations for improvements in the health of the British population and in reducing health inequalities. They advocate social and environmental changes, such as increased child benefits and improved road safety particularly strongly, viewing this as more important than changes in the health service. Other measures advocated are a fairer distribution of wealth, greater educational and employment opportunities, safe play areas for children, pre-school education and child care facilities, accident prevention programmes, improved housing and working conditions and a comprehensive disability allowance. Similar strategies have been put forward by Jacobson *et al.* (1991) and Whitehead (1995) including an environment where healthy food is available to all, safe and accessible forms of transport for all members of society, the control of environmental hazards and the reduction of unnecessary medical interventions during pregnancy. The reduction of inequalities in health is the first aim of the World Health Organization's European 'Targets of Health for All'. By the year 2000 the aim is to reduce health inequalities by 25%.

This is not to imply that health education or medical intervention are useless though health education has been of greater benefit to the advantaged than the disadvantaged (Fox and Benzeval, 1995). Jacobson *et al.* (1991) stress the interdependence of professional, political and individual strategies and believe that the best results occur when various groups pool their efforts and resources.

Physiotherapists are in a position to promote action in many areas within their traditional role and by engaging in broader strategies. Using the reduction of tobacco consumption as an example, physiotherapists can give help and support to those trying to give up the habit and can publicize the risks of smoking by broadening their health education role to institutions such as schools and by using the media. They can become involved in self-help organizations and work towards changing their own work environment and that of the wider society.

Such involvement requires a thorough understanding of smoking behaviour, including the external pressures which help to create and sustain it. Counselling skills, teaching skills and a willingness to engage in social and political action and to work with other interested groups are all important. Morris (1995) urges health professionals to become involved in organizations such as the Child Poverty Action Group and SHELTER and points out that the British Medical Association has shown impressive political skills which would be welcomed in these areas. Benzeval *et al.* (1995b) advocate a much wider role for health professionals than treating disease including joining with other agencies to empower people to assess the health needs of their own communities, the mapping of socioeconomic conditions and health and the monitoring of access to health services of homeless people. Physiotherapists can also create new knowledge in this area by engaging in research. Some of these skills are now being developed in undergraduate and postgraduate education.

It is clear from the evidence that health inequalities will not be reduced by focusing solely on existing disease or trying to change people's habits. The question for physiotherapists is whether they should continue in their traditional role of treating symptoms and attempting to change people's behaviour or whether they would be more effective in bringing about change by broadening their sphere of influence.

References

Aggleton P. (1990) *Health*. London: Routledge.

ASH (1993) *Tobacco Advertising: The Case for a Ban*. London: Action on Smoking and Health.

Baird D. (1974) Epidemiology of congenital malformations of the central nervous system in (a) Aberdeen and (b) Scotland. *Journal of Biosocial Science*, **6**, 113.

Benzeval M., Judge K., Whitehead M. (1995a) Introduction. In *Tackling Inequalities in Health: An Agenda for Change* (Benzeval M., Judge K., Whitehead M., eds). London: King's Fund.

Benzeval M., Judge K., Whitehead M. (eds) (1995b) The role of the NHS. In *Tackling Inequalities in Health: An Agenda for Change*. London: King's Fund.

Best R. (1995) The housing dimension. In *Tackling Inequalities in Health: An Agenda for Change*. (Benzeval M., Judge K., Whitehead M., eds.) London: King's Fund.

Blane D. (1991) Inequality and social class. In *Sociology as Applied to Medicine* (Scambler G., ed.), 3rd edn. London: Baillière Tindall.

Blaxter M. (1984) Equity and consultation rates in general practice. *British Medical Journal*, **288**, 1963–1967.

Blaxter M., Paterson L. (1982) *Mothers and Daughters: A Three Generational Study of Health Attitudes and Health Behaviour*. Oxford: Heinemann.

Campkin M. (1987) Why don't you listen to me for a change? In *While I'm Here Doctor* (Elder A., Samual O., eds). London: Tavistock Publications.

Cochrane R. (1983) *The Social Creation of Mental Illness*. London: Longman.

Durward L. (1984) *Poverty in Pregnancy*. London: Maternity Alliance.

Fogelman K., Fox J., Power C. (1987) Class and tenure mobility: Do they explain the social inequalities in health among young adults in Britain? Cited in Whitehead M. (1988) *The Health Divide*. Harmondsworth: Penguin Books.

Fox J., Benzeval M. (1995) Perspectives on social variations in health. In *Tackling Inequalities in Health: an agenda for change* (Benzeval M., Judge K., Whitehead M. (eds). London: King's Fund.

Fox A. J., Goldblatt P. O., Jones D. R. (1986) Social class mortality differentials: artefact, selection or life circumstances? In *Class and Health*, (Wilkinson R. G., ed.) London: Tavistock.

Goldblatt P. (1989) Mortality by social class 1971–1985. Cited in Jacobson B., Smith A., Whitehead M. (1991) *The Nation's Health: A Strategy for the 1990s*. London: King Edward Hospital Fund for London.

Graham H. (1986) *Caring for the Family*. Research Report Number 1. London: Health Education Council.

Hart N. (1985) *The Sociology of Health and Medicine*. Ormskirk: Causeway Press.

Hendricks J., Hendricks D. C. (1978) Ageing in advanced industrialised societies. In *An Ageing Population* (Carver V., Liddiard P., eds). Milton Keynes: The Open University Press.

Illsley R. (1986) Occupational class, selection and the production of inequalities in health. *Quarterly Journal of Social Affairs*, **2**(2), 151–165.

Jacobson B., Smith A., Whitehead M. (1991) *The Nation's Health: A Strategy for the 1990s*. London: King Edward's Hospital Fund for London.

Jones K., Brown J., Bradshaw J. (1983) *Issues in Social Policy*. London: Routledge and Kegan Paul.

Knight I. (1984) *The Height and Weight of Adults in Great Britain*. London: OPCS/HMSO.

Leviatan U., Cohen J. (1985) Gender differences in life expectancy among Kibbutz members. *Social Science and Medicine*, **21**, 245–251.

Lewis O. (1967) *The Children of Sanchez*. New York: Random House.

Ley P. (1988) *Communicating with Patients*. London: Croom Helm.

Lynch P., Delman B. J. (1981) Mortality from CHD in the British Army compared with the civil population. *British Medical Journal*, **283**, 405–407.

Morgan M. (1991) The doctor–patient relationship. In *Sociology as Applied to Medicine*, (Scambler, G., ed.), 3rd edn. London: Baillière Tindall.

Morris J. (1991) *Pride Against Prejudice*. London: The Women's Press.

Morris J. (1994) Gender and disability. In *On Equal Terms: Working with Disabled People* (French, S., ed.) Oxford: Butterworth-Heinemann.

Morris J. N. (1985) Inequalities in health: ten years and little further on. In *Health and Disease: A Reader* (Davey B., Gray A., Seale C., eds). Buckingham: Open University Press.

Pilgrim D., Rogers A. (1993) *A Sociology of Mental Health and Illness*. Buckingham: Open University Press.

Ridley S. (1993) Sudden death from suicide. In *Death, Dying and Bereavement*, (Dickenson D., Johnson M., eds). London: Sage.

Ryan W. (1976) *Blaming the Victim*. New York: Vintage Books.

Sagan L. A. (1987) *The Health of Nations*. New York: Basic Books.

Townsend J. (1995) The burden of smoking. In *Tackling Inequalities in Health: An Agenda for Change*, (Benzeval M., Judge K., Whitehead M., eds). London: King's Fund.

Townsend P., Davidson N. (eds) (1982) *Inequalities in Health*. Harmondsworth: Penguin Books.

Waldron L. (1980) Why do women live longer than men? In *Readings in Medical Sociology* (Mechanic D., ed.). New York: The Free Press.

Whitehead M. (1988) *The Health Divide*. Harmondsworth: Penguin Books.

Whitehead M. (1995) Tackling inequalities: a review of policy initiatives. In *Tackling Inequalities in Health: An Agenda for Change*. (Benzeval M., Judge K., Whithead M., eds). London: King's Fund.

Whitehead M., Dahlgren G. (1995) What can be done about inequalities in health? In *Health and Disease: A Reader* (Davey B., Gray A., Seale C., eds). Buckingham: Open University Press.

3

Institutional and community living
Sally French

Before discussing institutional and community living, it is necessary to explore what is meant by 'institution' and 'community'.

Institutions

The term 'institution' has various meanings, for example the family and marriage are institutions as are religious orders and the armed forces. More specifically, and in the context of this chapter, the term 'institution' is used to refer to social entities such as schools, prisons, hospitals and day centres (Reber, 1985). Institutions are very varied, ranging from those which are well integrated within society to those which are totally isolated. The latter are referred to as 'total' or 'closed' institutions. They are characterized by rigid routines with little or no attention being paid to individual needs. Daily activities such as working, eating, sleeping and exercise are carried out in groups within the same environment, and the many rules and regulations exist more for the benefit of the staff than the residents.

According to Humphries and Gordon (1992) the underlying purpose of closed institutions is to crush people's individual personalities in order to ensure conformity. Goffman (1961), in his famous book *Asylums*, describes a total institution as: 'A place of residence and work where a large number of like situated individuals, cut off from the wider society for an appreciable period of time, together lead an enclosed, formally administered round of life'. Examples of closed institutions are top security prisons and old style psychiatric and 'mental handicap' hospitals.

The incarceration of people considered to be deviant became commonplace in the nineteenth century and expanded rapidly in the first half of the twentieth century (Jones, 1993). Since then there has been an overall decline, although Hunt (1992) points out the marked growth of segregated facilities for disabled people in the 1960s and 1970s; the residents of Cheshire homes, for example, rose from 457 in 1961 to 1402 in 1970 (Hunt, 1992). Finkelstein (1991) remarks on the many honours which have been showered on non-disabled people, by other non-disabled people, for removing disabled people from mainstream society. He states:

> 'There is a singular lack of awareness that there may be something profoundly undemocratic about able-bodied people supporting the systematic removal of disabled people from their communities, that it is only able-bodied people who write glowingly about each other for having

done this to disabled people, and that it is able-bodied people who give themselves awards for this contribution to the isolation of disabled people from the mainstream of life'.

In the nineteenth century conditions labelled 'mental handicap' and 'mental illness' were 'medicalized' and the institutions where such people were detained adopted strict hospital rules and routines, often in the absence of any meaningful treatment; indeed the health needs of the 'patients' were frequently neglected (Oswin, 1978; Jones, 1993). It was common to incarcerate physically disabled people, including children, in these institutions too. It was not until the 1960s that any serious challenge to these practices was made. This followed several damning theoretical analyses of total institutions by sociologists such as Goffman (1961) and Townsend (1962), and later the uncovering of considerable abuse and cruelty. At the same time people such as Szasz (1961) and Laing (1967) were attacking the very concept of insanity, and advances in drug therapy made it more feasible to discharge people with schizophrenia and depressive illness from hospital; the growing Civil Rights movement may also have had an effect. Along with these changes, the large institutions were becoming difficult to staff and maintain, and were increasingly recognized as expensive, out-dated and stigmatizing. However, government policy explicitly advocating 'community care' did not gain momentum until the 1980s.

In contrast to total institutions, there are those which attempt to integrate into society. They are generally small and well staffed with residents having more autonomy over their lives, as well as opportunities for involvement in policy making. This type of institution has become more common as total institutions have declined.

Precisely when an 'institution' should be regarded as a 'community home' or part of 'the community', is impossible to say, but it certainly has less to do with size than the style of management, the attitudes and behaviour of staff, and the availability of resources. An institutionalized atmosphere can be created in a small group home, or even a family, just as a homely atmosphere can be created in a large institution, albeit with difficulty. Davidson (1987) is of the opinion that relationships in the community may be '... almost as debilitatingly dependent and institutional as any relationship in a long-stay hospital', and Morris (1993a) makes the point that, rather than being dismantled, institutions can be dispersed within the community. Holmes and Johnson (1988) give a detailed account of the deprived lives of old people living in private nursing homes, many of which are very small.

One of the major criticisms of institutions is their geographical isolation. This creates problems for residents who want to socialize outside the institution and for staff who are encouraging them to do so. It makes regular visiting by families and friends more difficult, and inhibits other people from becoming involved. It is also one of the factors giving rise to staffing problems. This physical isolation was sometimes planned, as in the case of psychiatric hospitals built in the nineteenth century, and sometimes a matter of convenience. Following the 1944 Education Act, for example, many large, isolated houses in the countryside were used as special residential schools, simply because they were available. To compound this situation, many people are socially isolated before entering institutions and any contacts and relationships they have tend to be unstable. This was recognized in the Warnock Report of 1978 with regard to children in special residential schools.

This social and geographical isolation, together with the powerlessness of the residents, can lead to considerable neglect and abuse which often remains undiscovered and unchallenged (Westcott, 1991; French, 1992; Humphries and Gordon, 1992; Marchant and Page, 1992; Westcott, 1993; Sobsey, 1994). Potts and Fido (1991), in their interviews with people detained in mental handicap hospitals, give graphic evidence of abuse perpetrated by professional staff; the inmates were totally controlled by the system while at the same time suffering severe neglect. French (1996) has similarly documented the abuse of visually impaired children in a residential school in the 1950s and 1960s.

It is generally believed that abuse is less likely to occur in community settings as 'the community' provides its own watchdog, but some people have argued that abuse is more likely in the community because systematic inspection is so difficult. Morris (1993b), in her study of independent living, found that most of the disabled people she interviewed could recall instances where helpers were patronizing and verbally or physically abusive. One of the reasons that abuse of disabled people, both inside and outside institutions, remains uncovered, is that many people have difficulty believing it exists, whereas in reality, disabled people appear to be at greater risk from abuse than others (Westcott, 1993).

Because of the lack of facilities to overcome physical and social barriers, as well as their social isolation, the residents of institutions are often unduly dependent on staff for their social and emotional, as well as their physical, needs. Thus any opposition to the treatment they receive may result in adverse labelling, which in turn may lead to greater isolation or harsher treatment. In this situation it is impossible for residents to complain without making themselves more vulnerable. Talking of disabled children in special schools during the first half of the twentieth century, Humphries and Gordon (1992) state that, 'The opportunity for children to resist such a harsh system of control and punishment was extremely limited. They were under immense psychological pressure to obey the rules at all times'. Morris (1993a) also found that disabled people living in institutions found it difficult to complain. As an ex-pupil of a residential school for visually impaired children explains:

> 'We were afraid of the abusers and knew that any complaints would lead to more abuse. We were afraid to tell our parents because of subtle pressure to pretend we were happy. Children with additional disabilities were the main targets for abuse as they couldn't fit into the rigid institutional routine'. (Marchant and Cross, 1993)

Although many staff working in institutions do their utmost for the welfare of the residents, often against tremendous odds, institutions sometimes attract inadequate people who find it difficult to cope in mainstream society themselves. Vaizey (1959) believes that people attracted to working in institutions are inadequate, unfulfilled, insecure and authoritarian, with a lust for power and control; over the years they become increasingly institutionalized themselves. Such people are often untrained, poorly educated, and underpaid. They frequently develop low expectations of the residents in their charge and a hostile attitude to outsiders. The influence of the environment on the behaviour of staff must not, however, be under-estimated, the staff of institutions are often working in a depressing and stressful environment with inadequate resources and support. Even well-meaning staff may have inappropriate attitudes and behaviour patterns, for example they may have low expectations of people's abilities.

Staff who have direct contact with residents are usually at the bottom of an authoritarian hierarchy where they are under considerable pressure to behave in the way that they do (Orford, 1980). Sedgwick (1989) believes that nurses '... frequently find themselves up against sets of rules and social mores which do not seem to have changed since the last century'. Oswin (1978) found that young nurses working with children with learning difficulties were discouraged, against their better judgement, from mothering them. In time the attitudes and behaviour of staff may become custodial and punitive in order to conform and reduce psychological conflict which tends to occur if a person's behaviour and attitudes are at variance. Despite the harshness of the environment, some staff do, however, manager to maintain their humanity (Potts and Fido, 1991).

The behaviour of people in institutions may also be affected by the environment. People have a tendency to live up to what others expect of them, a process known as the 'self-fulfilling prophecy'. People in institutions may emulate the expectations of the staff, reinforcing erroneous stereotypes and prejudices which justify the institution's existence. The social, emotional and intellectual deprivation which can result from institutional living may also lead residents to become 'institutionalized' themselves. Harriet, a visually impaired woman interviewed by French explains the effects of being in a special residential school for the whole of her schooldays:

> 'The most damaging thing was the way they destroyed your self-confidence. The way they said you couldn't do things because you were 'such and such' a person or because of your background. They really put you down. When you went out into the world you weren't your own person you were what they said you were. You had it drummed into you all the time 'you're a delinquent, you're no good for anything'. It made you feel you had to keep in the background all the time because you weren't as good as other people. I used to think 'I'm nothing, I'm nobody, I can't do it' but I gradually found that I could.' (French, 1996)

People with learning difficulties or psychiatric illness may, in particular, suffer from the ill-effects of a barren or hostile environment as they may be unable to create their own stimulation or form their own ideas;

thus psychological problems can be caused by the system of 'care' itself. Ford (1987) explains that after years of incarceration residents need considerable assistance in coping successfully with life in mainstream society. Thus the presence of institutions tends to confirm their need and inhibit the adoption of other, more creative approaches.

The lack of flexibility within some institutions hinders independence as everything must be done by a certain time and in a specific way. Wilkinson (1987) notes how the independence of mentally ill people is reduced by nurses who do too much for them, and Cooke (1987) believes that the independence of old people in geriatric wards is sometimes restricted to the extent of infringing their civil liberties. Many severely disabled people, who leave institutions for a life in the community, are surprised at how much they are able to achieve (Davis, 1981; Shearer, 1982; Briggs, 1993). Even institutions which express a specific aim to encourage independence may in reality be restrictive because any attempt to enhance self-sufficiency is offset by institutional rules and regulations.

The institutionalization of people and their removal from mainstream society, has the tendency to increase the stigma attached to their impairments and to worsen the fears and prejudices of the general public. The education of the public is often put forward as a major reason for the closure of institutions and the integration of residents in 'the community'. It is believed that people will never accept differences in their fellow citizens unless they are fully informed and have contact with them on an equal basis from an early age. Whether this acceptance actually occurs, however, is open to question. With regard to deaf children, Meadow (1980) and Ladd (1990) are very sceptical. The attitudes and feelings of disabled children attending special and mainstream schools are also very mixed (Booth and Statham, 1982; Madge and Fassam, 1982; Wade and Moore, 1993).

Some people believe it is immoral to subject ill and disabled people to an unsatisfactory community situation just to serve the function of educating the public, though they would obviously stand to gain eventually if attitudes and behaviour towards them became more positive. The knowledge and attitudes of the general public towards people living in institutions tends to be poor (McConkey, 1987); this obviously mitigates against a happy and successful 'community' experience, at least in the short term. Davidson (1987) believes that because of the attitudes of society and the pressure this puts on people who do not match society's expectations and standards, there may, in some circumstances and for some individuals, be a need for well run asylums. Davidson (1987) believes that even if the inadequacy of institutional living is accepted, it can still be inhumane to eject people into 'the community' when they have known no other home for many years.

An infrequently expressed view is that people with impairments may prefer to live with those who are similarly affected. Indeed the emphasis on integration may disguise a deep-rooted negativism, for there is an implicit assumption that ill and disabled people will be happier and more fulfilled in the 'normal' community, that they prefer the life style and company of those without impairment, and that they wish to be as 'normal' as possible. There is rarely any reference to the frustrations and disadvantages that striving for independence and 'normality' may create, or the benefits derived from being with similarly affected people in terms of empathy, friendship and the wealth of knowledge to be shared.

Harrison (1987) gives many examples of disabled people living in institutions who prefer the life style to that of more independent living. Morris (1993a) found that some disabled people she interviewed viewed residential care as giving them freedom because of the constant availability of staff, while others saw it as a stepping stone to independence from the parental home. It is likely, however, that these views were expressed in the light of inadequate community services and facilities.

Tully (1986) makes many suggestions for improving institutional life for disabled people. He believes that the principle of 'the least restrictive alternative' should operate at all times. This means that the environment must present the smallest possible restraint and disruption to the disabled person's well-being and preferred life style. He believes that residents should be fully involved in decision-making, including any concerning their own treatment and assessment, and that any records which are kept should be fully accessible to residents and reflect their own perspectives. Residents should not be prevented from taking risks and should be provided with sufficient privacy for relationships to develop. Every attempt should be made to integrate fully the institution with the community, according to the wishes of the residents.

Tully (1986) stresses the concept of 'normalization' which stresses the importance of disabled people having the same opportunities and conditions for living as any other citizen, so making their lives as 'normal' as possible. The concept of normalization must be used cautiously, however. For example, if activities such as dressing and eating take a long time and are difficult to achieve, it may make more sense for the person concerned to ask for assistance or to accomplish the task in a unconventional way. Having more time and being more efficient may be far more important to the disabled individual than being physically independent (French, 1991).

It should also be remembered that many non-disabled people have life styles considered 'abnormal' or deviant by mainstream standards. Thus ill and disabled people should not necessarily be expected to adopt a conventional way of life, nor should the criteria for their discharge from institutions be based on whether they can cook a meal, clean a room, or make a bed; there are many people living independently who do none of these things. Non-disabled helpers should not impose their definitions of 'normality' on residents but rather, in most circumstances, normality should be defined by the residents themselves.

The function of institutions

There are various views regarding the major functions of institutions. Professional rhetoric is usually in terms of 'treatment' and helping residents to reach their full potential, but others believe that they exist in order to enable mainstream society to run smoothly. Certainly many concerns have been expressed about the effects on non-disabled people of closing institutions and integrating ill and disabled people within society. For example, there are fears that the inclusion of disabled children in mainstream schools may adversely affect non-disabled children because of the amount of time the disabled children may require of teachers. This is unlikely to be a problem, however, if sufficient resources are available, indeed it has the potential to bring about favourable outcomes for all children, just as wheelchair access helps other groups such as those with young children in pushchairs. If, for example, a teacher talks very clearly, being sure to face the class in order to accommodate a hearing impaired child, then all children are likely to benefit. At a more subtle level, by paying attention to the needs of ill and disabled people, a greater atmosphere of tolerance to the needs of every individual may be created.

Institutions may also have the function of socializing disabled people to play a specific role. Scott (1969) gives a graphic account of rehabilitation centres for newly visually impaired people, where they are taught the behaviour and attitudes thought necessary to play the role of 'blind person'. The underlying philosophy of the majority of institutions is that disability is contained within the individual rather than within society, it is therefore viewed as a problem for the individual to 'overcome'. The staff of institutions are rarely in the business of encouraging people to challenge disabling physical and social barriers and attitudes which stand in their way.

The initial encounter with the service provider may occur at a time when the ill or disabled person is particularly vulnerable, either physically or psychologically. At a time such as this people may, understandably, be uncritical and unusually trusting, only later realizing that measures to solve the difficulties they are experiencing have been instigated and may be inappropriate. A further problem is that there is generally a lack of rehabilitation options which force people to accept whatever is on offer. As Davis (1993) puts it, '... the choice available to us amounts to little more than Hobson's choice'.

One of the justifications for the existence of institutions is that scarce and expensive resources, in terms of equipment and staff expertise, can be pooled. However, many people believe that such resources and services can and should be available within the community and that institutions should not be justified on these grounds. It is easy to over-estimate the importance of resources, the attitudes of ordinary people and their willingness to consult with and learn from those they wish to assist, is just as important. It is often the case that a reallocation of resources, rather than more resources, is all that is needed.

Without doubt one of the factors which has hindered the closure of institutions is the vested interests of the staff who work in them. If they close staff will have to work in a different way, in new surroundings, or may lose their jobs altogether. Professionals have defined and maintained institutions according to their own perspectives and interests, often viewing residents as less like others than they really are. They may welcome neither closure or a shift to 'the community' (Ryan and Thomas, 1987). Professionals are part of the institutional environment and it is therefore not always in their own interests to question that environment too closely (McConkey, 1987). Illich (1976), and many others, have argued that practices claimed by professionals to benefit clients, often serve their own interests more.

The large institutions have been inherited from a time when ideas about illness, disability and deviance were different from those held today. People with learning difficulties, for example, were thought to be dangerous, promiscuous, and a threat to society. No large and complex social system is easy to dismantle and will frequently persist even though those working within it, as well as the wider society, view it as divisive or have ceased to believe in its value. In order to reduce the psychological conflict this creates, people tend to find justifications for the existence and continuance of institutions which often have little in common with the original philosophy, or the reality of how they came to be.

Community

Abercombie *et al.* (1988) believe the concept of 'community' is 'one of the most elusive and vague within sociology' and that it is now 'without specific meaning'. Richman (1987) refers to the concept as one of 'infinite elasticity'. The notion of 'community' can refer to a group of people within a given geographical area, a collection of people living within a particular social structure, or a psychological entity; for example we talk of 'community spirit' and 'a sense of community'. When it comes to the concept of 'community care', Jones *et al.* (1983) point out the multitude of possible interpretations:

> 'To the politician 'community care' is a useful piece of rhetoric, to the sociologist it is a stick to beat institutional care with, to the civil servant it is a cheap alternative to institutional care which can be passed to the local authority for action or inaction, to the visionary it is a dream of the new society in which people really do care, to social service departments it is a nightmare of heightened public expectations and inadequate resources to meet them'.

Bayley (1973) made the distinction, more than 20 years ago, between care 'in' the community and care 'by' the community. During the 1980s to the present time, there has been increasing emphasis on care 'by' the community. Government now refers to the 'mixed economy of welfare', meaning that care of people deemed to be dependent must be the shared responsibility of statutory services, voluntary services, neighbours and family (Caring for People, 1989).

Illness and disability frequently result in extra expense in terms, for example, of diet, heating, transport, washing, special toys, and alterations to the home. This can lead to additional stress, especially as ill and disabled people and those who assist them are often excluded from the employment market. Inadequate community resources frequently leads to 'the revolving door syndrome' where people continually move between hospital and home.

Although discussion of 'community care' usually focuses on the closure of large institutions, in reality most ill and disabled people have always lived within the community, being assisted by their families. This caring role usually falls to close female relatives who receive little or no assistance from formal or informal services (Parker, 1993), although the role which men play in caring is now being recognized (Arber and Gilbert, 1989). Beardshaw (1988) refers to services for younger disabled people as the 'Cinderella of Cinderella services'.

Women, in particular, often feel compelled to become carers, and tend to feel guilty if they reject the role. This is due to the widespread belief, not only that it is their duty, but that to care is a central, almost biological, aspect of the female character. Parker (1993) found that informal help was limited when a carer was present, and that statutory help was given to male carers more readily than female carers.

Dalley (1988) believes that the liberation of one disadvantaged group, for example disabled people, can lead to the exploitation of another, for example women. Morris (1991) and Keith (1992), however, think that views such as these alienate disabled people by disregarding their experiences and viewing them as 'the problem'. There is little recognition that people are dependent on each other, physically and psychologically, or that those who need care are frequently carers themselves. Ryan and Thomas (1987) and Potts and Fido (1991) describe how the more able residents of mental handicap hospitals played a large role in caring for the less able residents, and Atkinson and Williams (1990), and Walmsley (1993) describe how people with learning difficulties often play a large role in caring for others in the community. This is frequently because they are 'trapped' in the family home with no socially sanctioned reasons, such as work commitments, not to care. Walmsley (1993) states:

> 'It is easy to over-simplify caring, to see a "carer" and a "dependent" in every caring relationship ... this is not always the case. There may be giving and taking, exploitation and opportunity, on both sides of the caring relationship.'

For these and other reasons disabled people have rejected the terms 'care' and 'carers' in favour of 'enablers' and 'personal assistants'. Disabled people are often under tremendous strain when forced to rely on a single helper, especially if that person would rather be somewhere else, they may also be at risk of emotional and physical abuse (Morris, 1993b).

'Community' is an emotive word which, like 'family', conjures up a nostalgic picture of warmth, friendship and neighbourliness. Politicians exploit this image when talking of 'care in the community', though in reality ill and disabled people discharged from institutions often end up in hotel rooms, inadequate hostels, or on the streets; Hudson (1991) provides a detailed analysis of the failure of deinstitutionalization for people with learning difficulties. It should be appreciated that the situation of disabled people in 'normal' society is frequently highly abnormal due to prejudice, adverse stereotyping, and the difficulty of adapting to an environment designed for non-disabled living. For life in 'the community' to be successful, therefore, the wider social and economic environment, in terms of housing, employment, transport, education and leisure facilities, must change to accommodate disabled people. Hicks (1988) states:

'A bridge needs to be built between the invisible world of family care and the public one of long-stay, institutional care. A middle way needs to be found which neither confines each carer to her private hell nor condemns our elderly and disabled population to being looked after exclusively by the state and its institutions'.

Independent living

For ill and disabled people who require help in everyday living, solutions other than institutions or assistance by relatives, do exist and ought to be expanded. Day hospitals and day centres have gone some way to providing assistance, and schemes where ordinary families live independently of, but in close proximity to, disabled people and assist them in exchange for a wage, operate in some parts of the country (Davis, 1981). Community Service Volunteers provide young people to assist disabled people on a 24-hour basis. Sheltered accommodation, where a warden is available, is another example.

Although solutions such as these can be a considerable improvement on both institutional living and total assistance by relatives, they still leave ill and disabled people fitting in with other people's schedules with little control of their own lives. Straughair and Fawcitt (1992), found, for example, that most of the young people they interviewed with arthritis felt it was not possible for them to leave the parental home because there was no substitute for the support and flexibility their parents provided. Others felt they could not move because of the financial benefits their parents would lose and the money they had expended on adaptations.

Many disabled people have found that the only way of achieving a satisfactory life style is to hire and train their own assistants. The Independent Living Fund, set up in 1988, provided disabled people with this opportunity, but the applications made drastically exceeded government expectations and the fund was closed to new applicants in 1992. Some disabled people use their own income, along with disability benefits, to buy their own assistance, but this option is out of the question for people whose income is low (Barnes, 1991). A few imaginative local authorities have, however, enabled disabled people to buy their own assistance and to do so has recently become law.

Morris (1993b) interviewed 50 disabled people between the ages of 19 and 55, who were living in the community. Some were relying on statutory services while others received direct payment to hire their own assistants. Those who relied on statutory services found that these were unresponsive to their needs and created major restrictions in their lives, dictating, for example, the time they went to bed and how frequently they bathed. Professional workers created barriers too by the specificity of their roles. Morris (1993b) states:

'A failure of statutory bodies to provide services which enabled disabled people to carry on their daily lives and engage in ordinary personal relationships creates a very poor quality of life and undermines human and civil rights'.

The interviewees in Morris's study who received direct payments for hiring and training their own assistants, had an entirely different experience. It enabled them to participate in society as they wished, and for some it permitted them to engage in paid employment, to support their parents, and to bring up their own children. Receiving some paid help from outside the family was seen by most disabled people as crucial to maintaining equality of relationships within the family. Some of the disabled people interviewed stressed that they did not want assistants with professional qualifications because they preferred to train them in their own way.

The only way of enabling disabled people to have the choices which non-disabled people take for granted is to introduce a fully comprehensive direct payment system, but as Morris (1993b) points out this has no place in the community care reforms which advocate resource-led assessments of disabled people by professionals, and the purchase of 'care' by managers. Morris (1993b) states:

> 'The ideology of caring which is at the heart of current community care policies can only result in institutionalisation within the community, unless politicians and professionals understand and identify with the philosophy and aims of the independent living movement. Independent living is a human and civil rights issue; community care confines people to the four walls of their own home, preventing them from fully participating in personal relationships and society, condoning the emotional and physical abuse which goes on behind closed doors'.

(For personal accounts of disabled people hiring and managing their own assistants, the reader is referred to Briggs (1993) and Macfarlane (1993).)

Oliver and Zarb (1992) carried out some similar research among 16 disabled people in Greenwich who were receiving direct payment for personal assistance. Employing their own workers improved the quality of their lives enormously, enabling them to work and to expand their social and leisure activities. Thirteen people had found out about the scheme through the Greenwich Association of Disabled People and only one through a social worker. The Greenwich Association of Disabled People also helped half of the disabled people to recruit their assistants. Considerable help may be required to manage personal assistants on an interpersonal as well as a practical level, for as Rae (1989) points out disabled people '... are conditioned not to structure other people's lives'.

Oliver and Zarb (1992) demonstrate by detailed analysis that money can be saved by providing disabled people with direct payments, and that the necessary resource can easily be found by switching it from other areas. They state:

> 'The success of Personal Assistance Schemes in allowing users to control how their support needs are met, provides a good model for the empowerment of disabled people by demonstrating that – given genuine choice and adequate resources – disabled people are able to exercise control over their lives and reduce for themselves their enforced dependency on inadequate services'.

Morris (1993a) is also of the opinion that current working practices tie up money in ways which are incompatible with independent living. (For further information on community care, the reader is referred to Bornat *et al.*, 1993.)

Conclusion

Physiotherapists work with ill and disabled people in a wide variety of institutional and community settings. It is important that they are aware of the full range of options possible and the advantages and disadvantages for each individual person. They need to think and act broadly and flexibly, outside the medical model of illness and disability, to avoid inadvertently restricting and alienating the very people they are trying to assist.

It is very important that physiotherapists become fully acquainted with illness and disability from the perspective of the client and to think very carefully about the ideas and wishes of ill and disabled people before proclaiming them unrealistic or impossible; most innovations, in independent living for example, have come from disabled people themselves not professionals. This level of understanding can only be achieved by consultation and cooperation with ill and disabled people themselves as well as the organizations which represent them.

Physiotherapists need to have a full understanding of the process of institutionalization. The civil rights of ill and disabled people, including their rights to take risks and lead unconventional life styles, should not be forgotten. Physiotherapists must take care that their own attitudes and practices are not influenced adversely by the institutional environment or based on erroneous stereotypes. They should be prepared to act as advocates and attempt to bring about change in management and policy if this would improve their clients' lives. Such an approach is a far cry from the traditional role of the physiotherapist and requires courage, especially of junior staff and students who lack influence and status themselves. Managers should be prepared to support them, for people new to the profession sometimes have a sharper perception of the situation than those who have worked within the system for many years.

It is important for physiotherapists to have a full understanding of the role and needs of carers. The expertise and knowledge of carers should be valued and their needs and limitations respected without making moral judgements. Hicks (1988) gives many examples of carers who found the help and support of professionals invaluable. Finkelstein's (1990) view that 'care' is frequently only necessary because disability is individualized, rather than being viewed as a product of society, should be considered and the physiotherapist should attempt, in full consultation and collaboration with the disabled person, to reduce disability by the provision of suitable aids, appliances and adaptations. A broad knowledge and understanding of where to refer the ill or disabled person and who to contact for help and advice, as well as the ability to work collaboratively is vital. Beardshaw (1988) believes that a major shift in the balance of power from professional to client needs to take place before any real progress can be made and that partnership approaches between professionals and disabled people have achieved nothing of significance. Physiotherapists may wish to join one of the many self-help and pressure groups concerned with improving the quality of life for ill and disabled people and those who assist them.

The Manchester Coalition of Disabled People state that: '... everyone has a right to choose how and where they want to live, and who they live with' and that 'Nobody should have to choose between being a burden to their family or living in a residential institution'. They believe that: 'Those who support and look after disabled people have rights and needs' and that 'disabled people and people who provide them with care do not have to suffer at each other's expense'. The assistance provided for ill and disabled people in Britain today is inadequate, restrictive, patchy and largely unimaginative.

A suitable place to live is of the utmost importance to the happiness and well-being of ill and disabled people. Yet in reality, despite many innovative schemes and considerable improvement, the choice is still too often between the family and an institution. This is unacceptable and a situation which physiotherapists can play their part in changing.

References

Abercrombie N., Hill S., Turner B. (1988) *Dictionary of Sociology*. Harmondsworth: Penguin Books.

Arber S., Gilbert N. (1989) Men: the forgotten carers. *Sociology*, **23**(1), 111–118.

Atkinson D., Williams F. (1990) *Know Me As I am: An Anthology of Prose, Poetry and Art by People with Learning Difficulties*. Sevenoaks: Hodder and Stoughton.

Barnes C. (1991) *Disabled People in Britain and Discrimination*. London: Hurst and Company.

Bayley M. J. (1973) *Mental Handicap and Community Care*. London: Routledge and Kegan Paul.

Beardshaw V. (1988) *Last on the List: Community Services for People with Physical Disabilities*. London: King's Fund Institute.

Booth T., Statham J. (1982) *The Nature of Special Education*. London: Croom Helm.

Bornat J., Pereira C., Pilgrim D., Williams F. (eds) (1993) *Community Care*. London: Macmillan.

Briggs L. (1993) Striving for independence. In *Disabling Barriers – Enabling Environments* (Swain J., Finkelstein V., French S., Oliver M., eds). London: Sage.

Caring for People: Community Care in the Next Decade and Beyond (1989) London: HMSO.

The Coalition and Care in the Community. Greater Manchester Coalition of Disabled People.

Committee of Enquiry into the Education of Handicapped Children and Young People (1978) *Special Educational Needs* (Warnock Report). London: HMSO.

Cooke M. (1987) Part of the institution. *Nursing Times*, **83**(23), 25–27.

Dalley G. (1988) *Ideologies of Caring*. London: Macmillan.

Davidson N. (1987) Community care or community neglect? In *A Question of Care*, (Davidson N., ed.). London: Michael Joseph.

Davis K. (1981) 28–38 Grove Road: accommodation and care in a community setting. In *Handicap in a Social World*, (Brechin A., Liddiard P., Swain J., eds). Sevenoaks: Hodder and Staughton.

Davis K. (1993) The crafting of good clients. In *Disabling Barriers – Enabling Environments*, (Swain J., Finkelstein V., French S., Oliver M., eds). London: Sage.

Finkelstein V. (1990) Home study text. *Disability – Changing Practice*. Milton Keynes: Open University Press.

Finkelstein V. (1991) Disability: an administrative challenge. In *Social Work, Disabled People and Disabling Environments*, (Oliver M., ed.). London: Jessica Kingsley.

Ford S. (1987) Into the outside. *Nursing Times*, **83**(20), 40–42.

French S. (1991) What's so great about independence? *The New Beacon*, **75**(886), 153–156.

French S. (1992) Memories of school 1958–1962. In *Living Proof*, (O'Keefe S., ed.). London: The Royal National Institute for the Blind.

French S. (1996) Out of sight, out of mind: the experience and effects of a 'special' residential school. In *Feminism and Disability*, (Morris J., ed.). London: The Women's Press.

Goffman I. (1961) *Asylums*. Harmondsworth: Penguin Books.

Harrison J. (1987) *Severe Physical Disability*. London: Cassell.

Hicks C. (1988) *Who Cares?* London: Virago Press.

Holmes B., Johnson A. (1988) *Cold Comfort*. London: Souvenir Press.

Hudson B. (1991) Deinstitutionalisation: what went wrong? *Disability, Handicap and Society*, **6**(1), 21–36.

Humphries S., Gordon P. (1992) *Out of Sight: The Experience of Disability 1900–1950*. Plymouth: Northcote House.

Hunt J. (1992) The Disabled People's Movement between 1960–1986 and its effect upon the development of Community Support Services. *Dissertation by Independent Study*. London: University of East London.

Illich J. (1976) *Limits to Medicine*. Harmondsworth: Penguin.

Jones K., Brown J., Bradshaw J. (1983) *Issues in Social Policy*. London: Routledge and Kegan Paul.

Jones K. (1993) *Asylums and After*. London: The Athlone Press.

Keith L. (1992) Who cares wins? Women, caring, and disability. *Disability, Handicap and Society*, **7**(2), 167–176.

Ladd P. (1990) Language oppression and hearing impairment. In the book of readings of the disability equality training pack *Disability – Changing Practice*. The Open University. Milton Keynes: Open University Press.

Laing R. D. (1967) *The Politics of Experience and the Bird of Paradise*. Harmondsworth: Penguin Books.

McConkey R. (1987) *Who Cares? Community Involvement with Handicapped People*. London: Souvenir Press.

Macfarlane A. (1993) The right to make choices. In *Community Care*, (Bornat J., Pereira C., Pilgrim D., Williams F., eds). London: Macmillan.

Madge N., Fassam M. (1982) *Ask the Children*. London: Batsford.

Marchant R., Page M. (1992) *Bridging the Gap*. London: National Society for the Prevention of Cruelty to Children.

Marchant R., Cross M. (1993) Places of safety? Institutions, disabled children and abuse. In the Reader of the *ABCD Pack Abuse and Children who are Disabled: training and resource pack for trainers in child protection and disability*. The National Deaf Children's Society, NSPCC, Way Ahead Disability Consultancy and Chailey Heritage.

Meadow W. P. (1980) *Deafness and Child Development*. London: Arnold.

Morris J. (1991) *Pride Against Prejudice*. London: The Women's Press.

Morris J. (1993a) *Independent Lives? Community Care and Disabled People*. London: Macmillan.

Morris J. (1993b) *Community Care or Independing Living?* London: Joseph Roundtree Foundation.

Oliver M., Zarb G. (1992) *Personal Assistance Schemes*. London: Greenwich Association of Disabled People.

Orford J. (1980) Institutional climates. In *Psychology and Medicine*, (Griffiths D., ed.). London: Macmillan.

Oswin M. (1978) *Holes in the Welfare Net*. London: Bedford Square Press.

Parker G. (1993) *With This Body: Caring and Disability in Marriage*. Buckingham: Open University Press.

Potts M., Fido R. (1991) *A Fit Person to be Removed: Personal Accounts of Life in a Mental Deficiency Institution*. Plymouth: Northcote House.

Rae A. (1989) Enablers not carers. *Disability Now*, October, p. 6.

Reber A. S. (1985) *The Penguin Dictionary of Psychology*. Harmondsworth: Penguin Books.

Richman J. (1987) *Medicine and Health*. London: Longman.

Ryan J., Thomas F. (1987) *The Politics of Mental Handicap*. London: Free Association Books.

Scott R. A. (1969) *The Making of Blind Men*. New York: Russell Sage Foundation.

Sedgwick J. (1989) Dressed with dignity. *Nursing Times*, **85**(48), 30–31.

Shearer A. (1982) *Living Independently*. London: Centre for the Environment of the Handicapped and The King's Fund Centre.

Sobsey D. (1994) Sexual abuse of individuals with intellectual disability. In *Sexuality and Learning Difficulties*, (Craft A., ed.). London: Routledge.

Straughair S., Fawcitt S. (1992) *The Road Towards Independence: The Experiences of Young People with Arthritis in the 1990s*. London: Arthritis Care.

Szasz T. S. (1961) *The Myth of Mental Illness*. New York: Harper and Row.

Townsend P. (1962) *The Last Refuge*. London: Routledge and Kegan Paul.

Tully K. (1986) *Improving Residential Life for Disabled People*. London: Churchill Livingstone.

Vaizey J. (1959) Scenes from Institutional Life. Cited in Jones K., Brown J., Bradshaw J. (1983) *Issues in Social Policy*. London: Routledge and Kegan Paul.

Wade B., Moore M. (1993) *Experiencing Special Education*. Buckingham: Open University Press.

Walmsley J. (1993) Contradictions in caring: reciprocity and interdependence. *Disability, Handicap and Society*. **8**(2), 129–141.

Westcott H. L. (1991) *Institutional Abuse of Children – From Research to Policy. A Review*. London: National Society for the Prevention of Cruelty to Children.

Westcott H. L. (1993) *Abuse of Children and Adults with Disabilities*. London: National Society for the Prevention of Cruelty to Children.

Wilkinson D. (1987) Busy doing nothing. *Nursing Times*, **83**(23), 30–31.

4

Sex, gender and health care

Helen Roberts

Women go to the doctor more often than men, they take more medicines than men, and they spend more time looking after other people's health than do men (Foster, 1995; Roberts, 1985).

The organization of health care and the care of sick people have a long history of sex differentiation. This is true on a routine, day-to-day basis, as well as in acute and chronic illness and disabling conditions.

It is not only in the gender structure of service delivery that we can see differences between men and women. As McPherson (1988) has pointed out, there have always been differences between the health problems of men and women. Even in early hunter-gatherer societies, the major causes of death are likely to have been different according to gender. What is of interest to us is not just the epidemiology of these differences, but the context in which they arise and are treated now.

This chapter falls into three sections. The first is largely descriptive, and is based mainly on 'hard' data. This section describes some differences between the sexes in morbidity (ill health) and mortality (death rates) and then discusses sex differences in the work force of the medical profession and the professions allied to medicine. Of course, the vast majority of health care, and the care of sick people, is not performed by professionals at all, but is carried out in the home. Sex differences among unpaid carers are discussed below, as is the problematic notion of 'caring', objectifying as it does those who are 'cared for' (Keith and Morris, 1995).

Statistical data give us one type of information about the health of men and women, and the relative proportions of men and women in different health care professions but they do not tell us about the experience of good or poor health, what it is like to be a woman in a male dominated profession, or a man in female dominated work. Some attention will be given to this, and to the differential respect accorded to 'care' and to 'cure'

The second section covers two areas of health care where physiotherapists are likely to have a significant presence. In the first, childbirth, women make up 100% of the clientele, and in the second, the area of spinal cord injuries, women patients are in the minority for reasons evident when one considers the sex differentiation in the kinds of activities where spinal cord injuries may arise.

The final section is speculative and focuses on the gender structure of the physiotherapy profession and the kinds of research, particularly in the area of physiotherapy, which might be fundable, feasible and useful in addressing the different needs of men and women patients.

Sex differences in health state and health status

What kinds of data do we have on men, women and health? Physiological variation between men and women and the process of reproduction account for some of the differences between the sexes in rates of death and illness. The social contexts within which women and men live also help us to understand some of these differences. Young men, for instance, are more prone to drive fast cars and are considerably more likely than young women to be seriously injured in road traffic accidents, rugby games or as a result of violence.

MacFarlane (1990), whose work provides a comprehensive discussion of sex differences in health statistics, with examples of the main data sources available in the UK, points out that while women can expect to live longer than men, statistics about the use of health services give the impression that women make greater use of these. Admission rates for men and women in acute non-psychiatric hospitals are higher among women than men overall, even when admissions to maternity wards are excluded. However, in people under 15 and over 45 years of age, more boys and men are admitted, and in the age group 15 to 44 MacFarlane shows that once admissions due to reproduction (abortions, miscarriages and so on) are excluded differences in admission rates between men and women virtually disappear. Sex differences in attendance at out-patient clinics are negligible.

There are a number of areas where rising levels of surgical intervention in relation to women have caused concern. One is Caesarian section; a large and increasing number of women are having their babies delivered in this way. Another is hysterectomy. Both of these procedures involve major abdominal operations and in many cases there is a lack of professional consensus over whether they are strictly necessary (Teo, 1990). More than 20 years ago in a much quoted editorial, it was suggested that 'after the last planned pregnancy, the uterus becomes a useless, bleeding, symptom producing, potentially cancer bearing organ and should be removed' (Wright, 1969). Would this sort of view of women's bodies be acceptable today? In some quarters, it would though it might not be so blatant. An editorial in the *British Journal of Obstetrics and Gynaecology* on the prophylactic removal of the ovaries (oophorectomy) concluded, '(their removal) should be offered to all women over the age of forty having an abdominal hysterectomy'. It is a sign of the times that the author adds: '(It) should only be performed after adequate discussion, understanding and of course consent. The woman has the ultimate choice. If she exercises what is perhaps the only worthwhile argument against prophylactic oophorectomy, namely a *sentimental desire to keep her ovaries* (my emphasis) then it would be a foolish and insensitive gynaecologist who would ignore this compelling argument' (Studd, 1989). It is interesting in this context that a recent legal case in which a woman of 35 had a hysterectomy during which, without her consent, an 11-week fetus was aborted, found in favour of the obstetrician concerned: 'During surgery, (the obstetrician) noticed a swelling of the womb and realised there was a possibility that his patient was pregnant. He decided to go ahead with the operation after failing to contact her husband ... He added that her age, then 35, also influenced his decision' (Veash, 1995).

In terms of primary health care, women consult general practitioners more often than men, and the sharpest differences are again in the child-bearing age group. MacFarlane (1990) presents data which show that once consultations which are not for illness are removed, for instance those for contraception, the differences are much smaller, and when consultations for pregnancy, childbirth and diseases of the male and female genitourinary systems are excluded, the differences virtually disappear.

Of course, data about the use made of health services are not necessarily the best measures of health. Consultation rates and hospital admission rates tell us about the use of services, not the state of people's health. Blaxter (1985) makes the distinction between temporary states of health, 'Am I ill today?' and longer term health status reflected in answers to the question, 'Am I basically a healthy or unhealthy person?' In a survey in Glasgow, women aged 35 to 54 were asked to report on their health (McIlwaine et al., 1989). When asked how they considered their own state of health, more than 60% replied that it was about the same as that of other women of their acquaintance. At the same time, over 50% described themselves as lacking in energy, over 40% had trouble sleeping and about 40% reported feeling depressed.

Sociologists have described how the process of defining oneself as ill, or acting on symptoms, depends in part on how common such symptoms are in a society or group. If a symptom is common, it is likely to be considered normal and therefore not defined as illness. Zola (1966), in his study of illness behaviour, found that tiredness was often considered normal. Some researchers have argued that women will report more ill health than men because they are in a better position to act on symptoms and adopt the 'sick role'. Verbrugge and Wingard (1987) have suggested that the crucial feature of women's social roles may be flexibility but as Popay (1991) points out, in her study of health and health care in families with vastly different levels of income, that flexibility was missing from women's daily experience of life as mother, housewife or paid employee.

We do not know very much about the differences in the ways health professionals view their male and female patients, but research by Walton (1968) suggests that women medical students are more patient orientated. Roos et al. (1977) found that they have more interest in people's emotional problems and Cartwright (1967) that they are more sensitive to 'relationship values'. Stimson (1976) asked doctors about the patients whom they considered least and most troublesome. Among patients considered 'least trouble' were men, those with organic, easy to diagnose medical problems and those who have confidence in the doctor, accept that there are limits to the doctor's skill, are cooperative and have good homes and circumstances. Among those considered 'most trouble' were women, those with vague symptoms and those who do not follow advice, are unable to cope and are in poor social circumstances.

Women as providers and users of health care

Women are both the main users of the health service, and the main providers of health care. Sex differences in the organization of both paid and unpaid health care and the care of sick people are not new as an article as century ago in the *British Medical Journal* makes clear: 'In the truest interest of women it is better that they should not practice the medical profession ... it is scarcely possible for a woman to go through a course of medical education without losing that simplicity and purity of character which we so much value ...'.

In case it should be thought that this would leave women with nothing to do, the authors suggest that unpaid health care may be the solution, '(We) have frequent reason to lament that there is no spinster aunt or sister at hand to take charge of some poor invalid' (*British Medical Journal*, 1977).

Women as colleagues in medicine still face stiff opposition from some quarters. When the Sex Discrimination Act came into force in the mid 1970s, one consequence was that the doors of all physiotherapy schools, some of which until that time had run courses exclusively for women, were open to men. Another consequence was the opening up of medical schools to women. A week after the new law came into force, an editorial in the *British Medical Journal* suggested: 'Any woman doctor who decides to make a career in a prestigious specialty such as neurology or cardio-thoracic surgery will find that she is competing with men who give one hundred percent of their effort to their work: she cannot expect to succeed if she tries to combine her specialist training with bringing up a family herself' (*British Medical Journal*, 1976).

In response to this, one might point to an article in *The Lancet* which notes that while women doctors who temporarily or permanently drop out of full-time practice have been studied frequently, men, who are just as expensive to train, have not, despite their disappearance from National Health Service practice through emigration, death, alcoholism, suicide or removal from the medical register. The authors point out that, 'in a working lifetime of forty years, a woman doctor with an average family is likely to do seven eighths of the work of a doctor who has not had to carry the primary responsibility for bearing and rearing children (Bewley and Bewley, 1975). While the 1976 *British Medical Journal* article did not speculate on the problems of *male* neurologists or cardiothoracic surgeons attempting to combine family and professional life, it is heartening to note that in the intervening years, there has been an increasing tendency for young men in medicine to explore ways of combining family and work life. (As with women attempting the same juggling act, their aspirations in this direction have frequently been the triumph of hope over experience.)

Although there had been a gradual erosion of male quotas in medical school entrance in the years preceding the new law, one result of the Sex Discrimination Act of 1975 has been that at least 50% of entrants to British medical schools are now women. Men have not rushed into physiotherapy with quite the same enthusiasm as women have entered medicine, and some possible reasons for this are discussed below.

How are men and women distributed within health care employment?

Graham (1990) points out that overall 11% of white women in paid employment work in the health services (public and private), for black and ethnic minority women, the proportion is 17%, and within the National Health Service about 75% of the workforce are women. While about one-quarter of all hospital doctors are women, only 14% of these are in the consultant grade. About 14% of unrestricted principals in general practice are women although women comprise about 35% of trainees. About 90% of nurses are women, 73% of chiropodists, 89% of dieticians and occupational therapists and 76% of physiotherapists (Buchan and Pike, 1989).

Efforts are currently being made to encourage more men into physiotherapy. Leaflets on physiotherapy as a career from the Chartered Society of Physiotherapy include pictures of both men and women practitioners and one leaflet explains: 'both men and women work as physiotherapists. In addition to having academic and practical ability, you need to be a good communicator, tolerant, patient and caring' (Chartered Society of Physiotherapy, 1990). It might be worth readers asking themselves what sort of person springs to mind when they read the adjectives 'tolerant, patient and caring'. While women by no means have the monopoly on these characteristics, they are adjectives frequently applied to the ideal mother. Industrial psychologists have shown the different values attached to characteristics like 'forceful', 'caring' or 'ambitious' when they are applied to men or to women. It may be that in spite of the efforts made to encourage men into the physiotherapy profession, there are all kinds of attributes attached to the skills felt to be desirable for physiotherapists which are seen as feminine.

An early (1984) version of the pamphlet *How to Become a Chartered Physiotherapist*, refers to both short and tall stature as possible problems for physiotherapists. While the contraindication for very tall people is apparently physiological since they 'are particularly susceptible to the occupational hazard of back injuries', in relation to short stature, there is an additional problem, 'whereas small people may often acquire the strength and skill to cope with (lifting and support of heavy patients), *they must also be able to gain the confidence of patients*' (my emphasis) (Chartered Society of Physiotherapy, 1984). It is a welcome sign of the times that the possible disqualification of being less than 1.57 metres tall, a height which is considerably more common among women than among men, does not appear in recent pamphlets.

The problem which the Chartered Society of Physiotherapy identified in the earlier leaflet is a realistic one. Some patients may lack confidence in short people, just as some patients may lack confidence in Black people, or disabled people. The solution is not to turn these prejudices into disqualifying characteristics. Practitioners, irrespective of height, ethnicity, sex or physical disability need to be taught the skills needed to gain the confidence of patients and to cope in a dignified way with those patients who lack confidence in their carers. Misplaced confidence by patients in treatment which has not been evaluated, or carers who do not in fact care very much, is quite another matter.

The pay for people who work in the professions allied to medicine within the National Health Service is not high. The management structure of the NHS does afford some relatively well paid posts as district physiotherapy managers but, by definition, these are few. The majority of practising physiotherapists are under the age of 30, and since the majority of physiotherapists are women, we can relate patterns of employment to family formation. The final section, which discusses working for change, comes back to this point.

Of course the majority of health care and a good deal of care of sick people, is not performed by health professionals at all, but is done in the home usually, but not always, by women as mothers, wives and daughters. Graham (1984, 1987, 1990), who has worked extensively on women's 'health work' describes and analyses some of the components of this work. Among those caring for children, about three out of every four women in households with pre-school children are full-time carers, and in single parent households, women outnumber men by nine to one. Piachaud (1985) points out that the 'principal carers' of able bodied children up to 2 years of age, spend about 8 hours a day in health behaviours directed to their children; getting them up and dressed, toileting, feeding, bathing and so on. Of those providing at least 20 hours a week of personal care for elderly people; disabled people and those suffering from long-term illness, research suggests that over 60% are women (OPCS, 1988).

While women predominate in health care, the high status and highly paid jobs continue to be overwhelmingly occupied by men. Lower paid and unpaid care are more likely to be undertaken by women. It is sometimes said that doctors cure and nurses care. Certainly with the exception of surgery, those who do the 'hands on' care tend to be the least rewarded in terms of pay and status.

Women's experiences of health care: examples from childbirth and motor impairment

This section describes some of the qualitative aspects of health care in two areas where physiotherapists have a significant presence. One is pregnancy, childbirth and the immediate post-partum period, which are transient physiological events, and the other, long-term disability. Different kinds of data can give us very different perspectives on the same subject. Knowing all there is to know about the physiology of normal labour, for instance, tells us nothing about what it is like to become a mother. Similarly, knowing all there is to know about spinal cord injuries does not tell us what it is like to be a healthy disabled person, and the recipient (or not) of others' caring activities.

Pregnancy, childbirth and maternity

Kitzinger (1984) points out that it was the work of Dick Grantly-Read in the 1930s, combined with advances in obstetric physiotherapy stemming largely from the office of Helen Heardman, which formed the basis for most types of preparation for childbirth that many midwives and obstetricians today accept as smoothing the path of women in labour.

In the area of childbirth, there is a level of 'official' concern about women's satisfaction with maternity services. The Maternity Services Advisory Committee which was set up by the Secretary of State for Social Services and the Secretary of State for Wales in 1981, was concerned with the number of consumer complaints about the impersonal nature of care in hospitals. This committee published three reports and one of their recommendations was that the satisfaction of parents with these services should be explored at a local level.

Quantitative work in obstetrics can tell us important facts about the number of instrumental births, the number of Caesarian sections, the use of induction and drugs to accelerate labour and so on. The maternity services have tended to be more inclined than some other clinical specialities to audit their work at a local level in order to monitor perinatal deaths, and in some cases to look more broadly at service provision.

Women's attitudes and feelings about their experiences of pregnancy, childbirth and early motherhood are more difficult to measure, though research instruments may be used to rate on a scale of 1 to 5 whether they found a particular procedure, such as episiotomy, very unpleasant (5) unpleasant (4) neither pleasant nor unpleasant (3) pleasant (2) or very pleasant (1). Attitudinal data collected in this way are naturally simpler to analyse than open-ended questions, but important work can be done by collecting information from patients in a systematic way by talking to them. Oakley's accounts of pregnancy, childbirth and the first months of motherhood for instance, provide grounds for thinking about the sorts of maternity services which women would find helpful, and some of the problems of becoming a mother (Oakley, 1981). Oakley's work is based very firmly on women's own accounts rather than on 'expert' views of how women feel or should feel. The majority of her data were obtained through careful face to face interviewing.

Questionnaires may also elicit some aspects of women's experiences of pregnancy; Mason (1989) describes how 'open' answers in women's own words may be used and analysed as part of a more formal survey. For readers interested in carrying out a survey into patient satisfaction *Women's Experience of Maternity Care: a Survey Manual* by Mason (1989) is essential reading, though physiotherapists might like to add questions on obstetric physiotherapy to the model questionnaire.

Some of the most important work on pregnancy and childbirth in recent years has been the move towards evidence-based medicine (a surprise to some that there was ever any other sort). The collection of data from randomized controlled trials – the gold standard of evaluation – on everything from episiotomy to pubic shaving; from trial labour in those who have undergone a previous Caesarian section to the prevention of premature labour, have revolutionized midwifery and obstetric practice, and given an important tool to women who want to influence the way they are treated in pregnancy and childbirth. One of the most important ways to empower people is through sharing knowledge and those working on evidence-based medicine (based in the UK at the Cochrane Collaboration in Oxford) are looking at different ways of ensuring a voice for 'users' as well as ensuring that the results of studies are well disseminated (Enkin *et al.*, 1990).

Women and disability

Physiotherapists will be aware of the important distinction between impairment and disability. Broadly, impairment refers to the injury or disease and disability to the consequences of impairment within a social context. People with impairments may be disabled by poor access to buildings, the prejudices of employers and others, and enforced dependency (see Chapter 23). Lonsdale (1990), who has written on women and disability, suggests that: 'Dependency has particular implications for women because of the important part which gender plays in determining whether someone is expected or encouraged or indeed even allowed to be independent. Since women are encouraged to play a more dependent role in society than men, disabled women often have a particular struggle to achieve control over their own destinies, although they are sometimes "allowed" out of the passive and dependent female role'.

One problem for women in general, but which takes on particular salience for disabled women, is that being 'good' may mean being passive and obedient. As Lonsdale points out, being a 'bad' patient could mean demonstrating precisely those characteristics of independence and activity which are necessary for coping and surviving. Lonsdale describes how it is not unusual for a disabled woman to be labelled 'unrealistic' if she wants to live independently, especially if her plans do not conform to the expected female role. Disabled women who are mothers face not only the challenges which all mothers face, but also the challenge of being a parent in a disabling society. In some cases, these challenges will be met by a response which supports the 'carers' of the disabled parent, without making those moves which would render the parent less dependent. Keith and Morris (1995) write ... 'the social issue of caring has been constructed on the assumption that unpaid work within the family ... will continue ... Colluding with the government's position that public resources will never be adequate to replace the practical assistance given within the family (mainly by women) to disabled and older people, many researchers and campaigners have focused on services which would 'ease the burden of caring'. As the authors point out, a statutory duty is imposed on social services authorities to carry out assessments by the 1986 Disabled Persons Act and to meet such needs by the 1970 Chronically Sick and Disabled Persons Act. Focusing on the needs of carers may obscure the rights which disabled people have to receive services.

Sometimes therapy can be considered more important than a disabled person's education and many disabled people have challenged this view. Before the 1981 Education Act disabled children would usually be educated at ordinary schools only if they had very insistent parents. One of the respondents in Lonsdale's study describes how physiotherapy disrupted her education at the special school she attended. She writes: 'If you are going to be disturbed from your maths class to go to physiotherapy, that's wrong. Physiotherapy and hydrotherapy should be a separate thing from school. It shouldn't affect your education ... It's bad enough being disabled but to have no qualifications either, then you're going into the world of work with nothing' (Lonsdale, 1990).

A book written by women with spinal injuries describes some aspects of their quality of life as workers, mothers, lovers and patients, after an accident or illness resulting in paralysis. One writes: 'I had regular physiotherapy and did occupational therapy, but there was no-one to discuss problems and personal feelings with, and no sort of counselling to help with the present or future. It seemed as if one was expected to be cheerful and "keep one's chin up" all the time' (Morris, 1989).

The book describes the problems women have in coping with the emphasis in spinal units on sport, competition and physical achievement, and suggests that this may be directly related to the fact that rehabilitation programmes have been geared primarily towards men with spinal cord injuries. This can mean people being pushed into an approach to physical achievement which they experience as oppressive and inappropriate. One woman wrote: 'Excellent though the physiotherapy was, I did find later that my performance improved with exercise done to music and for pleasure. Most things were sport orientated. I hate competition and have no eye for balls or arrows' (Morris, 1989).

In this section some of the qualitative research which provides us with a framework for understanding the experience of the patient as a person has been described. The translation of what can be learned from qualitative research into clinical practice may not be as straightforward as adopting a new drug which has been found effective through a randomized controlled trial, but it is as important.

Working for change

There has been a gradual change in the health professions in recent years in the extent to which they are willing to consult patients, and to see them as whole people rather than 'a tib and fib' or 'the paraplegic in bed five'. Some health professionals embrace this change while others are pushed more or less willingly towards it. The previous section described some of the ways in which we may begin to learn more about patients' needs and perspectives and how our differing views of men and women may affect the ways in which they are treated. We have different expectations of patients according to gender, and should be encouraged to question these and develop services in ways in which patients can describe to us if we listen. There are huge reservoirs of untapped knowledge among 'lay' people which professionals have been slow to access (Roberts *et al.*, 1995) and which we would do well to explore further (Beresford and Croft, 1995).

What of gender differentiation within the profession of physiotherapy? Much of the material above relating to sex differences in the health professions is based on literature concerning doctors, simply because this profession has been most frequently studied. What are the consequences of physiotherapy being a largely female profession in terms of the labour market?

According to a recent report by Buchan and Pike (1989) on the professions allied to medicine, the key characteristics of the work force are the comparatively low age profile and the predominance of women. There is a growing increase in the proportion of elderly people in our society which means that the demand for physiotherapists is likely to increase. Given the age and sex distribution of physiotherapists and what we know about family formation patterns however, problems are likely to arise as women take periods out of the labour market to bear and rear children. Research on female pharmacists currently working in the NHS revealed that better pay, more flexible hours and creche facilities were frequently given as factors important in the recruitment and retention of workers (Bevan *et al.*, 1989).

The Department of Health has made a number of recommendations, short of improving pay, aimed at the retention of staff. The Institute of Manpower Studies, which has considerable expertise in employment and training matters, reports that data are lacking on the extent to which these initiatives have been taken up. Meager *et al.* (1989) points out that where they have been taken up, in the area of job sharing for instance, there is some evidence that the increase has been as a result of pressure from individual employees rather than policy led management initiatives. Issues such as these, the European market and the organization and management of health provision within the NHS and the private sector, are likely to shape the way in which physiotherapy develops into the twenty-first century.

Conclusion

Female dominated professions have a number of strengths, although they tend to be short on industrial muscle. Ironically enough, some of these strengths are related to 'feminine' characteristics of caring, empathy and patience brought to the professional lives of many women through their female socialization. If men are to be encouraged into physiotherapy in greater numbers, it is important that these qualities are not lost. At the same time, it will be interesting to monitor the extent to which senior posts in physiotherapy are differentially occupied by men and women in proportion to their overall numbers in the profession, and for women to learn from men some of those characteristics which make them inclined to apply for, obtain, and function in those senior positions from which it is possible to have a wide-ranging influence on the way in which physiotherapy is practised.

In terms of service provision, we do not know exactly what patients need unless we ask them, and listen to their answers. Research need not be done in an academic library or a laboratory. Oakley (1981) points out that '... Experience does alter the way people (experts and others) behave: this is part of the scientific method that theories should be tested empirically, not just once under artificial conditions, but constantly in the real world'. Much of research is 'finding out' and physiotherapists, including students, are often in a position to find out from their patients and clients what their needs are, what they find satisfying about a particular service and in what ways they feel the service might be improved. Not all suggestions patients make have massive resource implications, and at a time when consumer satisfaction is said to be important, there should be management sympathy for carrying out this basic research.

Acknowledgements

I am grateful to Stuart Skyte of the Chartered Society of Physiotherapy for access to data on the physiotherapy profession.

References

Beresford P., Croft S. (1995) It's our problem too! Challenging the exclusion of poor people from poverty discourse. In *Critical Social Policy*, 44/45, pp. 75–95.
Bevan, S., Buchan J., Heyday S. (1989) *Women in Hospital Pharmacy*. Brighton: Institute of Manpower Studies, University of Sussex.

Bewley B., Bewley T. H. (1975) Hospital doctors' career structure and misuse of medical womanpower. *Lancet*, **ii**, August 9, 270–272.

Blaxter M. (1985) Self definition of health status and consulting rates in primary care. *Quarterly Journal of Social Affairs*, **1**(2), 131–171.

British Medical Journal (1976) Women in medicine (Editorial). *British Medical Journal*, **10**, January, 56.

British Medical Journal (1977) One hundred years ago (taken from *British Medical Journal* 1877). *British Medical Journal*, 30 April, 1149.

Buchan J., Pike G. (1989) *PAMS into the 1990s – Professions allied to medicine: the wider labour market context*. IMS Report No. 175. Brighton: Institute of Manpower Studies, University of Sussex.

Cartwright A. (1967) *Patients and their Doctors: A Study of General Practice*. London: Routledge and Kegan Paul.

Chartered Society of Physiotherapy (1984) *How to Become a Chartered Physiotherapist* (pamphlet). London: Chartered Society of Physiotherapy.

Chartered Society of Physiotherapy (1990) *Physiotherapy Career in a Caring Profession* (pamphlet). London: Chartered Society of Physiotherapy.

Enkin M., Keirse M. J., Chalmers I. (1990) *A Guide to Effective Care in Pregnancy and Childbirth*. Oxford: Oxford University Press.

Foster P. (1995) *Women and the Health Care Industry*. Buckingham: Open University Press.

Graham H. (1984) *Women, Health and the Family*. Brighton: Wheatsheaf.

Graham H. (1987) Women's poverty and caring. In *Women and Poverty in Britain*, (Glendinning C., Millar J., eds). Brighton: Wheatsheaf.

Graham H. (1990) Behaving well: women's health behaviour in context. In *Women's Health Counts*, (Roberts H. ed). London: Routledge, pp. 195–219.

Keith L., Morris J. (1995) Easy targets: a disability rights perspective on the 'children as carers' debate. In *Critical Social Policy*, London: Sage, 44/45, pp. 36–57.

Kitzinger S. (1984) *The Experience of Childbirth* (5th edn). Harmondsworth: Penguin Books.

Lonsdale S. (1990) *Women and Disability*. London: Macmillan.

Macfarlane A. (1990) Official statistics and women's health and illness. In *Women's Health Counts*, (Roberts H., ed.). London: Routledge, pp. 18–62.

McIlwaine G., Rosenberg K., Rooney I. (1989) The health of mid life inner city women. *Journal of Psychosomatic Obstetrics and Gynaecology*, **10** suppl. 1, 102.

McPherson A. (1988) Why women's health? In *Women's Problems in General Practice*, (McPherson A., ed.). Oxford: Oxford University Press, pp. 1–13.

Mason V. (1989) *Women's Experience of Maternity Care: A Survey Manual*. London: HMSO.

Meager N., Buchan J., Rees C. (1989) *Job Sharing in the NHS*. Brighton: Institute of Manpower Studies, University of Sussex.

Morris J. (1989) *Able Lives: Women's Experience of Paralysis*. London: The Women's Press.

Oakley A. (1981) *From Here to Maternity*. Harmondsworth: Pelican.

Office of Population Censuses and Surveys (OPCS) (1988) *Informal Carers: General Household Surveys*, 1985. London: HMSO.

Piachaud D. (1985) *Round About Fifty Hours a Week*. London: Child Poverty Action Group.

Popay J. (1991) Women's experience of ill health. In *Women's Health Matters* (Roberts H., ed.). London: Routledge.

Roberts H. (1985) *The Patient Patients*. London: Pandora.

Roberts H., Smith S. J., Bryce C. (1995) *Children at Risk: Safety as a Social Value*. Buckingham: Open University Press.

Roos M. P., Gaumont M., Colwill N. L. (1977) Female and physician: a sex role incongruity. *Journal of Medical Education*, **52**, 345–346.

Stimson G. (1976) General practitioners, trouble and types of patients. In *The Sociology of the NHS*, (Stacey M., ed.). Sociological Review Monograph no 2. Keele: University of Keele.

Studd J. (1989) Prophylactic oophorectomy. *British Journal of Obstetrics and Gynaecology*, **96**(5), 405–509.

Teo P. (1990) Hysterectomy: a change of trend or a change of heart? In *Women's Health Counts*, (Roberts H., ed.). London: Routledge.

Veash N. (1995) Doctor who carried out abortion without consent is cleared. *The Independent*, p. 5.

Verbrugge L. M., Wingard D. L. (1987) Sex differentials in health and mortality. *Women and Health*, **12**(2), 103–143.

Walton H. J. (1968) Sex differences in ability and outlook of senior medical students. *British Journal of Medical Education*, **2**, 156–162.

Wright R. (1969) Hysterectomy: past, present and future (Editorial). *Obstetrics and Gynecology*, **33**(4), 560–563.

Zola I. (1966) Culture and symptoms: an analysis of patients' presenting complaints. *American Sociological Review*, **31**, 615–630.

5 Health care for people from ethnic minority groups

Sally French and Ayesha Vernon

The ethnic minority population of Great Britain is approximately 4.5%. The main immigration occurred from the British colonies in the 1950s and 1960s. This was encouraged by Government as a way of rebuilding the infrastructure of the country following the Second World War. Over 40% of the current ethnic minority population were born in Great Britain (Kurtz, 1993) and their life styles are different from those of their elders. People from ethnic minority groups are more plentiful in some parts of the country than others; in Greater London, for example, about a quarter of the population are from ethnic minority groups and about half of the school population (Kurtz, 1993).

It has been shown beyond doubt that illness and impairment are positively correlated with low socioeconomic status including poor housing and higher rates of unemployment (Whitehead, 1988; Jacobson *et al.*, 1991; Hill, 1994a). People from ethnic minority groups are disproportionately represented in this section of society, and thus their level of illness and impairment is higher than that of the majority population (Kurtz, 1993; Hill, 1994a). Asian people, for example, have a higher incidence of diabetes (Patel, 1992), people of Afro-Caribbean origin have a higher incidence of stroke (Beevers and Beevers, 1993) and the babies of women from many ethnic minority groups are smaller than average, predisposing the infants to impairment (Jacobson *et al.*, 1991). There is, however, considerable variation in the level of illness and impairment among the ethnic minority groups with people of Afro-Caribbean origin being particularly adversely affected (Lonsdale, 1990).

As well as the link with poverty, there are a number of diseases which mainly affect people from specific ethnic minority groups; one of these diseases is sickle cell anaemia which is transmitted genetically and is confined mainly to people of Afro-Caribbean origin. It is estimated that one in ten people of Afro-Caribbean origin carries the defective gene, and one in four hundred has the disease. The disease is, however, also present in people of Mediterranean, Asian and Arabic origin (Louison and Dyer, 1994) and the incidence among other ethnic groups is rising (Sickle Cell Society, 1990; Davies *et al.*, 1993). At the present time there are approximately 5000 people in Great Britain with sickle cell anaemia (Davies *et al.*, 1993).

There is a higher than average incidence of tuberculosis, rickets and osteomalacia among Asian people (Donavan, 1984) and specific eye conditions, which can lead to severe visual impairment, are more common in some ethnic minority groups than others, for example, diabetic retinopathy is particularly common among Jewish people, and cataracts are prevalent among Asian people (Royal Association of Disability and Rehabilitation (RADAR), undated). White European people are, of course, similarly affected with a high incidence of specific diseases, such as cystic fibrosis and breast cancer, and thus any tendency to view people from ethnic minority groups in terms of 'problems' is unjustified and should be avoided.

This high incidence of illness and impairment is offset by the relatively low percentage of older people from ethnic minority groups in Great Britain, due to the fact that many people emigrated after the Second World War when they were young (Admani, 1993a). In a few years time many will reach old age and their health and social needs will become more urgent.

Despite these variations it must be borne in mind that low socioeconomic status, often resulting from racism, and leading to poor housing, diet, and unemployment, is far more influential than ethnic origin or cultural difference with regard to the incidence of illness and impairment (Confederation of Indian Organisations, 1987; Jacobson *et al.*, 1991). White people have traditionally emphasized cultural differences to explain racial inequalities, thereby avoiding the realities of white domination and power. However, people from ethnic minority groups should not be stereotyped as poor, unemployed and disadvantaged, and the enormous differences in terms of language, religion and social customs between people from different ethnic minority groups should be remembered; they do not form a homogeneous group and the majority population may resemble some ethnic minority groups in terms of culture more than the ethnic minority groups resemble each other.

Services for people with illnesses and impairments specific to their ethnic minority status have been neglected. Grimsley and Bhat (1988) point out that uncommon conditions which affect White European people, such as phenylketonuria, are screened, implying that diseases such as sickle cell anaemia would be if they affected the majority population. Bryan *et al.* (1985) and the Sickle Cell Society (1990) point out the general lack of interest in sickle cell anemia by health professionals. Screening is patchy and funding is low (People First, 1995). Tuberculosis, which is also more common in certain ethnic minority groups, has, in contrast, had a high profile, probably because of its threat to the majority population.

The lack of knowledge of diseases which specifically affect people from ethnic minority groups can easily interact with racist attitudes concerning illness behaviour leading to a lack of belief in symptoms, such as pain, of which a person is complaining. This is a common experience of people with sickle cell anaemia where they may be stereotyped as drug addicts and scroungers (Sickle Cell Society, 1990; Louison and Dyer, 1993; People First, 1995). Impairment can also interact with racial stereotyping; people with hearing impairments, for example, may be regarded as illiterate, unable to comprehend English, and stupid (Disability – Identity, Sexuality and Relationships, 1991).

Take up of services

It has frequently been noted that disabled people from ethnic minority groups tend not to use the health and social services which are available, such as meals on wheels, aids and equipment, rehabilitation, and preventative medicine (Greater London Association of Disabled People (GLAD), 1987). The uptake of benefits is also low (Baxter *et al.*, 1990). They are very often blamed for this behaviour, but on close inspection it is not difficult to understand the reasons for it.

Lack of knowledge of services

A general lack of knowledge about what services exist has been found among people from some ethnic minority groups (Confederation of Indian Organisations, 1987; Baxter *et al.*, 1990). This includes lack of awareness of statutory services, aids and equipment, disability organizations, community groups and benefits. There is also uncertainty, particularly among those who do not have British citizenship, regarding their rights, and perhaps a fear of enquiring into such issues too closely. One of the main reasons for this lack of knowledge is poor provision for people who do not speak English. In addition, Jeewa (1990) makes the point that Asian disabled people frequently believe that the services provided are simply not for them. This may, however, be due to the hostility and racism which they have experienced in the past when attempting to use these services (Disability – Identity, Sexuality and Relationships, 1991).

Inappropriate services

Even if people from ethnic minority groups do know of the existence of services, there are a variety of reasons why they may not take advantage of them. When talking of the NHS, Weller (1991) states: '… this service remains essentially geared to the attitudes, priorities and expectations of the majority population which is considered as white, middle class and nominally Christian'.

One of the biggest barriers for ethnic minority groups in accessing services results from the ethnocentric assumption that all those requiring services can speak English and the failure of the institutions to meet the linguistic needs of ethnic minority groups. The resulting lack of communication leads to many serious problems; treatments such as psychotherapy and counselling become impossible, and health education becomes inaccessible. Therapists cannot communicate with their patients and clients, and teachers and educational psychologists cannot communicate with disabled children or their parents.

Tomlinson (1990) and Baxter *et al.* (1990) point out that disabled children whose mother tongue is not English are assessed using tests written in English and may be placed in special schools inappropriately as a result. In addition, developmental tests are culture specific and based on white middle class norms which make them even more unsuitable. Children of Afro-Caribbean origin are over-represented in schools for pupils with learning difficulties which may be explained, at least in part, by these cultural biases (Crowley, 1991; Hill, 1994a). On the other hand, any genuine learning difficulties which children from ethnic minority groups have may go undetected or be interpreted as language problems.

With regard to special education, Tomlinson (1990) found that parents of disabled children from ethnic minority groups do not understand the complex assessment and referral procedures, lack knowledge of their parental rights, are confused by receiving conflicting advice from professionals, have problems in keeping in contact with special schools, and are dissatisfied with the ethnocentric nature of the curriculum. Some education departments now provide workers from ethnic minority groups to help and befriend parents of disabled children. They also provide literature in many languages giving parents practical advice.

The language problems of deaf and speech impaired adults and children and their families are compounded as speech and language therapists rarely operate in languages other than English. There is a need for speech and language therapists who speak such languages as Punjabi, Gujarati and Urdu (*Therapy Weekly*, 1991). Stokes (1988) states that 20% of people referred to speech and language therapy in the London Borough of Tower Hamlets are Bengali speakers and that it was impossible to treat them until a Bengali interpreter and assistant were employed.

The problems of communication do, however, run deeper than language; Hopkins (1993) believes that language should not be over-emphasized as a barrier at the expense of communication, and Farooqi (1993) points out that language is, as time goes by, a diminishing barrier. There is a lack of understanding among the majority population concerning the life styles, social customs and religious practices of people from ethnic minority groups (Weller, 1991; Admani, 1993a). This can lead to inappropriate service provision. Special bathing aids, for example, may be completely inappropriate for people whose washing methods are different from those of the indigenous population, child care practices may vary, ways of coping with terminal illness and death may differ (Green, 1989a,b,c,d), and it may be totally unacceptable for people from some ethnic minority groups to be treated by a person of the opposite sex or in view of other patients, in the hydrotherapy pool or gymnasium, for example.

Hospitals, day centres and residential homes are unlikely to attract disabled people from ethnic minority groups unless they provide suitable food, leisure activities, music and religious services; the decor, toys, books and magazines should also reflect the multi-ethnic society in which we live. Even though disabled people and those who assist them may be in desperate need of a break from each other, they are unlikely to accept assistance unless it caters for their particular needs. Javed (1993) found that 75% of visually impaired Asian people surveyed were in favour of a special day centre where their needs as Asian people would be met and respected. As Read (1988) reminds us, 'In an oppressive society unless you are actively countering the oppression you are perpetuating it. There is no neutral ground'.

Racism, prejudice and stereotyping

Institutional racism can be said to exist when institutions are not geared to meet people's needs and when a uniform culture is assumed (Watkins, 1987). In *Double Bind* (Confederation of Indian Organisations, 1987) racism is defined as:

'... all attitudes, procedures and practices – social and economic – whose effect, though not necessarily conscious intention, is to create and maintain the power, influence and well being of white people at the expense of black people'.

Weller (1991) refers to such an attitude as 'ethnocentrism' which she defines as '... the beliefs that the values and practices of one culture are superior or of greater worth than those of an alternative culture'. McDonald (1994) states:

'Black disabled people are marginalised in service provision by ethnocentrism because it requires that we alter our relationships to our culture of origin, to orientate ourselves towards the values of service providers'.

He points out the particular dangers of the concept of 'normalization' for people from ethnic minority groups.

Hugman (1991) believes that ethnocentric concepts of health underpin professional training and Connelly (1988) states that:

'... there is little hope that sensitive account will be taken of diversity and the experience of black people when policies, procedures and practices are seen as relatively fixed, when the responsibility of public authorities is seen as provision of standard service on a more-or-less "take it or leave it" basis, or when it is considered that constrained resources make this the only feasible course'.

For disabled people from the ethnic minority groups, institutional racism is combined with institutional disablism, whereby disabled people are barred from many public buildings and activities because of lack of access or rigid social practices which do not take their needs and rights into account (Hill, 1991). This dual disadvantage subjects people to a great deal of negative discrimination, for example in the employment market. McDonald (1991), who is black and has cerebral palsy, explains: '... to fight for black people is one thing, to fight for the rights of disabled people something else. There is not enough time and energy to fight two different wars'. Similarly Hill (1990) states: 'Black disabled people, I have found to my cost, are a discrete minority within a minority'.

There is, at present, very little empirical material on the ways in which ethnicity structures the experience of disability (Oliver, 1990), but Stuart (1993) believes that the concept of 'double discrimination' is simplistic, arguing that black disabled people are subjected to a unique type of oppression which is more than, and different from, the sum of racism and disablism. Begum (1994a) states:

'Notions of "double discrimination" or "triple jeopardy" do nothing to facilitate understanding of multiple and simultaneous oppression ... different forms of oppression are not lived out separately or in a hierarchical structure'.

It is the belief of the authors of *Double Bind* (Confederation of Indian Organisations, 1987) that most racism is institutionalized, but that is not to deny that disabled people from ethnic minority groups may experience racist attitudes directly from service providers. Hill (1991) states that, 'As far as disability is concerned, race and racism is rarely discussed. And all too often providers feel that they do not need to think any more specifically than in terms of disability alone'. Negative attitudes and a lack of understanding of cultural mores and norms of behaviour have led to serious consequences for people from ethnic minority groups, whose behaviour has often been considered odd or mad leading to an over representation of people from certain ethnic minority groups in psychiatric hospitals and hospitals for people with learning difficulties. People from the Caribbean, for example, are much more likely to be diagnosed as schizophrenic and admitted to psychiatric hospitals (Lipsedge, 1993), there are more compulsory admissions to psychiatric hospitals and secure units (Bahl, 1993a), and children of Afro-Caribbean origin are more likely to attend schools for children with emotional and behavioural problems (Kurtz, 1993). One explanation for this is overt and covert racism. Lipsedge (1993) states:

> 'The disproportionate number of compulsory admissions and the selective transfer of Afro-Caribbean people to locked wards indicate that the professional assessment of dangerousness is influenced by the colour of the patient's skin'.

Schizophrenia is diagnosed far more commonly in people of Afro-Caribbean origin than others, and people of Afro-Caribbean origin are often given a diagnosis of 'cannabis psychosis' although there is little evidence that cannabis plays any part in severe psychotic illness (Lipsedge,1993).

There are different beliefs about health, illness and disability among ethnic minority groups and different ways of responding which physiotherapists should understand. For example, Rack (1982) and Crowley (1991) have found that Indian and Pakistani people tend to describe emotional states in terms of physical illness; they may feel it is inappropriate to talk about emotional problems to health professionals. Lipsedge points out, however, that this may be little more than a response to poor communication. There are also cultural differences in people's responses to pain (Melzack and Wall, 1989) though this has probably been exaggerated. To assume that pain and other symptoms are inevitably of psychological origin in people from ethnic minority groups is racist (Ahmad, 1989).

Even pressure groups and organizations such as The British Council of Disabled People, have been accused of ignoring the needs and rights of disabled people from ethnic minority groups (Begum et al., 1994), and of a lack of understanding of racism (Disability – Identity, Sexuality and Relationships, 1991). Similarly, those who promote the rights of ethnic minority groups ignore the experience of disabled people from these groups. This situation has given rise to the formation of various groups of disabled people from ethnic minorities, such as the Association of Blind Asians and The Asian People's Disability Alliance. Groups such as these are usually chronically under funded and desperately over worked (Hill, 1994b).

Service providers often believe that the lack of service uptake among people from ethnic minority groups reflects a greater family and social network than the majority population enjoys. However, this can be used as an excuse for not providing an appropriate service and has been disputed (Confederation of Indian Organisations, 1987; Baxter *et al.* 1990; Disability – Identity, Sexuality and Relationships, 1991; Bahl, 1993b; Gunaratnam, 1993; Louison and Dyer, 1993; Begum, 1994b; Hill, 1994b; Vernon, 1994.). The Greater London Council of Disabled People (GLAD) (1987) believes that stereotyped beliefs that people of Afro-Caribbean origin are catered for by their families should be challenged. For example, GLAD's (1987) report, on a survey in Brent, revealed that 68% of elderly people of Afro-Caribbean origin live alone. Similarly McCalman (1990) studied Afro-Caribbean, Asian and Vietnamese/Chinese carers of old people in the London Borough of Southwark and found little evidence of an extended family network. People from ethnic minority groups are sometimes forced to live within the extended family against their will because of adverse circumstances (Admani, 1993a; Ghose, 1994).

Another common belief among health professionals is that the reason for the low uptake of services among people from ethnic minority groups is their attitude towards illness and disability. For example, it has been suggested that families can be very protective of disabled members, leading to lack of opportunity for their disabled relatives, especially for girls and women, outside the family (Association of Blind Asians, 1990). It has been argued that among Asian people, disability is sometimes looked upon as shameful or is viewed as a blessing or as a punishment from God (Baxter *et al.*, 1990). In *Double Bind* (Confederation of Indian Organisations, 1988) it is stated that, 'Disability is sometimes seen as a "curse" and this can cause the disabled person, particularly if a woman, to stay hidden away, or even worse to be hidden away'. Such feelings and beliefs are not, of course, confined to sections of the ethnic minority population and may be uncommon among them.

If there is any tendency to keep disability hidden it is certainly exacerbated by inappropriate services. It is stated in *Double Bind* (Confederation of Indian Organisations, 1987) that:

> 'Many disabled people now appear to find there is little point in trying to obtain benefits. As a consequence this gives the statutory authorities and administrators of benefits the excuse to maintain the stereotype of either Asian families and communities catering for the needs of their own disabled or, even worse, that disabled Asian people do not exist or reside in the United Kingdom'.

Simes (1990) believes that Asian people find it difficult to accept that disability cannot be cured. This is not, of course, uncommon among the majority population either. Simes states:

> 'Accepting that the handicap is not an illness but a condition that will last a lifetime is often very difficult for some of the parents. They frequently give for one of their reasons for settling in Britain the hope that because of better medical treatment the child will be cured of the handicap'.

There is also a lack of understanding of the concept of special educa-tion among some Asian parents (GLAD, 1987). Tomlinson (1990) believes that the word 'special' is sometimes interpreted as 'good' and 'better than' rather than 'different'. Misconceptions such as these, as well as language barriers, make high quality communication vitally important.

At a more profound level, many beliefs which are shared by the majority population, for example, the desirability for independence, may be viewed negatively in cultures which favour collectivism rather than individualism.

This all amounts to a tremendous lack of appropriate services for people from ethnic minority groups, although the situation is slowly improving. Where appropriate services do exist they tend to be found in areas with a high density of people from ethnic minority groups.

What should be done?

Section 20 of the 1976 Race Relations Act makes it unlawful to discrimi-nate against people on racial grounds in terms of facilities, goods and services, the manner in which they are delivered or their quality. The 1991 Patients' Charter highlights the needs for respect of privacy, dignity and religious and cultural beliefs, and makes it clear that hospitals must fulfil the cultural, dietary and spiritual needs of people from ethnic minorities (Bahl, 1993a,b). Education, high quality management, and adequate resources are all essential if health professionals, including physiothera-pists, are to abide by this Act and Charter.

'Race' equality training

Health professionals are predominantly white and non-disabled and receive very little training concerning the needs and difficulties of patients and clients from ethnic minority groups (Vousden, 1987). It is almost impossible to be entirely free of racist beliefs and attitudes when brought up in a racist society like our own. Some of these attitudes and behaviour patterns may be conscious while others are submerged. It may be that we attend to people from ethnic minority groups a little less than other people, that we do not expect as much of them, or that we give them a little less of our time. In many ways the more subtle and submerged racism becomes the more difficult it is to deal with. Read (1988) believes that, '… white people have to learn that, although it is not their fault, they are racist, however well intentioned they are, but that they can learn to change their behaviour'. Even the term 'race' can be crit-icized; it is not a scientific concept because there is more genetic differ-ence between people of the same ethnic origin than there is between different ethnic groups. 'Race' is a socially constructed term which high-lights and exaggerates biological differences.

'Race' equality training, when skilfully carried out by people from ethnic minority groups, can help people to become aware of their atti-tudes and behaviour in a relaxed and non-threatening environment. It is no longer acceptable to treat people from ethnic minority groups, 'just like everyone else' or to take a 'why can't they be like us?' approach, as this fosters prejudice (Eversley, 1988). The authors of *Double Bind* (Confederations of Indian Organisations, 1987), talking of Asian disabled people, state that: 'True integration is recognising that disabled Asians may have special needs. Treating everyone the same is not equality, because it does not take into account these needs. This would be assimilation and not integration'. Disabled trainers from ethnic minority groups must be sought and actively involved in the education of health professionals.

There also needs to be greater awareness and understanding of the cultural diversity of people from different ethnic minority groups and a sensitivity to these differences when communicating with and treating them. Physiotherapists should have a working knowledge of their likely health beliefs, dietary needs, religious practices and social customs, but above all should be prepared to learn from their patients and clients. Attempting to understand cultural differences must not, however, lead to simplification and stereotyping (McGee, 1992). Hugman (1991) believes that cultural knowledge can increase the power of professionals and can be used in a racist way. Concepts of culture can, for example, be used as a way of explaining pathology, for example notions of cultural conflict (Lipsedge, 1993), and focusing on 'special needs' rather than integrating the needs of people from ethnic minorities into mainstream services, can have a stigmatizing effect upon the people concerned (Hopkins, 1993).

Kroll (1990) and Baxter *et al.* (1990) believe that the training of health professionals fails to prepare them for work in a multi-ethnic society and that an awareness of racism and inequality should be a prominent strand which runs through the curriculum.

Interpreters

There is an urgent need for more trained interpreters. Their shortage is a major, but steadily diminishing, problem; in the London Borough of Tower Hamlets, for example, the 1988 census recorded 172 languages (Wilson, 1989). It is common practice in the Health Service to use relatives of people who cannot speak English as interpreters, including children, which is far from satisfactory. Such people are neither trained nor paid for their services, and their presence may be inappropriate when sensitive information is discussed. In addition child interpreters may not understand the complex issues raised. Watkins (1987) believes that it is '... quite inappropriate to expect people to discuss intimate medical problems through their children, relatives or friends'. Disabled people from ethnic minority groups deserve the same confidentiality as everyone else. Baxter *et al.* (1990) point out that interpreters must be matched carefully to the patient or client; for example, it may be inappropriate for an old person to talk through a young person or someone of the opposite sex.

A register of bilingual staff is helpful and can give rise to a dramatic uptake of services (Baxter, 1988), but Chaudbury (1990) believes that interpreters should ideally be independent of the organization. In relation to the education services she states: 'Interpreters who see their role as interpreting the LEA's wishes to the parent can very easily slip into putting pressure on to parents to go along with what is being proposed'. Ellis (1993) makes the point that interpreters are frequently used to pass on unpalatable information or to negotiate difficult decisions rather than to facilitate understanding.

It would also be helpful if more written information were translated into minority languages although this should not be regarded as a 'cure all'. Ley (1988) cites evidence, concerning patients and clients generally, that the written word is not always a very effective way of communicating information. Kroll (1990) believes that pamphlets should be used only to consolidate information which has been given orally, and Bahl (1993a) believes that people from ethnic minority groups should be involved in producing their own health education literature to ensure its accessibility.

Employment of health professionals from ethnic minority groups

In a survey of racial equality in the social services (Commission for Racial Equality, 1988) it is stated that: '… without equal employment opportunities it is unlikely that there will be equal opportunities in service delivery'. There is considerable evidence of lack of opportunities for training and employment in the health services (see Baxter *et al.*, 1990; French, 1992; Admani, 1993b) which can be viewed as a form of racism.

Holden (1988) reports that the social services department of Bradford Metropolitan Council found that the appointment of an Asian worker in a respite team brought a dramatic increase in the number of Asian people using it. In *Double Bind* (Confederation of Indian Organisations, 1987) it is recommended that outreach teams, comprising people from the Asian community, should attempt to reach Asian disabled people and their families who are not using statutory services. They believe that outreach teams should be of the same cultural background as the target groups.

In the programme *Mosaic* (BBC1 1991) the importance of advocates and initiatives coming from within the ethnic minority communities themselves was stressed. Unfortunately such projects often have great difficulty securing funding and what sometimes happens is that large numbers of people from the particular ethnic minority groups concerned are referred to whatever small facility exists. This results in less urgency being felt among mainstream services to adapt and tends to overwhelm existing services.

In today's climate of 'equal opportunities' it is to be hoped that more health professionals from ethnic minority groups will be recruited. Hugman (1991) makes the point, however, that equal opportunity policies can serve as a form of image management and that: 'Equal opportunity statements can be used as a smokescreen behind which racism remains intact'. The same can be said of disablism (French, 1994).

Consultation

In order to provide appropriate and culturally sensitive services to people from ethnic minority groups it is essential to consult the people concerned, and their organizations, at every stage of service planning and implementation. It is very important to avoid tokenism whereby just one or two people from ethnic minority groups (perhaps those already working in the organization) are asked for their opinions. The service should be regularly evaluated and an accessible complaints procedure put in place.

Conclusion

It is clear from the above account that although progress is slowly being made, a great deal still needs to be done to provide disabled people from ethnic minority groups with sensitive and effective health and social services. The attitudes and behaviour of individual practitioners is vitally important in bringing about change, but management backing and the development of policy relating to resources, staff recruitment, and working practices must be made at every level of the organization if meaningful progress is to be achieved. Connelly (1988) believes that:

> ' "Professional" has a number of different meanings. Some are to do with the practice of a particular body of knowledge, but with occupations concerned with social care it is at least as important that the emphasis should be on another meaning; competence – in this case competence in dealing with diversity. Humility and flexibility and willingness to ask questions thus become critical aspects of professional integrity. So too does the strength to take chances, to apply existing and increasing knowledge and skills to new situations'.

Acknowledgement

Many of the ideas in this chapter are based upon meetings, which took place in 1990 and 1991, with the following organizations: Association of Blind Asians; Sickle Cell Society; Disabled People with Disabilities Alliance; Jewish Blind Society; Association for the Support of Asian Parents of Handicapped People. Thanks are extended to these organizations for their time and assistance.

References

Admani K. (1993a) Special needs of elderly muslims. In *Access to Health Care for People from Black and Ethnic Minorities* (Hopkins A., Bahl V., eds). London: Royal College of Physicians.

Admani K. (1993b) Black and ethnic minority doctors in the National Health Service. In *Access to Health Care for People from Black and Ethnic Minorities* (Hopkins A., Bahl V., eds). London: Royal College of Physicians.

Ahmad W. T. U. (1989) Policies, pills and political will: a critique of policies to improve the health status of ethnic minorities. *Lancet*, **i**, 8630, 148–150.

Bahl V. (1993a) Access to health care for black and ethnic minority elderly people: general principles. In *Access to Health Care for People from Black and Ethnic Minorities* (Hopkins A., Bahl V., eds). London: Royal College of Physicians.

Bahl V. (1993b) Development of a black and ethnic minority health policy at the Department of Health. In *Access to Health Care for People from Black and Ethnic Minorities* (Hopkins A., Bahl V., eds). London: Royal College of Physicians.

Baxter C. (1988) *The Black Nurse: An Endangered Species.* London: National Extension College for Training in Health and Race.

Baxter C., Poonia K., Ward L., Nadirshaw Z. (1990) *Double Discrimination. Issues and Services for People with Learning Difficulties from Black and Ethnic Minority Communities.* London: King's Fund Centre/Commission for Racial Equality.

Beevers G., Beevers M. (1993) Hypertension: impact upon black and minority ethnic people. In *Access to Health Care for People from Black and Ethnic Minorities.* (Hopkins A., Bahl V., eds). London: Royal College of Physicians.

Begum N. (1994a) Mirror, mirror on the wall. In *Reflections: Views of Black Disabled People of their Lives and Community Care.* Paper 32.3 (Begum N., Hill M., Stevens A., eds). London: Central Council for Education and Training in Social Work.

Begum N. (1994b) Optimism, pessimism and care management: the impact of community care policies. In *Reflections: Views of Black Disabled People of their Lives and Community Care.* Paper 32.3 (Begum N., Hill M., Stevens A., eds). London: Central Council for Education and Training in Social Work.

Begum N., Hill M., Stevens A. (eds) (1994) *Reflections: Views of Black Disabled People of their Lives and Community Care.* Paper 32.3. London: Central Council for Education and Training in Social Work.

Bryan D., Denzie S., Scafe S. (1985) *The Heart of the Race: Black Women's Lives in Britain.* London: Virago.

Chaudbury A. (1990) Problems for parents – experiences of Tower Hamlets. In *Asian Children and Special Needs: A Report for ACE* (Orton C., ed.). London: Advisory Centre for Education.

Commission for Racial Equality (1988) *Racial Equality in Social Service Departments.* London: Commission for Racial Equality.

Confederation of Indian Organisations (1988), *Double Bind: To be Disabled and Asian.* London: Confederation of Indian Organisations.

Connelly N. (1988) *Care in the Multi-racial Community.* London: Policy Studies Institute.

Crowley J. (1991) Races apart. *Nursing Times,* **87**(10), 44–46.

Davies S. C., Modell B., Wonke B. (1993) the Haemoglobinopathies: impact upon black and ethnic minority people. In *Access to Health Care for People from Black and Ethnic Minorities* (Hopkins A., Bahl V., eds). London: Royal College of Physicians.

Deaf Minorities Need Speech Therapy (1991) *Therapy Weekly,* **17**(35), 20.

Disability – Identity, Sexuality and Relationships (1991) Video cassette of the disability equality training pack *Disability – Identity, Sexuality and Relationships (K665y).* Milton Keynes: Open University.

Donavan J. (1984) Ethnicity and health: a research review. *Social Science and Medicine,* **19**(7), 663–670.

Ellis K. (1993) *Squaring the Circle. User and Carer Participation in Needs Assessment.* London: Joseph Rowntree Foundation.

Ethnic Minority Groups and People with Disabilities (undated) London. Royal Association for Disability and Rehabilitation.

Eversley J. (1988) The same does not mean equal. *Therapy Weekly,* **16**(2), 3.

Farooqi A. (1993) How can family practice improve access to health care for black and ethnic minority patients. In *Access to Health Care for People from Black and Ethnic Minorities* (Hopkins A., Bahl V., eds). London: Royal College of Physicians.

French S. (1992) Health care in a multi-ethnic society. *Physiotherapy,* **78**(3), 174–180.

French S. (1994) Equal opportunities ... yes please. In *Mustn't Grumble: Writing by Disabled Women* (Keith L., ed.). London: The Women's Press.

Ghose A. (1994) The provision of housing for disabled Asian people. In *Reflections: Views of Black Disabled People of their Lives and Community Care.* Paper 32.3. (Begum N., Hill M., Stevens A., eds). London: Central Council for Education and Training in Social Work.

GLAD (1987) *Disability and Ethnic Minority Communities – A Study in Three London Boroughs.* London: Greater London Association of Disabled People (GLAD).

Green J. (1989a) Death with dignity: Islam. *Nursing Times,* **85**(5), 56–57.

Green J. (1989b) Death with dignity: Hinduism. *Nursing Times,* **85**(6), 50–51.

Green J. (1989c) Death with dignity: Sikhism. *Nursing Times,* **85**(7) 56–57.

Green J. (1989d) Death with dignity: Judaism. *Nursing Times,* **85**(8), 64–65.

Grimsley M., Bhat A. (1988) Health. In *Britain's Black Population: A New Perspective* (2nd edn.). Radical Statistics Race Group. (Bhat A., Currhill P., Ohri S., eds). Aldershot: Gower.

Gunaratnam Y. (1993) Breaking the silence: Asian carers in Britain. In *Community Care* (Bornat J., Pereira C., Pilgrim D., Williams F., eds). London: Macmillan.

Hill M. (1990) Independent living for black and ethnic minority disabled people In *Building Our Lives* (Laurie L., ed.). London: Shelter.

Hill M. (1991) Race and Disability. In the book of readings of the disability equality pack *Disability – Identity, Sexuality and Relationships (K665y).* Milton Keynes: Open University.

Hill M. (1994a) They are not our brothers: the disability movement and the black disability movement. In *Reflections: Views of Black Disabled People of their Lives and Community Care*. Paper 32.3. (Begum N., Hill M., Stevens A., eds). London: Central Council for Education and Training in Social Work.

Hill M. (1994b) Burn and rage: black voluntary organisations as a source of social change. In *Reflections: Views of Black Disabled People of their Lives and Community Care*. Paper 32.3. (Begum N., Hill M., Stevens A., eds). London: Central Council for Education and Training in Social Work.

Holden G. (1988) Why are people from ethnic minorities losing out? *Disability Now*, August, 8–9.

Hopkins A. (1993) Envoi. In *Access to Health Care for People from Black and Ethnic Minorities* (Hopkins A., Bahl V., eds). London: Royal College of Physicians.

Hugman R., (1991) *Power in Caring Professions*. London: Macmillan.

Jacobson B., Smith A., Whitehead M. (1991) *The Nation's Health: A Strategy for the 1990s*. London: King Edward's Hospital Fund for London.

Javed K. (1993) *Survey into the Needs of Visually Impaired Asians*. London: Association of Blind Asians.

Jeewa M. (1990) Asian people with disabilities alliance. In *Building Our Lives* (Laurie L., ed.) London: Shelter.

Kroll D. (1990) Equal access to care. *Nursing Times*, **86**(23), 72–73.

Kurtz Z. (1993) Better health for black and ethnic minority children and young people. In *Access to Health Care for People from Black and Ethnic Minorities* (Hopkins A., Bahl V., eds). London: Royal College of Physicians.

Ley P. (1988) *Communicating with Patients*. London: Croom Helm.

Lipsedge M. (1993) Mental health: access to care for black and ethnic minority people. In *Access to Health Care for People from Black and Ethnic Minorities* (Hopkins A., Bahl V., eds). London: Royal College of Physicians.

Lonsdale S. (1990) *Women and Disability*. London: Macmillan.

Louison E., Dyer P. (1994) Meeting the needs of people with sickle cell disease: an agenda for action. In *Reflections: Views of Black Disabled People of their Lives and Community Care*. Paper 32.3. (Begum N., Hill M., Stevens A., eds). London: Central Council for Education and Training in Social Work.

McCalman J. A. (1990) *The Forgotten People*. London: King's Fund Centre/Help the Aged/Standing Conference for Ethnic Minority Senior Citizens.

McDonald P. (1991) Double discrimination must be faced now. *Disability Now*, March 8.

McDonald P. (1994) Eurocentrism, ethnocentrism and social work concepts. In *Reflections: Views of Black Disabled People of their Lives and Community Care*. Paper 32.3. (Begum N., Hill M., Stevens A., eds). London: Central Council for Education and Training in Social Work, 99–109.

McGee P. (1992) *Teaching Transcultural Care*. London: Chapman and Hall.

Melzack R., Wall P. (1988) *The Challenge of Pain*. Harmondsworth: Penguin Books.

Mosaic (1991) BBC1 February 24.

Oliver M. (1990) *The Politics of Disablement*. London: Macmillan.

Patel K. (1992) On the margins: ethnic minority groups and services for visual impairment. *The New Beacon*, **76**(896), 90–93.

People First (1995) *Blood Count*. Channel 4 Television.

Rack P. (1982) *Race, Culture and Mental Disorder*. London: Tavistock.

Read J. (1988) *The Equal Opportunities Book*. London: Interchange Books.

Simes L. (1990) Partnership with parents – a positive example. In *Asian Children and Special Needs: A report for ACE* (Orton C., ed.). London: Advisory Centre for Education.

Stokes J. (1988) Breaking the Ethnic Language Barrier. *Therapy Weekly*, **14**(31), 7.

Stuart O. (1993) Double oppression: an appropriate starting point? In *Disabling Barriers – Enabling Environments* (Swain J., Finkelstein V., French S., Oliver M., eds). London: Sage.

Tomlinson S. (1990) Asian children with special needs – a broad perspective. In *Asian Children and Special Needs: A Report for ACE* (Orton C., ed.) London: Advisory Centre for Education.

Vernon A. (1994) Black and minority ethnic disabled people receive poorer quality social services. In *Reflections: Views of Black Disabled People of their Lives and Community Care*. Paper 32.3. (Begum N., Hill M., Stevens A., eds). London: Central Council for Education and Training in Social Work.

Vousden M. (1987) Racism in the Wards. *Nursing Times*, **83**(42), 918.

Watkins S. (1987) *Medicine and Labour*. London: Lawrence Wishart.

Weller B. (1991) Nursing in a multicultural world. *Nursing Standard*, **5**(3), 31–32.

Whitehead M. (1988) *Inequalities in Health. The Health Divide*. Harmondsworth: Penguin Books.

Wilson L. (1989) Dilemma of 172 recorded languages. *Therapy Weekly*, **16**(20), 3.

6

Ageism
Sally French

The term 'ageism' was coined by Butler (1975) who defined it as a process of systematic discrimination and stereotyping of people simply because of their age. Similarly, Hawker (1985) defines ageism as 'Society's negative and patronising attitudes towards its older members'. When people are treated in an ageist way they are viewed as a homogeneous group rather than as individuals. No age group is exempt from age-related stereotypes; thus children may be viewed as unreliable, teenagers as irresponsible, and middle-aged people as 'past it' by many potential employers. However, there can be no doubt that old people are affected by ageist attitudes more than any other age group.

Attitudes to old people vary over time and place which illustrates that our stereotypes are socially, rather than biologically, created (Scrutton, 1990). This chapter will examine attitudes to old people in British society today but it must be appreciated that in other societies, for example China, old people may be highly respected and afforded considerable status. It is often said that in Britain respect for old people has decreased, but Featherstone and Hepworth (1993) found little evidence that old people were ever respected unless they possessed wealth and power. The experience and knowledge of old people, which may have been valued in some parts of the world, has been made less relevant by rapid change and the loss of an oral tradition whereby information was passed on by word of mouth (Scrutton, 1990).

Abercrombie *et al.* (1988) define a stereotype as, 'a one-sided, exaggerated and normally prejudicial view of a group, tribe or class of people'. In the case of ageism many such beliefs, for example that old people are unadaptable, are potentially very harmful. Although sometimes containing an element of truth, stereotypical beliefs are over-generalizations which grossly simplify reality relieving us of the demanding task of viewing and relating to people as individuals. This is not to say that old people and other stereotyped groups may not benefit in various ways from such beliefs. They may, for example, be flattered by the notion that old people are exceptionally wise, or pleased that no one expects them to learn new skills. For most people, however, the disadvantages far outweigh any advantages.

Stereotyping frequently leads to discrimination which Reber (1985) defines as, 'the unequal treatment of individuals or groups based on arbitrary characteristics'. Discrimination is the behavioural component of prejudice. Thus old people may be denied access to employment, leisure activities, education and medical treatment simply because of their age.

As well as being evident in the attitudes and behaviour of individuals, ageism manifests itself within our culture in numerous ways. It pervades both literature and the media and is very easy to find in such items as birthday cards and postcards (Marshall, 1990). Old people very rarely feature in advertisements and we are constantly urged to spend time, money and effort preserving our youth and making ourselves appear younger (Townroe and Yates, 1987). Norman (1987) complains that charities portray old people as pathetic and dependent, and Johnson (1993) believes that negative images of old people are used when attempting to raise public awareness of their disadvantaged situation.

Ageism also manifests itself within the structures of society. It is firmly embedded in the practices of institutions and is reflected in government policy. An example of this is the inflexibility of retirement policy which forces people to cease paid employment at a given chronological age, whatever their wishes or abilities may be. Retirement thus fosters ageist stereotypes (Laczko and Phillipson, 1990; Featherstone and Hepworth, 1993).

Old people are denied many benefits to which younger people in a similar situation are entitled, such as the disability living allowance, and are forced into poverty and dependency by low pensions and the spurious notion that they need less money than younger people (Walker, 1990). Their lack of wealth reduces their social standing and personal resources, thus their dependency and status are socially constructed, at least in part. Old people may feel satisfied with their low pensions because they have lived through times of war and economic depression when poverty was even greater. Compared to their past lives and to the old people they remember, they may regard themselves as relatively affluent. It is likely that the next generation of old people will have very different attitudes to those of today. This is not to imply that all old people are poor; their personal resources and their social standing within society are likely to mirror earlier stages of their lives (Bond, 1993).

Ageist policy reflects the capitalist society in which we live which emphasizes youthfulness, energy, and technological innovation, perceiving our value in terms of our contribution to the production of wealth. People who are economically inactive are devalued and perceived as a burden. The social goods they have to offer, such as companionship and unpaid labour, are disregarded (Bond and Coleman, 1993). Old age can thus be perceived in terms of economic and political processes although it has generally been viewed in terms of biology and psychology. Most of the literature on ageing has taken a medical perspective where the problems of old age are individualized.

Ageist language

Barbato and Feezel (1987), French and Sim (1993) and Thompson (1993) point out that ageism frequently operates through language. Although it may seem trivial to focus on this, there can be no doubt that our attitudes are reflected in the language we use and are shaped by the language we hear. Knowles (1987) complains that it is not uncommon for nurses to refer to old people by such terms as 'dear', 'darling', 'love', 'poppet' and 'sweetie'. Knowles believes that old people find such terms patronizing and embarrassing and may not have been referred to in such a way since early childhood.

The tendency automatically to call old people by their first names, or by terms of endearment, such as 'Granny', is not uncommon. Payne (1989) believes that using first names can be demeaning when used by a stranger who has power over the person, especially when that person is expected to address the other formally. Even physical abuse towards old people is trivialized by the expressions 'Granny abuse' and 'Granny bashing', terms which are used in the professional literature (Eastman, 1988).

Norman (1987) believes that terms such as 'old girl' and 'old boy' are patronizing and tend to infantilize old people, as does the notion of a 'second childhood'. She complains of the way the word 'geriatric' is used as a noun and comments that we use many euphemisms to replace the word 'old', such as 'pensioner' and 'senior citizen'. It is as if we view old age so negatively that we cannot bring ourselves to refer to it in a straightforward way.

Terms such as 'the elderly' and 'the aged' can also be criticized for fostering the impression that old people form a homogenous group, whereas in reality they are as heterogeneous as any other large section of the population, even in terms of their age which may span 30 or 40 years. Such language is very common in employment advertisements for medical professions as well as in their journals and textbooks. Similarly Wertheimer (1988) and French (1994) criticize terms such as 'the disabled' and 'the handicapped'. Wertheimer (1988) questions the use of the word 'care' as it fosters a dependent and helpless image which is often quite inappropriate. Yet the term 'care of the elderly' has now been adopted in favour of 'geriatrics', which has almost been banned from medical vocabulary. The term 'geriatrics' is, in essence, neutral – referring to a medical speciality like 'paediatrics' or 'orthopaedics'. The term has taken on a derogatory quality because of our negative attitudes towards old people.

The word 'old' is frequently used as a term of abuse, for example 'old fool', 'old bag', 'old maid', and 'old dragon'. A fussy person is likewise referred to as an 'old woman' – a sexist as well as an ageist expression. Older women are, according to Fennell *et al.* (1988), in a particularly difficult situation. They state:

> 'Suffering from the double burden of ageism and sexism, older women have for too long been marginalised by society at large and by the literature stemming from sociology, gerontology and feminism: their visibility invariably restricted to the portrayal of negative stereotypes'.

Old people from ethnic minorities may also suffer multiple oppression. There are various incorrect, stereotyped views concerning people from ethnic minorities, for example, that they always belong to an extended family network which is ever ready to help and support them. Views such as these are disputed by McCalman (1990). Ageism interacts with sexism, racism and disablism. Thompson (1993) believes that, 'Anti-ageism needs to be part of the wider enterprise and challenge of anti-discriminatory practice'.

Terms such as 'dirty old man', 'mutton dressed as lamb' and 'cradle snatcher' indicate our distaste of any sexual behaviour in old people and the adage that, 'you can't teach an old dog new tricks' indicates the widespread and erroneous belief that old people are incapable of learning new skills, a view hotly disputed by Ellard (1988). Croft and Beresford (1991) complain of the patronizing way in which old people are referred to as 'crumblies', 'wrinklies' and 'pensioners' and believes they should be 'citizens' like everyone else rather than 'senior citizens'. The use of the word 'senile' as a synonym for 'dementia' is also ageist as 'senile' merely means, 'relating or belonging to old age' (*Butterworths Medical Dictionary*, 1978).

Joseph (1990) and Scrutton (1990) believes that society is far too inclined to concentrate on the 'problems' of old age. Concerns are constantly voiced regarding the increasing numbers of old people within society. However, Joseph makes the point that the population of the nineteenth century was abnormally youthful because few lived into old age. He comments, '... put this way the problem of old age appears already to be less of a problem'. Bond (1993) agrees that viewing old age as a problem perpetuates ageism. It is the social disadvantage that old people suffer which creates problems not the old people themselves. Ellard (1988) remarks that although much is spoken of the burden old people place on the young, little is said of the burden the young have already placed on old people.

Misconceptions of old age

Joseph (1990) points out the various misconceptions pertaining to old age.

The first misconception is that the number of years lived (chronological age) equates with biological, psychological and sociological ageing. There are tremendous individual differences in the ageing process and no straightforward correspondence between these different aspects of ageing. Thus at a chronological age of 75 a person may look older but in terms of mental agility and social roles appear younger. Or a person of 85 may look young but may be unable to look after him or herself because of depression or confusion. It is important not to judge people by their appearance alone.

Another misconception relates to ill health. Although it is true that illness and impairment are concentrated among older people more than any other age group, deterioration of health is not inevitable as we age and the majority of older people remain independent and healthy. Thompson (1993) contends that the extent of illness and disability in old age is grossly exaggerated and yet genuine symptoms can be disregarded, by health professionals and old people alike, as an inevitable consequence of old age. The idea that ill health is a natural part of ageing is dangerous because it may lead health professionals to under treat old people or to assume that nothing can be done for them, and as Day (1988) points out, it may lead old people to view themselves in a similar way. These ideas may be reinforced by the fact that health workers are in contact with a disproportionate number of old people who are ill and disabled (Marshall, 1990). The differences between old and younger people has been exaggerated; there is no medical condition exclusive to old age (Johnson, 1993) and most old people never need long-term institutional care (Bond, 1993).

A third misconception is that most old people suffer from senile dementia. According to Joseph (1990) 29% of people over 80 years of age show some signs of senile dementia, but although this is a sizeable minority it does leave 71% free of the condition and younger elderly people are far less likely to be affected. Bond (1993) claims that 80% of people over the age of 85 are not mentally frail. Depression is the most common mental illness in old age, as it is for younger people, but it is frequently confused with senile dementia, especially as depression can be a major cause of forgetting. Given the multiple losses old people tend to experience, for example loss of spouse, friends and employment, depression can often be explained in terms unrelated to ageing *per se*.

The behaviour of old people is often interpreted in terms of senile dementia. Thus if a 30-year-old goes to work leaving the gas on or the back door unlocked occasionally, it is considered to be normal forgetfulness, but if an old person does likewise he or she is apt to be suspected of 'going senile'. Carp (1969) devised a 'senility' scale and found that students were more inclined to demonstrate 'senile' signs than old people! Hasler (1989) points out that senile dementia is a disease and should not be regarded as part of the normal ageing process, and Davison and Neale (1990) remind us that the dementias are a group of illnesses with different causes. An old person may become demented due to a high temperature, lack of fluids and poor nutrition or as a side-effect of medications.

It is often assumed that old people are rejected and isolated, yet in reality only about 20% of people over the age of 65 live alone and one must assume that some of them choose to do so, as people from any other age group might. It is also incorrect to believe that families do not look after their older relatives, Hasler (1989) states that most old people remain in close contact with their families who provide care and support, and Joseph (1990) makes the point that the poorest old people, in financial and social terms, tend to be those who do not have families. The small proportion of old people who live in institutions are more likely to be unmarried, childless and without siblings. It is also wrong to equate living alone with loneliness (Thompson, 1993).

A further erroneous notion is that old people are unproductive and a burden upon society. This can be used as an excuse for not providing services and for giving preferential treatment to younger people (Thompson, 1993). It is not uncommon for employers to state that they require young people with those in middle age often being regarded as on the decline (Laczko and Phillipson, 1990). Yet many old people live busy and productive lives, forming, for example, the backbone of the informal caring services. There are many examples of people who have produced excellent work in old age, including Winston Churchill, Pablo Picasso, Mother Teresa, Sigmund Freud and Bertrand Russell, and it is not uncommon for retired people to succeed as students of the Open University and in many other areas of life. The fact that such people are singled out and admired only serves to emphasize our ageist attitudes, for successful old people are generally thought to be the exceptions.

Some decline of intelligence, as measured by intelligence tests, can be demonstrated in old age, especially for tasks which do not involve language, but, according to Gross (1993) and Ellard (1988) this is mainly due to a reduced memory span, and a slower rate of response. Any lessening of such abilities is not very important in everyday life and is probably compensated for in most situations by an increase in experience and knowledge. Coleman (1993) states:

> 'In really advanced age the negative effects of biological ageing upon psychological functioning may be more evident than the benefits of experience, but for the greater part of the life course the gains are likely to be as evident as the losses'.

Furthermore, comparing IQ scores of people in different age groups is fraught with problems as IQ is affected by experience. Today's young people generally have greater opportunities than their parents or grandparents in terms of education, employment, travel and leisure pursuits. There is also a danger in automatically viewing changes which may occur in old age as necessarily negative. Gadow and Berg (1978) point out the advantages of some aspects of ageing arguing, for example, that decreased speed of thought and action may give rise to experiences of greater depth. (For further information on the cognitive abilities of old people the reader is referred to Chapter 14.)

The words 'retire' and 'retirement' foster the image of decline. The *Concise Oxford Dictionary* (1975) defines 'retire' as 'withdraw, go away, retreat, seek seclusion'. Our expectations are that people will relax and wind down. Perhaps Cumming and Henry's theory of 'disengagement' (1961), where old age is viewed as a time of voluntary withdrawal from society, has helped to promote this view. The activities of older people, however, tend not to decline if they stay in good health and have an adequate income.

Another common belief about old people is that they have inflexible personalities. Joseph (1990) and Coleman (1993) however, point out that there is no sharp discontinuity of personality with age; thus an awkward old person may well have been awkward all of his or her life and any increase of cautiousness which may be evident in old age is probably due to past experience rather than the ageing process itself. The sort of life experience the person has had will obviously influence his or her personality and ability to cope in later life. Marshall (1990) states that ageing is not necessarily related to conservatism or inflexibility or rigidity of attitude. Felstein (1990) complains that we have negative stereotypes of old peoples' personalities and states: 'The truth is that there are as many varieties of personality among the old as in any other age group'.

It should also be remembered that the way people behave is determined not only by personality characteristics but by the situations they are in. Old people may talk of the past because their present lives offer so few opportunities and any anger or unwillingness to cooperate may well be justified and understandable in terms of their situation. The old person who no longer has to impress employers, set a good example to the children or worry about promotion, may feel free to be assertive or eccentric. Indeed the founder of The Gray Panthers, a pressure group of old people in the USA, urges all members to behave outrageously at least once a week because they have absolutely nothing to lose! The organization, which has been in existence for 25 years, has brought about many changes through direct action and civil disobedience. These include the introduction of anti-ageist legislation and the abolition of the statutory retirement age (Grey Power, 1995).

Old age is all too often viewed as a time of misery. This has been challenged by the organization Age Concern (Inequality and Old People, 1982), which found that only 7% of old people felt there was nothing for them to look forward to. Hasler (1989) remarks that the media concentrates on stories of poor care rather than good care of old people, putting over a bleak picture which serves to intensify negative attitudes towards old age as well as a fear of becoming old.

Felstein (1990) and Thompson (1993) mention another ageist stereotype, that of asexuality. In reality many old people remain sexually active until their death. Jerrone (1993) states:

'Contrary to popular assumption, old people are sexual beings. Sexual interest and activity are sustained throughout life though the volume of activity might diminish, and sexual expression take different forms'.

The self-fulfilling prophecy

Perhaps the most unfortunate outcome of ageism is the effect it may have on the self concept, beliefs and behaviour of old people (Marshall, 1990; Coleman, 1993). As Joseph (1990) states:

'Old people themselves act in ways expected of them and so collude in a social construction of reality in which society sets them apart and they in turn expect and accept that they are a group apart'.

This process, whereby oppression is internalized leading to low self-esteem, has been termed the 'self-fulfilling prophecy'.

Many old people believe or accept society's stereotypic ideas about them, just as the members of any oppressed group might before consciousness raising occurs. Thus they may delay seeking medical advice because they perceive their symptoms as the inevitable consequence of old age, they may feel it is futile to take up a new hobby because 'you can't teach an old dog new tricks', or they may be very grateful for their bus passes, failing to realize that such hand-outs are only necessary because their pensions are inadequate. They may believe that young people are more important than they are and that work is the principal good in society. Such beliefs tend to alter the behaviour of old people, thus the stereotype is confirmed and our negative attitudes justified.

Even if old people do not share these beliefs and attitudes they may act in accordance with them, for to oppose any stereotype requires determination and stamina and brings about its own negative effects. For example, if old people in hospital challenge the way they are being treated by staff, they may be avoided and thus forego the fulfilment of social and emotional needs. This is particularly likely if the person has few contacts outside the institution. In many ways the role of 'old person' is forced upon them by society, and their behaviour in this role only serves to reinforce ageist beliefs and to justify ageist practices.

Attitudes of professionals

Professional workers have also been accused of ageist attitudes and behaviour. Norman (1987) and Kenwood (1990) believe that gerontology tends to take a 'victim blaming' approach, looking for the problems within old people rather than within society. For example we are led to believe that old people are isolated and likely to suffer from hypothermia simply because of their age rather than because of their low incomes and poor housing conditions. Old age is thus viewed in biological terms rather than social and political terms.

Norman (1987) criticizes medical training for focusing on acute illness and points out that work with old people lacks prestige and attracts less skilled workers or those who are subject to discrimination themselves and cannot find alternative work. Kenwood (1990) and Blane (1991) comment that geriatric services are poorly funded when compared with other specialities and that geriatric medicine is not a popular option among medical professionals. Finn (1986) and Gregg (1991) report similar findings in relation to physiotherapists. Kenwood (1990) and Thompson (1993) believe that the lack of popularity of work with old people in the health professions is a reflection of ageism and Featherstone and Hepworth (1993) contend that the emergence of geriatric medicine as a distinct discipline raised age consciousness thereby differentiating 'ordinary' people from 'old' people. Thompson (1993) regards the medicalization of old age as an aspect of ageism.

Kvitek et al. (1986) report that physical therapists in San Francisco, who were presented with two hypothetical patients identical in every respect except for their age, set much more demanding goals for the younger patient in terms of walking aids, prostheses, general rehabilitation, endurance, return to work and living situation. Those who were more positive towards old people had more dynamic treatment aims. Knowledge of old age did not appear to be related to the vigour of the treatment, thus it appears that attitudes towards old people, not merely factual information about old age, need to be addressed in education.

Nieuwboer (1992) examined the responses of physiotherapists who had watched a video of post-amputation gait training involving a young patient and an older patient. The physiotherapists tended to interpret non-compliance in the older patient as being due to lack of motivation, whereas in the young patient they interpreted it as being due to the problems of adjusting psychologically to the amputation. They also tended to set less ambitious targets for the older patient. The majority of the physiotherapists had negative attitudes towards working with older people which were based on stereotyped beliefs about old age. These included beliefs that older people are inflexible, depressed, unhealthy, unintelligent and inactive.

Phillipson and Walker (1986) complain that the dependency of old people is fostered both in institutional and community settings. Talking of the community they state: 'People visit, or are transported, to day centres where programmes are often restricted and entirely within the control of social workers, physiotherapists and others to decide and organise'. Excessive 'care' by relatives can also lead to dependency and lack of morale (Scrutton, 1990). Thompson (1993) urges health professionals to empower old people by giving them control and helping them to bring about change rather than encouraging them to adjust to their situation.

Stevenson (1989) and Kenwood (1990) dislike the way in which medical professionals focus on the age of patients and are concerned by the widespread belief that such information is vital. Although it is frequently said that the age of a person is a determinant of the treatment he or she should receive, Stevenson believes that the ethics of this view should be examined. The emphasis on age is all too common in physiotherapy examination questions which so often start with phrases like, 'A 26-year-old lorry driver' or 'A 65-year-old housewife'. The ethics of emphasizing gender and occupation can also be challenged. Day (1988) suggests, as an exercise in challenging our own ageism, that we should try to get through a consultation without reference to age.

Kenwood (1990) points out that old people are frequently exempt from treatments and screening programmes which are available to younger people and that diseases which are common in old age, such as osteoporosis, are neglected. She highlights the fact that 40% of people who die from cervical cancer are 65 years and over but they are not entitled to use screening facilities.

The relevance of ageism to physiotherapists

Many physiotherapists are working with older people both in hospital and community settings. They often represent the interests of old people and are considered to be experts in this area of health care. It is vital, therefore, that any ageist attitudes or behaviour patterns that may have been acquired should be challenged in order that communication and treatments are really effective. We live in an ageist society and are probably all ageist to some extent. Changing such attitudes and behaviour takes both effort and practice.

Physiotherapists need to acquire knowledge and experience of older people who are well. There is a danger that by constantly interacting with those who are ill and disabled, their views of old people will be distorted. Howden and Baggaley (1989) explain how student nurses visit well old people as part of their education in order to change any misconceptions they may have.

By careful thought concerning the language they use, physiotherapists may gradually alter their own attitudes as well as those of their colleagues. This is a difficult area, however, as neutral words, such as the medical speciality 'geriatrics', tend to acquire negative meanings because of our underlying attitudes. Thus the vocabulary constantly needs revision.

Physiotherapists need to keep in mind that the various aspects of ageing – biological, social and psychological – do not necessarily correspond and that many everyday ideas concerning old people, to which we are all exposed, are incorrect. There needs to be a thorough understanding of the true situation and experience of old people.

Practising physiotherapists and tutors of physiotherapy, are in an ideal situation to pass on non-ageist attitudes and behaviour patterns to students both formally and by example. Stevenson (1991) believes that a huge educational programme is needed to combat negative attitudes towards old age among health professionals. Physiotherapists and tutors can also learn from students who have perhaps been exposed less to ageist attitudes, especially those relating to health care.

By non-ageist practice physiotherapists may help to avoid the 'self-fulfilling prophecy' in old people, whereby they live up to the ageist expectations of others and share the same ageist views. Day (1988) believes that medical personnel should take every opportunity to challenge ageist attitudes in old people themselves, and Thompson (1993) thinks that it is part of the health professional's role to give old people positive feedback to enhance their self-esteem.

Physiotherapists are in a position to reduce ageist practices in their work places. This can be achieved by offering old people choice, attempting to 'improve' the environment, involving old people in decision-making regarding their rehabilitation, and challenging the overall running of institutions and community services. Hasler (1989) points out that a non-ageist approach often involves risks as the old person has greater choice and is no longer so constrained and confined by others. Safety and the avoidance of accidents is heavily emphasized in physiotherapy education and some acceptance of risk, in the interest of the old person's happiness and fulfilment, may be difficult to accept. Thompson (1993) states:

> '... the more protective we become the more we challenge older people's rights to make their own decisions and be responsible for themselves. Anti-ageist practice needs to ensure that the protection offered is not at the expense of rights'.

Thompson contends that the assumption that old people are child-like and incapable of making their own decisions is patronising, and that treating old people like children is ageist and a form of abuse.

It is part of the physiotherapist's role to support relatives who are assisting older people in the community. These people are often beyond retirement age themselves and should be viewed and treated in a non-ageist way. Day (1988) believes that ageism demonstrated by carers, for example not involving the older person in decision-making, should be challenged. Physiotherapists, while supporting carers, also need to be aware of the possibility of old age abuse which may be physical, psychological or social and which, when compared with child abuse, has been greatly neglected (Scrutton, 1990).

All physiotherapists, be they in managerial or junior positions, have difficult decisions to make regarding time and treatment priorities. Making such decisions is never easy and is always fraught with ethical dilemmas. Blane (1991) points out that old people are often low on the list of priorities for medical as well as other services and that the reasoning behind this is frequently ageist in nature. Careful thought therefore needs to be given when such decisions are made. (For further information on ethical decision-making, the reader is referred to Chapter 22.)

Physiotherapists who are responsible for recruiting and promoting colleagues, need to avoid making global judgements on the grounds of age. A physiotherapist of 50 may have more energy and enthusiasm than one of 25 and, conversely, a physiotherapist of 25 may have a greater sense of responsibility than one of 50.

Finally, on a more self-interested note, any steps we can take to combat ageism will be doing ourselves an invaluable service, as most of us too will one day be old.

Conclusion

It is clear that there is much that can be done to reduce ageist attitudes and practices within the health care services. This can be achieved by the careful use of language, the dismantling of institutions, and ridding ourselves of ageist misconceptions. However, Stevenson (1991) believes that real change will only come about when the political will to tackle ageism at the social, economic and political level is present. As Scrutton (1990) states:

> 'If age discrimination was entirely a matter of individual attitudes it could be more easily tackled. It is when ageist attitudes become part of the rule of institutions, govern the conduct of social life and blend imperceptibly into everyday values and attitudes that they have a drastic effect on the way older people live their lives'.

Scrutton believes that legal action against ageism must become the major objective.

Perhaps it is this realization that leads Ellard (1988) to advise us to become politically involved on behalf of, or in collaboration with, older patients. However, if we accept that society, even at the level of government and the state, merely consists of the perceptions, attitudes and ideas of individuals, then there is some hope that ageist attitudes and practices can be eliminated. As the word 'ageism' enters everyday vocabulary and its meaning becomes well known, we will perhaps become more conscious of how we think and act towards old people, making ageist attitudes and behaviour less acceptable. Old people too may become more aware of their oppression and this, together with the growing increase in their numbers, has the potential to transform them into a powerful political force.

References

Abercrombie N., Hill S., Turner B. S. (1988) *Dictionary of Sociology.* Harmondsworth: Penguin Books.

Barbato C. A., Feezel J. D. (1987) The language of ageing in different age groups. *The Gerontologist*, **27**, 527–531.

Blane D. (1991) Elderly people and health. In *Sociology as Applied to Medicine.* (3rd edn) (Sambler D., ed.). London: Baillière Tindall.

Bond J. (1993) Living arrangements of elderly people. In *Ageing in Society: An Introduction to Social Gerontology* (2nd edn) (Bond J., Coleman P., Peace S., eds). London: Sage.

Bond J., Coleman P. (1993) Ageing into the twenty-first century. In *Ageing in Society: An Introduction to Social Gerontology* (2nd edn) (Bond J., Coleman P., Peace S., eds). London: Sage.

Butler R. N. (1975) *Why Survive? Being Old in America*. New York: Harper and Row.

Butterworths Medical Dictionary (1978) (2nd edn) (Critchley M., ed.). London: Butterworths.

Carp E. M. (1969) Senility or garden variety adjustment. *The Gerontologist*. April. Cited in Puner L. (1974) *To the Good Long Life*. London: Macmillan Press.

Coleman P. (1993) Adjustment in later life. In *Ageing in Society: An Introduction to Social Gerontology* (2nd edn) (Bond J., Coleman P., Peace S., eds). London: Sage.

Concise Oxford Dictionary (1975) (5th edn) (Fowler H. W., Fowler H. G., eds). Oxford: Oxford University Press.

Croft S., Beresford P. (1991) Old people 'are not a collection of deficits'. Cited in *Therapy Weekly*, Reporting on an Age Concern Conference, *The Human Factor* (1991) London. *Therapy Weekly*, **17**(29), 20.

Cumming E., Henry W. E. (1961) *Growing Old*. New York: Basic Books.

Davison G. C., Neale J. M. (1990) *Abnormal Psychology* (5th edn). New York: John Wiley.

Day L. (1988) How ageism impoverishes elderly care and how to combat it. *Geriatric Medicine*, **18**, 14–15.

Eastman M. (1988) Granny abuse. *Community Outlook*, October, 15–16.

Ellard J. (1988) Growing old: What it is, and what it is not. *Geriatric Medicine*, **18**, 71–77.

Featherstone M., Hepworth M. (1993) Images of ageing. In *Ageing in Society: An Introduction to Social Gerontology* (2nd edn) (Bond J., Coleman P., Peace S., eds). London: Sage.

Felstein I. (1990) Old age is not a disease. *Therapy Weekly*, **16**(30), 6.

Fennell G., Phillipson C., Evers H. (1988) *The Sociology of Old Age*. Milton Keynes: Open University Press.

Finn A. M. (1986) Attitudes of physiotherapists towards geriatric care. *Physiotherapy*, **77**(3), 129–131.

French S. (1994) What is disability? In *On Equal Terms: Working with Disabled People* (French S., ed.). Oxford: Butterworth-Heinemann.

French S., Sim J. (1993) *Writing: A Guide for Therapists*. Oxford: Butterworth-Heinemann.

Gadow S., Berg G. (1978) Towards more human meanings of aging: ideals and images from philosophy and art. In *Aging and the Elderly: Humanistic Perspectives in Gerontology* (Spicker S. F., Woodward L. M., Van Tassel D. D., eds). New Jersey: Humanities Press.

Gregg M. (1991) Factors affecting the attitudes of final year physiotherapy students in Ireland and Northern Ireland towards a career with elderly people. *Physiotherapy Ireland*, **12**(1), 14–20.

Grey Power (1995) *People First*. Channel 4. September 16th.

Gross R. D. (1993) *Psychology: The Science of Mind and Behaviour* (2nd edn). London: Edward Arnold.

Hasler P. (1989) Tackling ageism. *Nursing Standard*, **4**(9), 51.

Hawker M. (1985) *The Older Patient and the Role of the Physiotherapist*. London: Faber and Faber.

Howden C., Baggaley S. (1989) Learning from the experts. *Nursing Times*, **85**(25), 42–44.

Inequality and Old People (1982) Report of the Age Concern Scottish Conference. Cited in Joseph M. (1990) *Sociology for Everyone* (2nd edn). Cambridge: Polity Press.

Jerrome D. (1993) Intimate relationships. In *Ageing in Society: An Introduction to Social Gerontology* (2nd edn) (Bond J., Coleman P., Peace S., eds). London: Sage.

Johnson M. (1993) Dependency and interdependency. In *Ageing in Society: An Introduction to Social Gerontology* (2nd edn) (Bond J., Coleman P., Peace S., eds). London: Sage.

Joseph M. (1990) *Sociology for Everyone* (2nd edn). Cambridge: Polity Press.

Kenwood M. (1990) No sense of urgency: age discrimination in health care. In *Age: The Unrecognised Discrimination* (McEwen E., ed.). London: Age Concern.

Knowles R. (1987) Who's a pretty girl then? *Nursing Times*, **23**, 58–59.

Kvitek S. D. B., Shaver B. J., Blood H., Shepard K. F. (1986) Age bias: physical therapists and age bias. *Journal of Gerontology*, **41**(6), 706–709.

Laczko F., Phillipson C. (1990) Defending the right to work: age discrimination in employment. In *Age: The Unrecognised Discrimination* (McEwen E., ed.). London: Age Concern.

McCalman J. A. (1990) *The Forgotten People*. London: King's Fund Centre and Help the Aged.

Marshall M. (1990) Proud to be old: attitudes to age and ageing. In *Age: The Unrecognised Discrimination* (McEwen E., ed.) London: Age Concern.

Nieuwboer A. E. (1992) Attitudes towards working with older people: Physiotherapists' responses to video presentations of post-amputation gait training for an older and a younger patient. *Physiotherapy Theory and Practice*, **8**(1), 27–38.

Norman A. (1987) *Aspects of Ageism*: a discussion paper. London: Centre for Policy on Ageing.

Payne R. (1989) First impressions count. *Therapy Weekly*, **15**(29), 6.

Phillipson C., Walker A. (1986) *Ageing and Social Policy*. Aldershot: Gower.

Reber A. S. (1985) *The Penguin Dictionary of Psychology*. London: Penguin Books.

Scrutton S. (1990) Ageism: the foundation of age discrimination. In *Age: The Unrecognised Discrimination* (McEwan E., ed.). London: Age Concern.

Stevenson D. (1989) Ageism is a prejudice which nurses perpetuate each and every day. *Nursing Times*, **85**(14), 13.

Stevenson O. (1991) Cited in *Therapy Weekly*, Challenge negativism. Reporting on an Age Concern Conference, *The Human Factor* (1991) London. *Therapy Weekly*, **17**(29), 20.

Thompson N. (1993) *Anti-discriminatory Practice*. London: Macmillan.

Townroe C., Yates G. (1987) *Sociology for GCSE*. London: Longman.

Walker A. (1990) The benefits of old age?: age discrimination and social security. In *Age: The Unrecognised Discrimination* (McEwen E., ed.) London: Age Concern.

Wertheimer A. (1988) *Images by Appointment*. London: the Campaign for People with Mental Handicaps.

7

The attitudes of health professionals towards disabled people

Sally French

Introduction

'Attitudes are enduring mental representations of various features of the social or physical world. They are acquired through experience and exert a directive influence on subsequent behaviour.' (Baron and Byrne, 1991)

This chapter will explain the nature and function of attitudes and will review the literature on the attitudes of health professionals towards disabled people. It will conclude by considering various strategies for attitude change.

The nature of attitudes

Most definitions of attitude comprise three components; cognitive, affective and behavioural. The cognitive component refers to our beliefs about the object or person to whom the attitude is directed. We may believe, for example, that blind people have a 'sixth sense', or that the number of patients referred for physiotherapy has increased; our beliefs may or may not be correct.

The affective component refers to our evaluation of the object or person to whom the attitude is directed. We may think, for example, that the 'sixth sense' of blind people makes them superior beings, or that the rise in patient numbers is placing an unfair burden on physiotherapists. These evaluations are based on the underlying values we hold which represent ethical codes and social and cultural norms; whereas beliefs represent what we know, values represent what we feel. Gross (1992) points out that in order to convert a belief into an attitude a value ingredient is needed. The more important or central our beliefs and values, the more difficult they are for ourselves or for others to change. This is because they tend to underpin our other attitudes and may influence the way we behave.

Our beliefs and values may, in turn, affect our behaviour. We may, for example, fail to assist the blind person when he or she needs it, or display resentment towards the patients queueing up for our services. These ideas are summarized below; our beliefs and values constitute our attitudes which may, in turn, influence our intentions and behaviour (Fishbein and Ajken, 1975).

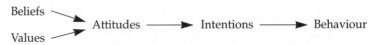

Beliefs
Values ⟶ Attitudes ⟶ Intentions ⟶ Behaviour

It can be seen that behaviour is sometimes viewed as a component of an attitude and sometimes as a separate entity.

Prejudice

Prejudice literally means to pre-judge or to form a strong attitude without sufficient information (Reber, 1985). Although, in its pure form, a prejudice can be either positive or negative, it usually refers to an extreme negative attitude. Reber (1985) defines prejudice as, 'A negative attitude towards a particular group of persons based on negative traits assumed to be uniformly displayed by all members of that group'.

Prejudices, like attitudes, have cognitive, affective and behavioural components. The cognitive component is a stereotype (an over-generalization) which is, in itself, neutral. The affective component is a feeling of liking or hostility, and the behavioural component may manifest itself as aggression, avoidance, discrimination, or preferential treatment. Holmes and Karst (1990) believe that professionals learn to rely on culturally acceptable stereotypes of disabled people as a way of handling their clients and serving the organizations where they work, they state:

> '... it may take less time to use a myth as a basis of action than it does to learn something firsthand from a client ... stereotyping allows humans to infer characteristics at the cost of distorting and restricting awareness of people and individuals'.

Stereotypes of disabled people may strengthen negative attitudes towards them. Disabled people may be expected to behave in various ways, as passive recipients of care for example, yet when they comply their behaviour may validate and reinforce prevailing attitudes that they are inferior or incapable of self-determination. A particular set of behaviours, often referred to as the disabled role, may be expected of disabled people so strongly that those who do not conform are viewed in negative terms (French, 1994a). Funk (1986) believes that self-advocacy is not generally considered part of the behavioural repertoire of disabled people, and Holmes and Karst (1990) maintain that disabled people who take control of their lives may be viewed as aggressive, while passive clients may be viewed as cooperative. As choice of rehabilitation facilities is usually non-existent, disabled people are frequently forced to conform to the stereotyped role prescribed for them.

Disabled people are, of course, members of society and the prejudices which are held against them may become part of their own self-identity and view of the world leading to the 'self-fulfilling prophecy'. These processes are rarely at a conscious level so health professionals do not necessarily guard against them or even think about them. This situation is exacerbated by the big, impersonal organizations where most health professionals work. Although professional ethics may demand the self-determination of patients and clients, bureaucratic organizations may insist that professionals remain in control (Holmes and Karst, 1990).

According to Brown (1986) two factors are particularly important in breaking down prejudice; non-competitive contact of an equal status, and the pursuit of common goals which are obtainable through cooperation.

The relationship between attitudes and behaviour

Our attitudes and behaviour tend to be poorly correlated; Wicker (1969) estimates that only 10% of the variance in our behaviour can be explained by our attitudes. This is because factors other than attitudes, such as habits, social norms, and group pressure, influence our behaviour. As Gross (1992) states:

> 'It is generally agreed that attitudes are only one determinant of behaviour; they represent predispositions to behave but how we actually act in a particular situation will depend on the immediate consequences of our behaviour, how we think others will evaluate our actions, and habitual ways of behaving in those kinds of situations'.

Although attitudes do predict behaviour to a limited extent, situational factors often have a stronger influence. It cannot be assumed, for example, that patients who faithfully attend every appointment have a positive attitude towards their treatment; they may simply feel that attendance is expected of them, or have nothing better to do. Similarly health professionals may behave impeccably towards their patients even though their attitudes may not always be positive. Discrimination may also arise from habit, social pressure, or group norms, rather than prejudice. Some people are more inclined to keep consistency between their attitudes and behaviour than others.

A problem when evaluating research which relates attitudes to behaviour, is that *general* attitudes have often been used to predict *specific* behaviour. Atkinson *et al.* (1993) state that attitudes predict behaviour best when they are strong and consistent, based on the person's direct experience, and specifically related to the behaviour in question. Fishbein and Ajken (1975) agree that general attitudes are poor predictors of specific behaviour, and that to obtain a positive correlation, both the attitude and the behaviour must be specific. Thus in order to infer a health professional's behaviour when confronted with a severely disabled person wishing to live independently, the attitude of the therapist towards that specific issue would be a better predictor than a measure of his or her general attitude towards severely disabled people.

It is also the case that various aspects of our attitudes may be inconsistent. We may, for example, be very attracted to someone yet have serious doubts about his or her integrity. Related attitudes may also conflict, we may be in favour of greater public spending yet object to tax increases. In situations such as these one of the attitudes, or attitude components, may be more related to behaviour than the others.

The function of attitudes

Social psychologists have demonstrated that our attitudes serve many important functions relating to our psychological well-being. For this reason attitudes are often very resistant to change. Below are listed the major functions that attitudes serve (Pennington, 1986; Atkinson *et al.*, 1993).

1. *Adaptive function* – We hold attitudes for practical reasons; to achieve our goals, to increase satisfaction and pleasure, and to avoid punishment. We may develop similar attitudes to those we like, or to those

with whom we work, in order to maintain the pleasure of their company and avoid conflict. In this way our attitudes help us achieve and maintain social adjustment, and avoid social isolation. Those living in isolated areas, where the choice of social contacts is small, would perhaps feel a greater necessity to alter their attitudes in this way than those living in cities with a more diverse population.

2. *Knowledge function* – In order to cope with the complexities of life, we impose a structure on the world making it a simpler and less uncertain place. In this way we may form stereotypes (over-generalizations) of groups of people to simplify our understanding of them and responses to them. We may believe, for example, that physiotherapists are out-going and confident, or that disabled people are in need of care and protection.

3. *Self-expressive function* – Our attitudes give expression to our underlying values and beliefs; by expressing our attitudes we are confirming the positive aspects of our self-concept. We need to tell others about ourselves in order to develop a strong self-identity. The reactions of others may also lead us to modify or strengthen our attitudes.

4. *Ego-defensive function* – Our attitudes give us protection from anxiety and threats to our self-esteem, both from ourselves and from others. If, for example, we value ourselves and believe we are basically good, we are better able to reject or to cope with the criticisms and evaluations of others, and to dismiss or accept our own behaviour when it fails to meet the expectations we have of ourselves. In dealing with threats to our self-esteem we may deny or distort information, or project our conflicts and failings on to other people.

It is clear that in order to change an attitude its function must be known. If, for example, the attitude is serving an ego-defensive function, providing the person with information would be unlikely to bring about change.

Measuring attitudes towards disabled people

There are many ways of measuring attitudes towards disabled people. Most measures focus on disability in general terms, rather than on specific impairments. The survey, using various questionnaires, is by far the most common method, though sociometric measures, to investigate behaviour, and instruments involving video and picture presentation have also been used. The most widely used instrument is the *Attitudes Towards Disabled Persons Scale* (ATDP) developed by Yuker *et al.* in 1960. It measures attitudes in terms of perceived differences between groups of disabled and non-disabled people.

The Interaction with Disabled Persons Scale (IDP) is a new instrument which was developed in Australia in the late 1980s and early 1990s (Gething, 1993); it is used to measure community attitudes towards disabled people. The scale explores the motivations and emotions considered to underlie negative attitudes towards disabled people, rather than focusing on the perceived differences between disabled and non-disabled people. Gething (1993) explains that the IDP scale is based upon the notion that negative attitudes reflect strangeness, or lack of familiarity, which creates uncertainty or anxiety.

The Disability Social Distance Scale (DSDS) was developed by Tringo in 1970. It measures how closely people wish to be associated with disabled people with particular impairments. In this way it can be seen to what extent people with particular impairments are viewed as acceptable or unacceptable. It is not, of course, possible accurately to predict behaviour from attitude measures.

It is interesting and enlightening to note that most research about disabled people has focused on impairment rather than on the social and environmental barriers which stand in the way of disabled people. Research into disability has been conducted mainly by non-disabled people and has not reflected the social model of disability, articulated by disabled people, which views disability as a civil rights issue rather than an individual tragedy (French, 1994b).

Attitudes of health professionals towards disabled people

'Health care professionals share the values and expectations of their society and show the same reactions that unstigmatised individuals have towards those with differences.' (Allen and Birse, 1991)

Research evidence regarding whether the attitudes of health professionals are more or less positive than those of the general public tend to conflict (Elston and Snow, 1986; Vargo and Semple, 1988). Studies concerning the change of attitudes of medical students throughout their training, for example, show that they may improve (Mitchell *et al.*, 1984), deteriorate (Rezler, 1974), or remain the same (Duckworth, 1988). Chubon (1982) concludes that after three decades of research regarding the attitudes of health professionals towards disabled people, the evidence is still indeterminate.

Although research findings do conflict, the weight of the evidence suggests that the attitudes of health professionals are not very different from those of the general public, and that they may become more negative as professional education proceeds (Brillhart *et al.*, 1990). Chubon (1982) found the attitudes of occupational therapists to be more negative towards disabled people than those of the general public, Brillhart *et al.* (1990) found that first year nursing students had more positive attitudes towards disabled people than graduating nurses, Diseker and Michielutte (1981) showed that empathy towards disabled people decreased during medical training, and Rezler (1974) discovered that medical education tends to increase cynicism. Elston and Snow (1986) used the ATDP scale with rehabilitation counsellors and found no difference between their attitudes and those of other occupational groups.

Duckworth (1988) used the ATDP scale to test the attitudes of first and fourth year medical students, house officers, and the general public. He also asked them to agree or disagree with the statement: *'Disabled people cause more problems to doctors than non-disabled people'*. No significant difference was found among the doctors with regard to age, sex, occupation, intended medical career, length of contact with disabled people, or personal knowledge of a disabled person. Those who agreed with the statement, however, had more negative attitudes.

Lyons (1991) used the ATDP scale to compare undergraduate occupational therapy students with undergraduate business students. No significant difference was found between the two groups or between junior and senior students. There was, however, a significant difference ($P \leq 0.01$) between those students who had had close contact with a disabled person and those who had not. Lyons and Hayes (1993) discovered that the attitudes of occupational therapy students did not change during their professional education, a finding consistent with that of Lyons (1991). De Poy and Merrill (1988) found that occupational therapy students learned to articulate the humanistic values presented to them but did not necessarily apply them; the students, in turn, believed that the faculty did not practice the values it expounded.

Gething (1992) studied undergraduate health professionals. They watched 12 different videotapes of people applying for a job where the use of a wheelchair, the applicant's manner, and the applicant's gender were manipulated. The presence of the wheelchair led to a general devaluing by the health professionals of the individual on characteristics having no necessary relationship to disability, for example psychological and social adjustment. Westbrook et al. (1988) found that student health professionals tended to view disability as more tragic and limiting than statistics indicate, and Gething (1993) found that health professionals make negative judgements of personality and adjustment on the basis of disability.

Lyons and Hayes (1993) found that junior and senior occupational therapy students and business students all identified the same most and least preferred disabilities. The most preferred disabilities were asthma, diabetes, arthritis, ulcer, amputation, and heart disease; the least preferred disabilities were, alcoholism, mental illness, mental handicap, and hunchback. Gordon et al. (1990) found that people with epilepsy were preferred by health care students over those with cerebral palsy, blindness, and amputation. There seems to be a preference for physical impairments, those which are not visible, and those which are perceived to be outside the person's control. Sim (1990) maintains that ascription of responsibility is a powerful determinant of stigma. He states:

'Any condition encountered in clinical practice liable to be seen as "self-inflicted" is potentially a target for stigmatisation on the grounds of moral failure. Somewhat less obviously, patients who fail to display appropriate courage or determination in coping with their disability may be regarded as morally deficient in a similar way'.

Paris (1993) believes that the negative attitudes of health professionals towards disabled people must be examined for the following reasons:

1. Negative attitudes may adversely affect the self-image and recovery of recently injured or disabled people.
2. Health professionals may influence the attitudes of the general public towards disabled people.
3. Negative attitudes may affect the delivery of services to disabled people.

4. Negative attitudes may influence funding decisions.
5. Negative attitudes may influence the attitudes of health care students, thus perpetuating a negative image of disabled people.

The attitudes of health professionals are influential in shaping services for disabled people and their life opportunities. Lyons (1991) doubts whether students with anything but highly positive attitudes towards disabled people should be accepted in the health professions. Talking of occupational therapy he states:

> 'Persons with disabilities have a right to expect that occupational therapy students will receive an education that prepares them to be professionals that are enabling rather than disabling by virtue of their attitudes'.

Other research evidence indicates that the attitudes of health professionals towards disabled people are more positive than those of the general public, and that their attitudes improve during professional education. Huitt and Elston (1991), using the ATDP scale, found attitudes of counsellors more positive than those of the general public, and Gething and Westbrook (1983) found that first year physiotherapy students had more positive attitudes to disabled people than students of other occupations. Paris (1993), using the ATDP scale, found that fourth year medical students had more positive attitudes than first year medical students. Lyons and Hayes (1993) used the DSDS scale to compare the attitudes of occupational therapy students and business students towards disabled people at an Australian University. The occupational therapy students showed much less social distance than the business students although there was no significant difference between the junior and the senior occupational therapy students.

These more positive attitudes may result, to some extent, from the curriculum the students study. Rosswurn (1980) found that the attitudes of a group of nursing students who had received a learning programme planned to promote positive attitudes towards disabled people, had a more positive attitude after the programme, although 6 months later the improvement was lost. Estes *et al.* (1991) used the ATDP scale to measure the attitudes of occupational therapy and medical technology students. The occupational therapy curriculum included content related to values and attitudes, contact with disabled people, and information about disability and disabling conditions. The medical technology curriculum did not cover these aspects. Fourth year occupational therapy students were found to have more positive attitudes than both first year occupational therapy students and first and fourth year medical technology students.

Some of the inconsistencies in the professional literature may be due to the differing nature of professional and personal attitudes. Leonard and Crawford (1989) observed that people's beliefs about the way disabled people should be treated by society, and their own personal reactions to disabled people, were often in conflict. Gordon *et al.* (1990) found that the attitudes of health professionals varied according to the social context; they were more favourably disposed to working with disabled people than dating or marrying them. Vargo and Semple (1988) studied a cohort of 40 physiotherapy students in their fourth year of study using the ATDP scale. The students were asked to respond firstly according to their professional reaction and secondly according to their personal reaction. The students were more positive when they responded professionally ($P \leq 0.5$).

Health professionals tend to show more positive attitudes when the IDP scale, rather than the ATDP scale, is used. Using the IDP scale, Gething found that nurses and nursing students (Gething, 1992), and physiotherapists (Gething, 1993) had more positive attitudes towards disabled people than the general public. Furthermore, those physiotherapists who had daily contact with disabled people had more positive attitudes than those who had less contact.

The fact that the majority of health professionals are women, may also be a factor in accounting for their positive attitudes when compared with the general public. Previous research is inconclusive, but many studies show that women have more positive attitudes towards disabled people than men (Furnham and Pendred, 1983; Potts, 1986; Brillhart et al., 1990). Lyons and Hayes (1993) used the DSDS scale to investigate the attitudes of junior and senior occupational therapy students towards disabled people. They found that males chose a far greater social distance from disabled people than females ($P \leq 0.001$). Similarly, Paris (1993) found that women health professionals were more positive towards disabled people than male health professionals. Disabled men tend to be viewed more positively than disabled women by both sexes (Weisel and Florian, 1990).

Attitude change

There are many theories of attitude change, but the one which has given rise to the most research is undoubtedly the theory of cognitive dissonance (Festinger, 1957). The theory of cognitive dissonance asserts that we seek a state of psychological balance and that our state of mind is negative if our attitudes, or our attitudes and behaviour, are inconsistent. Reber (1985) defines cognitive dissonance as:

> 'An emotional state set up when two simultaneously held attitudes or cognitions are inconsistent or where there is a conflict between belief and overt behaviour. The resolution of the conflict is assumed to serve as a basis for attitude change in that belief patterns are generally modified so as to be consistent with behaviour'.

Thus the health professional who is expected to carry out treatment procedures with which he or she disagrees, is likely to be in a state of cognitive dissonance. In a situation such as this there may be a shift of attitude to bring it in line with the expected behaviour, or the importance of the discrepancy between the attitude and the behaviour may be minimized by refuting or ignoring it. Alternatively, the health professional may decide to find employment elsewhere or attempt to convert the organization to his or her way of thinking; these are more difficult options, however, and Baron and Byrne (1991) believe that as human beings we tend to follow the path of least resistance. If there is external justification for our behaviour there is little need for attitude change as we are unlikely to experience cognitive dissonance.

It is necessary to be committed to an attitude or a way of behaving in order to experience cognitive dissonance. The harder someone works towards achieving a goal the more highly that goal is valued and the greater the cognitive dissonance if it turns out to be deficient in some way. Pennington (1986) states:

> '... any situation in which a person struggles to gain acceptance, is likely to result in the goal when achieved being seen as desirable and worthwhile, regardless of whether it actually is or not'.

The ideas of the growing Disabled People's Movement, which views disability as a civil rights issue rather than a medical problem, may give rise to cognitive dissonance in those health professionals willing to consider the arguments. Having gone through a long and arduous professional education, and having worked with the best of intentions for many years, it may be difficult to accept that fundamental changes of practice are needed.

Contact with disabled people

Contact with disabled people is an important ingredient in bringing about positive attitude change (McConkey and McCormack, 1983; Berrol, 1984; Sampson, 1991; Lyons and Hayes, 1993). Most people do not get to know about disability at first hand and may avoid disabled people because of feelings of fear and inadequacy. Interacting with a disabled person can place a strain on the encounter and may call into question many taken for granted assumptions about the process of communication. It may, for example, be disconcerting when the person with a learning difficulty fails to understand or when the deaf person needs to lip read. Clough (1982) highlights the discomfort of interacting with visually impaired people. He states:

> 'If someone doesn't look directly at us we feel uncomfortable. If he gazes intently at us we feel equally uncomfortable. If his face and especially his eyes don't immediately respond to what we say we feel slightly deterred, and wonder if he is in any way deficient – so we either speak louder or we get discouraged and turn our attention elsewhere'.

Simple contact, or contact on a professional level, does not, however, appear to be enough to bring about positive attitude change (Evans, 1976; Fichten et al., 1985), although the research evidence does, to some extent, conflict (Paris, 1993; Biori and Oermann, 1993). Gething (1993) points out that interaction between the health professional and the disabled person tends to focus on what the disabled person cannot do thereby highlighting the differences between them. Lyons and Hayes (1993), talking of occupational therapy students state:

> 'In our view much of students' clinical contact with persons with psychiatric disabilities occurs only in situations where, as patients, their problems, deficiencies, or distress are highlighted'.

One factor that consistently seems to promote positive attitudes towards disabled people is equal status contact (Anthony, 1977; Yuker and Block, 1979; McConkey and McCormack, 1983; Mitchell *et al.*, 1984). Contact on an equal level is more likely than professional/client contact to break down stereotypes and promote effective interaction. McConkey and McCormack (1983) found that personal contact on an equal level, where dependence was avoided and where the disabled person could demonstrate competence, was the most successful strategy in bringing about attitude change. This view is shared by Gething (1992) who believes that effective interaction between disabled and non-disabled people occurs when they are of equal status, where the contact is voluntary and mutually rewarding, and where the context allows the disabled person to present him or herself as capable and multi-faceted. He points out that these features rarely characterize interactions between health professionals and disabled people.

It is important that health professionals, particularly students, have greater equal status contact with disabled people. As well as changing their attitudes through interaction, contact with disabled people outside rehabilitation and other 'special' settings has the potential to change perceptions by drawing attention to the social and physical barriers which disabled people encounter (Allen and Birse, 1991). Gething (1993) believes that it is vitally important to monitor the quality of contact between health professionals and disabled people in order to bring about positive attitude change, and many writers advocate the training and employment of disabled health professionals as a means of changing attitudes within the professions (Turner, 1984; Bennet, 1987; French, 1988; Chinnery, 1991). Positive attitudes would also be promoted by a more equal relationship between health professionals and disabled clients (French, 1994c).

Information about disabled people

Giving information about disability and disabled people is also important in bringing about positive attitude change (McConkey and McCormack, 1938; Berrol, 1984). This may include specific information, such as how to guide a blind person, or broader information concerning the ways disabled people define their situation, and their substantial achievements within the growing Disabled People's Movement. Duckworth (1988) and Lyons and Hayes (1993) believe that there should be substantial input from disabled people throughout the education of health professionals. This is best achieved by comprehensive disability equality training conducted by qualified disabled trainers.

Some methods of imparting information are more conducive to attitude change than others. McConkey and McCormack (1983) and Dickson *et al.* (1991) believe that role play is a suitable method for changing attitudes, heightening sensitivity, and familiarizing learners with situations they may later encounter. Role playing is perhaps the next best thing to experiencing a genuine event. It does, however, have various advantages over real life situations in that timing can be made artificially rapid, situations rarely encountered can be enacted, and the learner can receive constructive feedback from supportive colleagues. Mistakes can also be made in a safe environment. Role play should not be confused with simulation exercises. Exercises which attempt to simulate disability have undergone considerable criticism, particularly by disabled people, because of their artificiality and the negative attitudes of disability they tend to induce (Finkelstein, 1991; French, 1992).

Lyons and Hayes (1993) advocate discussion of and reflection on feeling to bring about positive attitude change. According to Beard (1976), attitude change is facilitated by exposure to different points of view and from constructive criticism from other people. Even if attitudes are not changed discussion may help learners to become more tolerant of different view points and perspectives (Curzon, 1990). Discussion does need careful planning, however, or it can degenerate into a forum for the exchange of prejudices.

Social psychologists have discovered, through empirical investigation, many factors which improve the outcome of persuasive communication. These concern the person delivering the message, the message itself, the recipient of the message, and the context in which the message is delivered. It includes such factors as the status and credibility of the communicator, the intensity of the message, whether a one-sided or a two-sided argument is given, and the level of education of the recipients (Gross, 1992; French, 1994d).

Anthony (1984) concludes that neither information nor contact alone is sufficient to alter attitudes towards disabled people, but that a combination of both factors is required.

A supportive work environment

In order for attitudes and behaviour towards disabled people to change the work environment must be enabling and supportive to health professionals. Marsh and Fisher (1992) believe that managers and practitioners are under enormous pressure to take shortcuts and compromise principles, and that 'user-orientated practice requires user-orientated policies'. Chinnery (1990) states that:

'Individual workers may well act in non-disabling ways, but the structure of services which reaches far beyond that which is visible to disabled users, militates actively and very effectively against individual efforts to promote a helpful, non-disabling, client orientated service'.

Ellis (1993) notes that advocating for a client can put practitioners into conflict with employers, and Stevenson and Parsloe contend that, 'without a new culture there will be severe limitations on what workers can do'.

The organizational context and culture should not, however, be used as an excuse for doing nothing, Stevenson and Parsloe (1993) found many examples of excellent practice in the face of organizational opposition. It is also the case that once changes in policy and practice are initiated, shifts in attitude and behaviour are likely to follow (Kilbury et al., 1992).

Conclusion

This account indicates that although research evidence conflicts there is room for considerable improvement in the attitudes of health professionals towards disabled people. In order to promote positive attitudes and behaviour towards disabled people there need to be changes in both professional education and practice. It is important that health professionals receive high quality disability equality training, that they understand the meaning of disability as disabled people define it, and that they are informed about the important role disabled people have played in the development of services. Informal, equal status contact with disabled people, and the education and employment of disabled health professionals, would also help promote positive attitudes and improve services to disabled people. As Munro and Elder-Woodward (1992) state: 'The challenge for workers at all levels of community care is to make sure that the service user is in control of his own life style *and* in control of the services surrounding him which are designed to support that life-style'.

References

Allen M., Birse E. (1991) Stigma and blindness. *Journal of Ophthalmic Nursing and Technology*, **10**(4), 147–151.

Anthony W. A. (1977) Social rehabilitation: changing society's attitudes towards the physically and mentally disabled. In *Social and Psychological Aspects of Disability* (Stubbins J., ed.). Baltimore: University Park.

Anthony W. A. (1984) Societal rehabilitation: changing society's attitudes towards the physically and mentally disabled. In *The Psychological and Social Impact of Physical Disability* (Marinelli R. P., Dell Orto L. E., eds). New York: Springer.

Atkinson R. L., Atkinson R. C., Smith E. E., Bem D. J. (1993) *Introduction to Psychology* (11th edn). London: Harcourt Brace Johanovich College Publishers.

Baron R. A., Byrne D. (1991) *Social Psychology* (6th edn). London: Allyn and Bacon.

Beard R. (1976) *Teaching and Learning in Higher Education* (3rd edn). Harmondsworth: Penguin Books.

Bennet G. (1978) *The Wound of the Doctor.* London: Secker and Warburg.

Berrol C. (1984) Trainee attitudes towards disabled persons; effect of a special education program. *Archives of Physical Medicine and Rehabilitation*, **65**, 760–765.

Biori B. Oermann M. H. (1993) The effect of prior experience in a rehabilitation setting on students' attitudes towards the disabled. *Rehabilitation Nursing*, **18**(2), 95–98.

Brillhart B. A., Jay H., Wyers M. E. (1990) Attitudes towards people with disabilities. *Rehabilitation Nursing*, **15**(2), 80–82, 85.

Brown R. (1986) *Social Psychology* (2nd edn). New York: Free Press.

Chinnery B. (1990) Disabled people get the message: non-verbal clues to the nature of social work. *Practice*, **4**(1), 49–55.

Chinnery B. (1991) Equal opportunities for disabled people in the caring professions: window dressing or commitment? *Disability, Handicap and Society*, **6**(3), 253–258.

Chubon R. A. (1982) An analysis of research dealing with the attitudes of professionals towards disability. *Journal of Rehabilitation*, **48**, 25–29.

Clough E. (1982) Attitudes. *Inter-regional Review*, Summer, **71**, 324–37.

Curzon L. B. (1990) *Teaching in Further Education: An Outline of Principles and Practice* (4th edn). London: Cassell.

De Poy E., Merrill S. (1988) Value acquisition in an occupational therapy curriculum. *Occupational Therapy Journal of Research*, **8**, 259–274.

Dickson D. A., Maxwell A., Saunders C. (1991) Using role play with physiotherapy students. *Physiotherapy*, **77**(2), 145–153.

Diseker R. A., Michielutte R. (1981) An analysis of empathy in medical students before and following clinical experience. *Journal of Medical Education*, **56**, 1004–1010.

Duckworth S. (1988) The effect of medical education on the attitudes of medical students towards disabled people. *Journal of Medical Education*, **22**, 1023–1030.

Ellis K. (1993) *Squaring the Circle. User and Carer Participation in Needs Assessment.* London: Joseph Rowntree Foundation.

Elston R. R., Snow B. M. (1986) Attitudes towards people with disabilities as expressed by rehabilitation professionals. *Rehabilitation Counselling Bulletin*, **29**(4), 284–286.

Estes J., Deyer C., Hansen R., Russell J. (1991) Influence of occupational therapy curicula on students' attitudes towards persons with disabilities. *American Journal of Occupational Therapy*, **45**, 156–159.

Evans J. H. (1976) Changing attitudes towards disabled persons: an experimental study. *Rehabilitation Counselling Bulletin*, June, 172–179.

Festinger L. (1957) *A Theory of Cognitive Dissonance*. Stanford, CA: Stanford University Press.

Fichten C., Hines J., Amsel R. (1985) Public awareness of physically disabled persons. *International Journal of Rehabilitation Research*, **8**(4), 407–413.

Finkelstein V. (1991) It is insulting to trivialise disability. *Therapy Weekly*, **17**(25), 5.

Fishbein M., Ajken I. (1975) *Belief, Attitude, Intention and Behaviour*. Reading, MA: Addison-Wesley.

French S. (1988) The experiences of disabled health professionals. *Sociology of Health and Illness*, **10**(2), 70–88.

French S. (1992) Simulation exercises in disability awareness training: a critique. *Disability, Handicap and Society*, **7**(3), 257–266.

French S. (1994a) The disabled role. In *On Equal Terms: Working with Disabled People* (French S., ed.). Oxford: Butterworth-Heinemann.

French S. (1994b) Researching disability. In *On Equal Terms: Working with Disabled People* (French S., ed.). Oxford: Butterworth-Heinemann.

French S. (1994c) Disabled people and professional practice. In *On Equal Terms: Working with Disabled People* (French S., ed.). Oxford: Butterworth-Heinemann.

French S. (1994d) The art of gentle persuasion. *Therapy Weekly*, **20**(36), 13.

Funk R. (1986) Self-advocates push beyond civil rights. *Independent Living Forum*, **4**(1), 3–5. The Research and Training Center on Independent Living. University of Kansas.

Furnham A., Pendred J. (1983) Attitudes towards the mentally and physically disabled. *British Journal of Medical Psychology*, **56**, 179–187.

Gething L. (1992) Nurse practitioners' and students' attitudes towards people with disabilities. *Australian Journal of Advanced Nursing*, **9**(3), 25–30.

Gething L. (1993) Attitudes towards people with disabilities of physiotherapists and members of the general public. *Australian Journal of Physiotherapy*, **39**(4), 291–295.

Gething L., Westbrook M. (1983) Enhancing physiotherapy students' attitudes towards disabled people. *Australian Journal of Physiotherapy*, **29**, 48–52.

Gordon E., Minnes P., Holden R. (1990) The structure of attitudes towards persons with a disability, when specific disability and context are considered. *Rehabilitation Psychology*, **35**, 79–90.

Gross R. D. (1992) *Psychology: The Science of Mind and Behaviour* (2nd edn). London: Edward Arnold.

Holmes G. E., Karst R. H. (1990) The institutionalisation of disability myths: impact on vocational rehabilitation services. *Journal of Rehabilitation*, **56**, 20–27.

Huitt K., Elston R. R. (1991) Attitudes towards persons with disabilities expressed by professional counsellors. *Journal of Applied Rehabilitation Counselling*, **22**(2), 42–43.

Kilbury R. F., Bensoff J. J., Rubin S. E. (1992) The interaction of legislation, public attitudes, and access to opportunities for persons with disabilities. *Journal of Rehabilitation*, **58**(4), 6–9.

Leonard R., Crawford J. (1989) Two approaches to seeing people with disabilities. *Australian Journal of Social Issues*, **24**, 112–125.

Lyons M. (1991) Enabling or disabling? Students' attitudes towards persons with disabilities. *American Journal of Occupational Therapy*, **45**, 311–316.

Lyons M., Hayes R. (1993) Student perceptions of persons with psychiatric and other disorders. *American Journal of Occupational Therapy*, **47**(6), 541–548.

McConkey R., McCormack B. (1983) *Breaking Barriers: Educating People about Disability*. London: Souvenir Press.

Marsh P., Fisher M. (1992) *Good Intentions: Developing Partnership in Social Services*. London; Joseph Rowntree Foundation.

Mitchell K. R., Hayes M., Gordon J., Wallis B. (1984) An investigation of the attitudes of medical students to physically disabled people. *Journal of Medical Education*, **18**, 21–23.

Munro K., Elder-Woodward J. (1992) *Independent Living*. Edinburgh; Churchill Livingstone.

Paris M. J. (1993) Attitudes of medical students and health care professionals towards people with disabilities. *Archives of Physical Medicine and Rehabilitation*, **74**, 818–825.

Pennington D. C. (1986) *Essential Social Psychology*. London: Edward Arnold.

Potts M. J. (1986) Sex differences in medical students and house staff attitudes towards the handicapped. *Journal of the American Women's Association*, **41**, 156–159.

Reber A. S. (1985) *Dictionary of Psychology*. Harmondsworth: Penguin Books.

Rezler A. G. (1974) Attitude changes during medical school. *Journal of Medical Education*, **49**, 1023–1030.

Rosswurn M. (1980) Changing nursing students' attitudes towards persons with physical disabilities. *Journal of American Registered Nurses*, **5**, 12–14.

Sampson D. E. (1991) Changing attitudes towards persons with cerebral palsy through contact and information. *Rehabilitation Education*, **5**(2), 87–92.

Sim J. (1990) Physical disability, stigma, and rehabilitation. *Canadian Journal of Physiotherapy*, **42**(5), 232–238.

Stevenson O., Parsloe P. (1993) *Community Care and Empowerment*. London: Joseph Rowntree Foundation.

Tringo J. L. (1970) The hierarchy of preference towards disability groups. *Journal of Special Education*, **4**, 295–305.

Turner C. (1984) Who cares? *Occupational Health*, **36**(10), 449–452.

Vargo J. W., Semple J. E. (1988) Professional and personal attitudes of physiotherapy students towards disabled persons. *Australian Journal of Physiotherapy*, **34**(1), 23–26.

Weisel A., Florian V. (1990) Same and cross-gender attitudes towards persons with physical disabilities. *Rehabilitation Psychology*, **35**(4), 229–238.

Westbrook M., Adamson B. J., Westbrook J. I. (1988) Health science students' images of disabled people. *Community Health Studies*, **12**(3), 304–311.

Wicker A. W. (1969) Attitudes versus actions: the relationship of verbal and overt behaviour responses to attitude objects. *Journal of Social Issues*, **25**, 41–78.

Yuker H. E., Block J. R. (1979) *Challenging Barriers to Change; Attitudes Towards the Disabled*. Albertson, NY: Human Resources Center.

Yuker H. E., Block J., Campbell W. (1960) *A Scale to Measure Attitudes Towards Disabled Persons*. Albertson, NY: Human Resources Center.

Section 2

The Experience of Illness and Disability

8

Why do people become patients?

Sally French

Not everyone who feels ill decides to become a patient, in fact although most people experience unpleasant symptoms fairly regularly, the majority decide against assuming the patient role (Pitts, 1991; Scambler, 1991; Gillespie, 1995a). Thus patients do not form a cross-section of people with a given disease and those who reach consultants or physiotherapists may be an even more select group. Wadsworth *et al.* (1971) found that less than one-third of people who had experienced a distressing symptom in the previous 2 weeks had consulted a doctor and similar results have been found by Dunnell and Cartwright (1972), Hannay (1980), and many other researchers. Tuckett (1976) concludes that, 'for the majority of individuals visiting a doctor is a rather rare method of managing the symptoms of disease'. It is far more common to ignore symptoms or to buy medicines across the counter. Last (1963) used the term 'illness iceberg' to describe the situation where only a minority of people with symptoms become patients.

That only certain people decide to define themselves as patients raises important issues regarding our knowledge of disease, for most research is carried out on patient populations within orthodox medicine, which are clearly not representative of people with any particular condition. For example, it may be concluded that people with a certain disease are more anxious than normal, but an alternative explanation is that anxious people become patients more readily. If the illness iceberg is not considered, health professionals, including physiotherapists, can get a very distorted view of illness and impairment and the way people behave towards it. Patients are not a cross-section of people with any particular disease.

The seemingly obvious explanation of the 'illness iceberg' is that people with severe symptoms consult health professionals, whereas those with mild symptoms do not. Surveys show, however, that the reasons for becoming a patient cannot be explained in terms of symptom severity alone. Hannay (1980) interviewed a sample of people registered with a health centre and found that 11% who considered their symptoms not to be serious consulted their GPs, whereas 26% who considered their symptoms to be serious did not. Many people who know they are very ill and have unpleasant symptoms choose not to seek medical advice or care. Thus the severity of symptoms is just one factor among many which determine whether or not a person becomes a patient. As Pitts (1991) states:

'... there is a complex inter-relationship between the perception of symptoms of ill-health, the response to such symptoms and the decision to seek the opinion of a health professional'.

The ways in which people respond to illness and impairment and the type of help they seek, if they seek it at all, has been termed 'illness behaviour'. If they become patients they are said to be in the 'patient role' and if they define themselves as ill they are said to occupy the 'sick role'. Mechanic and Volkart (1961) define illness behaviour as, '... the way in which symptoms are perceived, evaluated and acted upon by a person who recognizes some pain, discomfort or other signal of organic malfunction'.

There is considerable discrepancy between the definitions of illness and impairment between health professionals and lay people (Helman, 1994). Cartwright (1967) found that GPs regarded about half of their work as trivial, unnecessary and inappropriate. Yet health professionals despair of people who ignore serious symptoms or who only consult when their disease is advanced. Although no similar work has been done with physiotherapists, it is likely that their definitions of illness and impairment also differ markedly from those of their patients.

Factors which influence how people perceive illness and impairment and how they respond to it will now be considered.

Characteristics of the symptoms

Before seeking medical advice the person must decide that he or she is ill and that the problem is an appropriate one for medical intervention. The person's decision will depend on many factors including cultural influences, personality, medical knowledge and past experience of medical care (Armstrong, 1994). The person may conclude, correctly or incorrectly, that medical intervention will be of no help. With the more chronic diseases which are typically seen today, such decisions are by no means straightforward as it can be very difficult distinguishing normality from abnormality, especially as people tend to accommodate symptoms if their onset and progression is gradual. Over time symptoms which would initially have been considered abnormal by the individual come to be viewed as normal.

Symptoms which appear suddenly are most likely to be regarded as serious or due to disease than those of gradual onset; and symptoms, whatever their nature, will be more alarming to some people than others, according to such factors as family background, personality and culture (Armstrong, 1994). Some may experience such intense fear at the discovery of a lump, for example, that they decide against seeking medical help, while others are motivated by the same degree of fear to seek help immediately. Some may avoid health services because they are afraid of diagnostic procedures or acutely embarrassed by medical examinations. Thus the nature of the symptoms and the way people respond to them are important factors concerning whether or not they become patients and how they behave in that role. It is important for the physiotherapist to realize that the anxiety and distress caused by a symptom are not necessarily related to its severity.

Social and cultural factors

Whether someone will become a patient or not depends in part on social and cultural factors. These will influence the person's perception of the symptoms and what type of help, if any, is sought. Jacobson *et al.* (1991), Gillespie (1995b) and many others, have found that women use the health service more than men and people in social class five (those employed in unskilled manual work and their families) are under-represented, particularly with regard to preventative medicine, when their high levels of disease and impairment are taken into account (see Chapter 2). Thus people have different ideas about what constitutes health, illness and impairment and what action, if any, should be taken. Attitudes change over time so the views of young and old people are likely to differ and our expectations of good health tend to rise if we become more affluent.

Having said this the influence of broad cultural and social factors should not be exaggerated. There is more variation within social and cultural groups than between them. Tuckett (1976) states: '... it is unlikely that socio-cultural factors of the broad demographic type will be found to play a major role in determining who does, and does not, seek medical aid'. Although broad demographic indices give us some information regarding who will become patients and how they will behave in that role, it is important that physiotherapists and other health professionals do not form rigid stereotypes of social, cultural and ethnic groups from which to interpret their behaviour.

Differences in patient referral, diagnosis and treatment may in part be due to the biases and stereotyped behaviour of medical staff. Jeffery (1984) found that even in accident and emergency departments staff varied the treatment according to their moral evaluations of patients. For example patients perceived to be alcoholic did not receive the same quality of treatment as those judged to be sober. Treatment may also differ according to the gender and race of the patient. Health professionals have often been accused of sexist and racist attitudes and behaviour (Roberts, 1985; Pilgrim and Rogers, 1993; Doyal, 1995; Gillespie, 1995b). Macintyre and Oldman (1984), for example, believe that women who suffer from migraine tend to be viewed as neurotic, whereas male sufferers are usually thought to be under severe occupational stress. Similarly the problems experienced by people from ethnic minorities with sickle cell anaemia tend to be under-estimated and misunderstood (Louison and Dyer, 1993).

Factors within the individual's life may trigger entry to the patient role (Scambler, 1991; Armstrong, 1994). The person may become a patient when the symptoms begin to interfere with work or social activities, or when an important aspect of support, such as the help provided by a neighbour, is lost. Tuckett (1976) states that: '... considerable accommodation may develop between individuals, their symptoms and the pattern of relationships and activities they are involved in'. Thus the individual's social network may accommodate symptoms to the extent that the person experiencing them does not need or desire to become a patient. Conversely a change in the person's social network can precipitate entry to the patient role, even if there is no deterioration of symptoms. Stewart *et al.* (1995) argue that being sick is a social state of affairs which cannot be understood in terms of the biochemical malfunction of organs.

Traditionally physiotherapy education and practice has followed the 'medical model' of disease which views it in terms of signs, symptoms and pathology. This is now recognized as constituting a very narrow perspective, ignoring or minimizing social and psychological factors. By taking a broader view of health, illness and impairment the physiotherapist is likely to be more effective in his or her role and have a more satisfactory relationship with patients, as their concerns will be acknowledged, taken seriously and acted upon.

The 'lay referral system'

When deciding whether or not to seek medical help the person with the symptom will frequently consult others, usually family members and friends, who will help him or her to decide what course of action, if any, to take. This network has been referred to by Freidson (1970) as 'the lay referral system'. Friends and relatives may persuade the person to see the doctor or even insist upon it. Scambler (1989) found that, in the case of people with epilepsy, four out of five first medical consultations were organized by someone else. On the other hand, relatives and friends may discourage the person from seeking medical help or suggest self-medication or the services of 'alternative' practitioners. People may be greatly inconvenienced if a relative becomes a patient and may be strongly motivated to stop him or her from doing so. The 'lay referral system' also operates after receiving professional advice; the patient will consult lay advisers on the wisdom of taking drugs, doing the exercises or modifying life style. This, together with his or her own evaluation, can lead to low levels of compliance.

Weighing up the costs and benefits

When deciding whether or not to become a patient the costs and the benefits are assessed. The person with the symptom may be too busy to become a patient, may have just started a new job and be eager to create a good impression, may live too far away from the medical facilities, have young children to care for or be reluctant to lose money by staying away from work. Commonly, people who are in most need of medical help are the ones least able to receive it. Tudor Hart (1971) has referred to this situation as the 'inverse care law'. Disease and impairment are concentrated among the poorest members of the society, yet these are the very people who find it most difficult to become patients. The lack of a car can make access to the medical facilities tedious or impossible, employers may be less sympathetic than those of professional workers and poor people are more likely to be single parents and less able than others to afford help. In addition deprived neighbourhoods usually have the worst health facilities (See chapter 2). In such circumstances good health may not be the person's main goal in life, a fact which Scambler (1991) believes should not be viewed as irrational.

The 'inverse care law' has important implications for physiotherapists. It is all too easy to blame people when they do not attend for treatment or fail to carry out advice. However, their behaviour is often quite rational when a broader perspective of their situation is taken. It is important that the physiotherapy service is run flexibly so that people who may benefit from it can use it with ease and convenience.

The 'inverse care law' may operate during interaction with the doctor or other health professionals. Research concerning doctor/patient interaction has shown that working class people tend to find communication difficult because they do not share the same culture, vocabulary or experience of life as the doctor. The doctor, in turn, may have various erroneous beliefs about working class people regarding their intelligence and ability to understand medical information (Gillespie, 1995b). Fitzpatrick and Scambler (1984) state: 'Middle-class patients are more likely to be confident in meeting middle-class doctors and hence more likely to be successful in achieving their objectives from the consultation'.

It has been found that doctors spend considerably longer in consultation with patients in social classes one and two (the professional classes) than with those in social classes four and five. They are more likely to refer professional people to a specialist and provide them with more information and explanation (Blaxter, 1983). In addition, the way in which people in social classes one and two view health, illness and impairment tends to tally closely with those of health professionals making communication easier and the consultation a more satisfactory experience for all concerned.

There has been no work on this theme concerning physiotherapists but it is likely that similar social dynamics operate. It is easier to communicate with people we judge to be similar to ourselves and good communication gives rise to a more satisfactory consultation. The people we find most difficult to communicate with are often the ones in most need of help so it is important that physiotherapists take extra care when communicating with these patients in order to enhance their practice and understand the patient's illness or impairment from his or her perspective.

Psychological distress

Sometimes people become patients not primarily because of the presence of a physical symptom but because of psychological distress (Scambler, 1991; Armstrong, 1994). This is not to imply, of course, that the physical symptoms do not exist. Zola (1973) found that people with physical illness often consult a doctor following a stressful event like a row. This situation is complicated by the fact that both depression and anxiety tend to heighten the perception of symptoms such as pain and the increased intensity of symptoms can, in turn, heighten anxiety and depression, thus creating a vicious circle (see Chapter 10). Stress may also be an aetiological factor in conditions such as stomach ulcer, asthma and coronary heart disease, and clinical depression often gives rise to numerous physical symptoms which cannot be explained physiologically (Rose, 1995).

A stressful event can break down the patient's own accommodation and the accommodation of his or her family and friends to the symptoms. This breakdown in the containment of the symptoms, may lead to the person becoming a patient even at a time when the illness or impairment is not particularly severe. The health professional often seems the most appropriate person to consult with emotional and social problems. This is culturally determined, many of the problems now taken to health professionals were, in the past, taken to the priest or dealt with within the family. Loneliness may motivate people to become patients, particularly perhaps for those who find communication in an informal, social setting difficult and demanding. Anxiety can give rise to either extreme help-seeking behaviour or alternatively to denial.

Medical professionals, including physiotherapists, can mediate symptoms by relieving depression and anxiety, though how far they are prepared to do so depends in part on the perception they have of their role and their definitions of illness and impairment. It is important for physiotherapists to realize how effective they can be in this regard. For example by allowing someone to attend physiotherapy primarily for 'social reasons', depression may be lifted to the extent that pain or other symptoms are reduced. Distinguishing stress and psychophysiological illness from malingering is fraught with problems, however, and health professionals sometimes feel they are being manipulated by patients (Asher, 1995).

Secondary gain

The role of patient may be one which is desired by the person. There are important secondary gains attached to being a patient in terms of increased sympathy and care from others and exemption from customary roles such as work. People sometimes occupy the patient role in order to escape failure, evade a difficult situation, avoid a stigmatizing label such as 'lonely', 'inadequate' or 'criminal' or simply to get a bed for the night. Williams (1989) believes that behaviours which bring about reward will be repeated and that in this way illness behaviour is learned, and Peck (1982) points out that symptoms such as pain may enable the person to avoid other problems. She states:

> 'One problem may work to help a person escape or avoid having to confront one or more other problems ... The first problem serves a useful function in allowing the other to be avoided. This is not to say that pain is created for the purpose of getting the patient out of something. Rather it is simply that when pain and other problems exist side-by-side, the pain may eventually come to serve such a function'.

Some people view their illness and impairment in terms of gain rather than loss, as a challenge and an opportunity for personal growth. It is not unusual for those who become ill or disabled to find the experience a positive one, at least in part (Morris, 1989; Morris, 1991; Magee and Milligan, 1995). It may force them to view life from a different and more satisfying perspective, to escape the 'rat race', change direction or meet new and interesting people. Alternatively people may believe their illness or impairment to be a punishment for misdeeds in this life or a past one, while others may view it as a sign of personal weakness and failure. Such views frequently coexist and may change over time (Rieser, 1995). Thus illness and impairment are viewed in diverse ways both by people experiencing it and the society in which they are placed. Such beliefs have a large effect on the ways in which people respond to illness and impairment.

The patient role is itself stigmatized and rather than seeking it many people will avoid it at all costs, particularly with such conditions as epilepsy and mental illness which are not well accepted by society and may cause enormous disadvantage in terms of relationships and employment prospects. Other people positively dislike being dependent, being physically handled, being in close proximity to others and being outside the mainstream of life, and for these and other reasons will avoid the patient role.

The person's role as patient may be desired by another family member. It is sometimes the case that relationships work best if one person is in a dependent position (Hanson and Gerber, 1990). This situation may suit both partners or may give rise to conflict. The relationship may always have functioned in that way or, if a family member has been ill or disabled for some time, life may become organized around that situation and behaviour and attitudes may be difficult to change if the person becomes well. Rogler and Hollinghead (1965) studied families in Puerto Rico where one family member had schizophrenia. They found that schizophrenia among the males was valued by their wives as it gave them more freedom than they had in their traditional role. Similarly a woman interviewed by Swain and Thirlaway (1994) admits to being dependent on her son with learning difficulties. She states:

> 'Actually, I needed Martin more to be honest. I only realised it later. I could see that I needed Martin more than he needed me. And if you are honest about it, you do as you get older'.

A family member may be motivated to keep a relative in a hospitalized patient role if he or she is threatened with having to take on the responsibility of caring. On the other hand, the relative may hinder the person's attempts at independence if he or she wants the caring role to continue. Keeping someone in the patient role or preventing him or her from entering it, is usually entirely rational behaviour which can be readily understood.

The sick role can be used in families as a powerful tool to manipulate others and may legitimate behaviour which would not otherwise be acceptable. For example a child with asthma may have attacks of breathlessness in order to avoid school or helping with domestic chores, a woman may refuse all offers of help from the social services because she wants her daughter to be with her all the time, and a person in pain may create feelings of guilt in other family members in order to get his or her own way. This type of manipulation is not necessarily premeditated and is frequently under-pinned by considerable stress and anxiety.

It is important that physiotherapists understand the gains and losses patients and their relatives experience when they become ill, how successful relationships may be destroyed if the patient role is disturbed and how severe pressure can be put on family members when someone leaves hospital. Dalley (1988) goes so far as to suggest that when one group of people is liberated, for example disabled people from long-term care, another group of people is oppressed, usually women in 'the community'. (For further discussion of community care the reader is referred to Chapter 3.)

Past experience of medical services

A person's past experience of being a patient is an important factor when considering whether to assume the role again. The person who experiences no improvement or only minimal improvement from a past course of treatment is less likely to return, as is the patient who found his or her treatment painful. The relationship with the health professional is very important, it has been found that people are more ready to return to some doctors than others, findings which cannot be explained by factors such as age or social class (Tuckett, 1976). Zola (1973) found that people tend to discontinue treatment if the doctor fails to take account of the reasons why they came. There is a large literature on the problematic nature of communication between patients and health professionals (Elder and Samual, 1987; Scambler, 1991; Stewart *et al.*, 1995). Scambler (1991) believes that the rapid growth of self-help groups in the last decade, serves in part to compensate for poor relationships with professionals. Thus the relationship the physiotherapist has with his or her patients is likely to influence their behaviour during future episodes of illness. (For further discussion of patient/therapist communication the reader is referred to Chapter 17.)

Legitimating illness

Frequently people go to the doctor with the sole aim of having illness legitimated, in this situation the contact is largely administrative. The role and power of the doctor is widespread and sometimes motives for making contact are not directly associated with an impairment or illness, but rather such visits are part of a procedure which people are obliged to go through. For example, it may be necessary to make contact with a doctor in order to be put on a waiting list for a ground floor flat, obtain the Disabled Living Allowance, claim compensation or be proclaimed fit for a new job. Even if the patient does have symptoms, for example a sore throat and raised temperature, he or she may not expect the doctor to prescribe any medications, the purpose of the visit being simply to have the illness legitimated in order to stay away from work for a while.

Professionals' definitions of illness and impairment

Whether someone is permitted to become a patient will depend in part on the professionals' definitions of illness and impairment, how they define their particular clients, how they define their own role and the resources available to them. Thus someone of over 65 years of age may be denied access to a rehabilitation centre, someone with a persistent chronic illness may be deemed unsuitable for physiotherapy and someone whose symptoms are thought to result from stress and depression may be considered an inappropriate candidate for physical treatment.

Such criteria change over time and according to circumstances. Although professional rhetoric is almost always in terms of patient care, all organizations, including the professionals, are in the business of self-survival and are often eager to expand (Hugman, 1991). Thus if patients are in short supply people not previously permitted entry may be encouraged to become patients and if, on the other hand, patients become very plentiful or staffing levels depleted, then people who had once been allowed to take on the role of patient may be denied it. If one source of work ceases to exist or is reduced, for example acute illness, then professionals will tend to extend their services to other groups, for example mentally ill people and those with learning difficulties. Not everyone views such 'medicalization' as helpful or appropriate (see Illich, 1976) and physiotherapists should be clear as to why their services have developed in various directions, what they are trying to achieve and whether they are the most appropriate people to intervene.

Specific functions of the sick role

The sick role may have functions specific to particular individuals and institutions. For example, prisoners may use it in order to meet people from whom they are isolated or to bring a little variety into a life full of tedium. They may hoard any drugs they receive and use them as currency. Children may use the sick role in order to avoid meeting a bully at school and adults may use it to have a day off from work, perhaps just for a rest or to make time for domestic tasks which have built up or become urgent.

Entering the sick role for reasons such as these often reflects underlying psychological and social stress. Physical illness is less stigmatizing and more readily accepted than many other states, for example depression and anxiety. Although the person may be taking the day off from work because of the illness of a friend, the behaviour of a child, the death of a family pet or the failure of an examination, this will not be revealed or if it is may be met with scorn or ridicule. Although the excuse of physical illness is not always believed, it tends to be accepted as it creates less disruption to organizational routines than complaints about stress or work practices.

McKinlay (1972) listed six approaches to the utilization of health care which summarize much of what has been said:

1. Economic – the availability of medical care and whether or not people have the resources to use it depends in part on economic considerations.
2. Sociodemographic – gender, class, race, social networks, etc. all influence how people feel and behave when ill.
3. Geographic – proximity to the medical facilities is an important factor when considering whether or not to become a patient.
4. Sociocultural – values, beliefs, norms, and life styles are important factors which determine whether someone will become a patient and how he or she will behave when ill.
5. Sociopsychological – perception of symptoms, motivation, personality, social situation, knowledge and the ability to learn, will all influence a person's response to illness and impairment.
6. Organizational – the way in which health facilities are organized, for example how convenient they are and how humane the organizational practices are, will influence the degree to which people make use of them.

It is clear that our perception of symptoms and how we behave towards them are highly subjective and based on many factors including personality, past experience, our situation at the time and the influence of family and friends. Individuals differ greatly one from another in their response to illness and impairment as does the same person at different times according to circumstances. Orthodox medicine too, including physiotherapy, is far less objective than people commonly believe with very different courses of action being suggested by equally well qualified and committed health professionals. Bond and Bond (1986) state:

> '... if health care professionals are to understand their patients – why they discontinue breast feeding within a few weeks, fail to bring children for immunization, wish to discharge themselves from hospital or do not prac- tise their exercises – it is necessary to find out the patient's version of events rather than impose their own views'.

Patient compliance and non-compliance

Much of what has been discussed so far in this chapter concerns compli- ance and non-compliance of patients to medical advice. Compliance can be defined as 'Disposition to yield to others' (McLeod, 1986), 'Action in accordance with request or demand' (McIntosh, 1964) and 'A type of conformity' (Evans, 1978). There has been an increasing interest in the topic of compliance over the years. Ley (1988) notes that in the 1950s there were only 25 publications on compliance in the whole of the medical literature in Britain but that this had risen to 810 by the 1970s. There is now a whole journal devoted to the topic of compliance, *Journal of Compliance in Health Care*.

The term 'compliance' has been criticized for having authoritarian overtones (Ley, 1988; Pitts, 1991). It implies that people should go along with the wishes of others whether they agree or not. Compliance denotes passivity which physiotherapists rarely require of their patients and clients. Other words such as 'adherence' and 'partnership' are now being used. Pitts (1991) states:

> 'Compliance tends to carry the connotation of a passive adherence on the part of the patient to the doctor's wishes and other rather more positive terms such as co-operation and collaboration are perhaps to be preferred since they imply a more active relationship on both sides'.

The extent of compliance

Studies vary markedly in their findings but typically compliance is low with only approximately 50% of patients and clients complying with medical advice (Weinman, 1981; Ley, 1988; Mathews and Steptoe, 1988; May, 1991; Ley and Llewelyn, 1995). O'Carroll and Hendriks (1989) found that only five out of 14 patients with rheumatoid arthritis wore their wrist splints and that compliance with home exercise was also low. Compliance is low even with serious diseases like diabetes and heart disease (Ice, 1985; Pitts, 1991). Diagnosis and severity of disease are not good indicators of compliance (Mathews and Steptoe, 1988).

The degree of compliance found in studies depends, in part, on how it is measured. Self-report is the easiest and most commonly used measure but it tends to over-estimate compliance when compared with other measures such as pill counts and physiological measurements such as urine and blood analysis (Mathews and Steptoe, 1988; Belanger and Noel, 1991; Pitts, 1991). Ways of defining compliance also vary. If a patient is defined as compliant when he or she adheres to the treatment regimen

75% of the time then compliant behaviour will be greater than when it is defined more stringently (Ley and Llewelyn, 1995).

It should be appreciated, however, that non-compliance is perfectly normal behaviour among human beings and does not apply to medical advice alone (Thompson, 1984). We tend not to do what other people tell us to do; indeed a totally compliant person would probably seem very strange. Ley (1988) has documented that health professionals do not comply to recommended procedures when administering medical interventions within their professional role. Hyland and Donaldson (1989) state:

> 'One should certainly question whether it is beneficial for patients to behave in a way in which they relinquish all sense of self-determination in health care to "the experts" … a tendency not to comply with instructions unless convinced may be psychologically healthy'.

Factors contributing to compliance and non-compliance to health advice

Features of the patient

O'Carroll and Hendriks (1989) highlight the following four categories of variables relating to compliance to medical advice:

Patients who do not comply are often blamed and viewed as deviant. This is, however, to individualize the problem. Research which has attempted to find links between personality charactristics and non-compliant behaviour have been largely unsuccessful (Pitts, 1991), and no consistent association has been found between compliance and age, compliance and socioeconomic class and compliance and psychiatric illness. There are many good reasons why patients and clients do or do not follow medical advice. Shillitoe (1995) states:

> 'The abandonment of terms such as "compliance", which also carries overtones of "doctor's orders" and which sees non-compliance in terms of some deficit in the patient, is long overdue'.

Compliant behaviour tends to reduce with the time the patient has had the illness or impairment. It also reduces if the benefits of carrying out the advice are not immediately obvious to the patient, or if the advice is given in order to prevent ill health rather than deal with an existing problem (Ashworth and Hagan, 1993). The patient's views of his or her illness or impairment, as well as the treatment suggested, will influence the level of compliance. If there is a large discrepancy between the patient's and the therapist's views and beliefs then compliance is likely to be low. Overcoming the health problem may not be of central importance to the person or may not be high on his or her list of priorities. The more behavioural change that is expected of the patient, the less he or she is likely to comply. This can be a problem with diseases such as diabetes and heart disease where the degree of behavioural change demanded is quite large. In addition people are less likely to comply with advice if they are depressed or anxious or if the information they receive has a high fear content.

Some patients may value a particular activity so much that they are psychologically unable to comply with advice to refrain from engaging in it. This is not an uncommon situation with sportsmen and women (see

Chapter 11). Satterfield *et al.* (1990) suggest that in cases such as these an alternative programme of activity should be instigated.

Features of the illness

Although there is no close association between the severity of the symptoms and compliance to medical advice, patients are more likely to comply when the symptoms are acute. Compliance will, however, tend to decrease if pain or discomfort are increased by carrying out the advice. O'Carroll and Hendriks (1988) found that patients with rheumatoid arthritis were less inclined to wear wrist splints if they were awkward or uncomfortable.

Features of the treatment programme

Good communication by the health professional has been consistently found to improve patient satisfaction and compliance to medical advice (Weinman, 1981; Thompson, 1984; Ley, 1988; Mathews and Steptoe, 1988; Hyland and Donaldson, 1989; Terpstra *et al.*, 1992; Niven, 1994; Walker, 1995). As well as providing a friendly, empathic atmosphere the quality of the professional's communication when giving instructions and information will affect how much the patient can understand and recall; it is helpful to back up verbal with written instructions and to ensure that information provided is clear and accessible to the patient.

The therapist must also become attuned to the patient's values and beliefs. Mathews and Steptoe (1988) state:

'... if doctor–patient contact satisfies the patient's psychological and social needs, then otherwise poor rates of patient adherence will be significantly improved. A good doctor–patient relationship is therefore not just desirable, it is essential for the effective practice of medicine'.

Compliance to medical advice is also affected by the quality of the service given (Weinman, 1981; Thompson, 1984; O'Carroll and Hendriks, 1989; Niven, 1994). Patients are more likely to comply if they see the same health professional on each occasion, if they are seen on time and if the service is convenient. Patients are also more likely to comply if they are given a simple, rather than a complicated, regimen of treatment and if their progress is monitored (Mathews and Steptoe, 1988; Niven, 1994).

Social and environmental background

There are numerous factors in the patient's social environment which may reduce or increase compliance. Compliance has been found to increase if the patient has a supportive social network of family and friends (Mathews and Steptoe, 1988; Ley and Llewelyn, 1995). Vasey (1990) and Brookes (1992) found that patients failed to attend physiotherapy for a range of social and environmental reasons including work commitments, family pressures and problems with transport. As noted above constraints such as these are more likely to affect poor people.

Models of professional–patient relationships

Parsons (1951) was the first sociologist to elaborate the concept of the 'sick role'. Role is a sociological concept not a medical concept. All our roles contain certain rights and obligations. The student, for example, has the right to receive a good standard of education but is obliged to hand in

Parsons' (1951) consensus model of the doctor–patient relationship

essays on time and prepare for examinations; the employee has the right to work in a safe environment but is obliged to be punctual and to follow the instructions of supervisors. Most people occupy multiple roles; for example mother, employee, neighbour, daughter and friend. The person defined as ill occupies the 'sick role' and the person who becomes a patient occupies the 'patient role'. Bond and Bond (1986) state: 'The behaviour of the sick person and the behaviour of others around him must conform to the particular pattern of expectations that surround the sick role'. Parsons believed the 'sick role' to contain two major rights and two major obligations:

Right one
The sick person is not responsible for his illness.

Right two
The sick person is relieved of normal social responsibilities.

Obligation one
The sick person must view his condition as undesirable.

Obligation two
The sick person must seek and cooperate with competent medical help.

Parsons thought that the second right, to be relieved of normal social responsibilities, was potentially desirable and that as this threatens social order, entry to the sick role must be controlled. The sick role legitimates illness, and behaviour viewed as deviant under some circumstances, but it also regulates it so that social obligations are not evaded unnecessarily. Hart (1985) explains:

> 'If outbreaks of sickness were left to the whims of individuals in the private sphere of domestic life they might gradually erode people's sense of duty to work, to family life, to community. Only by bringing sickness into the public sphere and encasing it in a system of social control would the risks of role evasion be kept to a minimum'.

The official control of illness behaviour is medical certification. Parsons (1951) saw medicine as serving a social control function aimed at stabilizing society. People who occupy the sick role, yet appear to enjoy it and fail to seek medical help are not keeping to their side of the bargain and are likely to meet with great disapproval from friends, family, employers and health professionals.

Criticisms of Parsons' model

Parsons' model does not account for the fact that most illnesses never reach the doctor, thus it fails to distinguish between the 'sick role' and the 'patient role'. It does not take social and psychological factors into consideration, but concentrates instead on physical signs and symptoms. It is not concerned with the individual's experience of illness or impairment. A person's entry or withdrawal from the sick role is probably influenced more by friends, relatives and employers than medical professionals.

Medicine is so uncertain that doctors tend not to bar entry to the patient role very often for fear of making a mistake; although it is dangerous to label someone ill when he or she is well, most doctors feel it is worse to label a person well when he or she is ill, thus medical certification is not difficult to achieve.

The model assumes an ideal patient, one who brings along appropriate symptoms and is perfectly compliant. Yet Ley (1988) points out that the professional–patient relationship is more often characterized by negotiation, conflict and non-compliance. There is no recognition in Parsons' model that the interests of the patient and the doctor may not be in accord.

The model fits acute illness best, people with chronic conditions or psychiatric illnesses, may not be allowed to terminate their usual social duties or may never be able to resume them. Sutherland (1981) and French (1994), talking of disabled people, believe that they are expected to 'adjust' to their limitations, 'overcome' their difficulties and be as 'normal' as possible. Other conditions of medical concern, such as pregnancy and child development, do not fit this model either.

Times have changed since Parsons formulated his model of the sick role. People are better educated, doctors are more likely to work in teams with other health professionals and consumer organizations, self-help groups and alternative medicine have developed. This has changed the nature of the professional–patient relationship to some extent making medical professionals, including physiotherapists, less authoritarian. Medicine is now characterized by chronic rather than acute disease which means that the sick role concept, as formulated by Parsons, is less relevant. The patient with a chronic condition may become an expert in his or her own right by virtue of living with the condition for so long. This, together with the lack of a cure, tends to erode the professional's status and authority. Parsons' sick role concept relates to a particular society at a particular time, ignoring broader cultural, temporal and social factors.

Szasz and Hollander's (1956) typology of doctor–patient relationships

Szasz and Hollander (1956) believe there are several types of doctor–patient relationships:

1. Activity–passivity. In this type of relationship the doctor is active and the patient is passive. This would exist if the patient were in a coma or very seriously ill.
2. Guidance–cooperation. In this situation the doctor advises and the patient is willingly compliant. It is most commonly seen when the patient has an acute disease of short duration.
3. Mutual participation. This relationship is characterized by partnership. It is most commonly seen when the patient has a long-term, chronic illness or impairment.

The Parsonian model fits the 'guidance–cooperation' relationship most closely. In recent years there has been a shift from this type of relationship to that of mutual participation.

Stewart and Roter's (1989) model of conflict and control

Stewart and Roter highlight four types of doctor–patient relationships based upon the amount of control given to the patient and the doctor. When the professional has high control and the patient has low control a paternalistic relationship results similar to that described by Parsons. When the patient has high control and the professional has low control a consumerist relationship results. This type of relationship is present in private medicine and is increasing in the National Health Service with its more 'market-orientated' philosophy. When the professional and the patient both enjoy high control a relationship of mutuality results where both parties are involved in decision-making. With the default relationship neither the patient nor the professional are taking control, this situation may arise when the professional wants the patient to take control but the patient is unwilling to do so or vice versa.

There is no such thing as an 'ideal' professional–patient relationship though the qualities of empathy, competence and trust are probably always necessary. The type of relationship will depend on numerous factors relating to the illness or impairment, the patient, the professional and the situation in which they interact.

Conclusion

Physiotherapy education and practice have traditionally focused on an understanding of disease and the interpretation of signs and symptoms. Such an understanding is vitally important to the physiotherapist but becoming a patient or, conversely, failing to do so is influenced by a multitude of other factors. By understanding these factors the physiotherapist will be in a position to help and influence people both to become patients, when that seems beneficial to their health, and to leave the patient role when health and fitness are maximized.

References

Armstrong D. (1994) *Outline of Sociology as Applied to Medicine* (4th edn). Oxford: Butterworth-Heinemann.

Asher R. (1995) Malingering. In *Health and Disease: A Reader* (2nd edn) (Davey B., Gray A., Seale C., eds). Buckingham: Open University Press.

Ashworth P. D., Hagan M. T. (1993) Some social consequences of non-compliance with pelvic floor exercises. *Physiotherapy*, **79**(7), 456–471.

Belanger A. Y., Noel G. (1991) Compliance to and effects of a home strengthening exercise program for adult dystrophic patients: a pilot study. *Physiotherapy Canada*, **43**(1), 24–30.

Blaxter M. (1983) Health services as a defence against the consequences of poverty in industrialised societies. *Social Science and Medicine*, **17**, 1139–1148.

Bond J., Bond S. (1986) *Sociology and Health Care*. London: Churchill Livingstone.

Brookes C. (1992) Loss of treatment time due to non-attendance for physiotherapy out-patient appointments in a district general hospital. *Physiotherapy*, **78**(5), 249–252.

Cartwright (1967) *Patients and Their Doctors*. London: Routledge and Kegan Paul.

Dalley G. (1988) *Ideologies of Caring*. London: Macmillan.

Doyal L. (1995) *What Makes Women Sick: Gender and the Political Economy of Health*. London: Macmillan.

Dunnell K., Cartwright A. (1972) *Medicine-takers, Prescribers and Hoarders*. London: Routledge and Kegan Paul.

Elder A., Samual O. (1987) *While I'm Here Doctor: A Study of The Patient–Doctor Relationship*. London: Tavistock Publications.

Evans C. (1978) *Psychology: A Dictionary of the Mind, Brain and Behaviour*. London: Arrow Books.

Fitzpatrick R., Scambler G. (1984) Social class, ethnicity and illness. In *The Experience of Illness* (Fitzpatrick R., Hinton J., Newman S., Scambler G., Thompson J., eds). London: Tavistock Publications.

Freidson E. (1970) *The Profession of Medicine.* New York: Dodd, Mead and Co.

French S. (1994) The disabled role. In *On Equal Terms: Working with Disabled People* (French S., ed.). Oxford: Butterworth-Heinemann.

Gillespie R. (1995a) Health behaviour and the individual. In *Society and Health: An Introduction to Social Science for Health Professionals* (Moon G., Gillespie R., eds). London: Routledge.

Gillespie R. (1995b) The lay–professional encounter. In *Society and Health: An Introduction to Social Science for Health Professionals.* London: Routledge.

Hannay D. (1980) The 'iceberg' of illness and 'trivial' consultations. *Journal of the Royal College of General Practitioners,* **30**, 551–554.

Hanson R. W., Gerber K. E. (1990) *Coping with Chronic Pain.* London: Guildford Press.

Hart N. (1985) *The Sociology of Health and Medicine.* London: Causeway Books.

Helman C. G. (1994) *Culture, Health and Illness* (3rd edn). Oxford: Butterworth-Heinemann.

Hugman R. (1991) *Power in Caring Professionals.* London: Macmillan.

Hyland M. E., Donaldson M. L. (1989) *Psychological Care in Nursing Practice.* London; Scutari Press.

Ice R. (1985) Long term compliance. *Physical Therapy,* **65**(12), 1832–1839.

Illich I. (1976) *Limits to Medicine.* Harmondsworth: Penguin Books.

Jacobson B., Smith A., Whitehead M. (1991) *The Nation's Health: A Strategy for the 1990s.* London: King Edward's Hospital Fund for London.

Jeffrey R. (1984) Normal rubbish: deviant patients in casualty departments. In *Health and Disease: A Reader* (Black N., Boswell D., Gray A., Murphy S., Popay J., eds). Milton Keynes: Open University Press.

Last J. (1963) The iceberg: completing the picture in general practice. *Lancet,* **ii**, 28–31.

Ley P. (1988) *Communicating with Patients.* London: Croom Helm.

Ley P., Llewelyn S. (1995) Improving patients' understanding, recall, satisfaction and compliance. In *Health Psychology: Processes and Applications* (Broome A., Llewelyn S., eds). London: Chapman and Hall.

Louison E., Dyer P. (1993) Meeting the needs of people with sickle cell disease. In *Reflections: views of black disabled people on their lives and community care* (Begum N., Hill M., Stevens A., eds). London: Central Council for Education and Training in Social Work.

McIntosh E. (1964) *The Concise Oxford Dictionary* (5th edn). Oxford: Oxford University Press.

Macintyre S., Oldham D. (1984) Coping with migraine. In *Health and Disease: A Reader* (2nd edn) (Davey B., Gray A., Seale C., eds). Buckingham: Open University Press.

McKinlay J. (1972) Some approaches and problems in the study of the use of services: an overview. *Journal of Health and Social Behaviour,* **13**, 115–152.

McLeod W. T. (1986) *The Collins Paperback English Dictionary.* London: Collins.

Magee B., Milligan M. (1995) *On Blindness.* Buckingham: Open University Press.

Mathews A., Steptoe A. (1988) *Essential Psychology for Medical Practice.* Edinburgh: Churchill Livingstone.

May B. (1991) Diabetes. In *The Psychology of Health: An Introduction* (Pitts M., Phillips K., eds). London: Routledge.

Mechanic D., Volkart E. H. (1961) Stress, illness behaviour and the sick role. *American Sociological Review,* **5**, 51–58.

Morris J. (1989) *Able Lives: Women's Experience of Paralysis.* London: The Women's Press.

Morris J. (1991) *Pride Against Prejudice.* London: The Women's Press.

Niven N. (1994) *Health Psychology: An Introduction for Nurses and Other Health Care Professionals.* Edinburgh: Churchill Livingstone.

O'Carroll M., Henriks O. (1989) Factors associated with rheumatoid arthritis patients' compliance with home exercises and splint use. *Physiotherapy Practice*, **5**, 115–122.

Parsons T. (1951) *The Social System*. London: Routledge and Kegan Paul.

Peck C. (1982) *Controlling Chronic Pain*. London: Fontana.

Pilgrim D., Rogers A. (1993) *A Sociology of Mental Health and Illness*. Buckingham: The Open University Press.

Pitts M. (1991) The medical consultation. In *The Psychology of Health: An Introduction* (Pitts M., Phillips K., eds). London: Routledge.

Rieser R. (1995) The history of disabling imagery. In *Invisible Children: Report of the Joint Conference on Children, Images and Disability* (Rieser R., ed.). London: Save the Children and the Integration Alliance.

Roberts H. (1985) *Patient Patients; Women and Their Doctors*. London: Pandora Press.

Rogler L., Hollinghead A. (1965) *Trapped Families and Schizophrenia*. New York: John Wiley.

Rose N. (1995) Psychiatric illness. In *Physiotherapy in Mental Health: A Practical Approach* (Everett T., Dennis M., Ricketts D., eds). Oxford: Butterworth-Heinemann.

Satterfield M. J., Dowden D., Yasumura K. (1990) Patient compliance for successful stress fracture rehabilitation. *Journal of Orthopaedic Sports Physical Therapy*, **11**(7), 321–325.

Scambler G. (1989) *Epilepsy*. London: Routledge.

Scambler G. (1991) Health and illness behaviour. In *Sociology as Applied to Medicine* (3rd edn) (Scambler G., ed.). London: Baillière Tindall.

Shillitoe R. (1995) Diabetes mellitus. In *Health Psychology: Processes and Applications* (Broome A., Llewelyn S., eds). London: Chapman and Hall.

Stewart M., Brown J. B., Weston W. W. *et al.* (1995) *Patient-centred Medicine: Transforming the Clinical Method*. London: Sage.

Stewart R., Roter D. (1989) *Communicating with Medical Patients*. New York: Sage.

Sutherland A. T. (1981) *Disabled We Stand*. London: Souvenir Press.

Swain J., Thirlaway C. (1994) Families in transition. In *On Equal Terms: Working with Disabled People* (French S., ed.). Oxford: Butterworth-Heinemann.

Szasz T. S., Hollander M. H. (1956) A contribution to the philosophy of medicine: the basic models of the doctor–patient relationship. *American Medical Association Archives of Internal Medicine*, **97**, 585–592.

Terpstra S. J., de Witte P. L., Diederiks J. P. M. (1992) Compliance of patients with an exercise program for rheumatoid arthritis. *Physiotherapy Canada*. **44**(2), 37–41.

Thompson J. (1984) Compliance. In *The Experience of Illness* (Fitzpatrick R., Hinton J., Newman S., Scambler G., Thompson J., eds). London; Tavistock Publications.

Tuckett D. (1976) Becoming a patient. In *An Introduction to Medical Sociology* (Tuckett D., ed.). London: Tavistock Publications.

Tudor Hart J. (1971) The inverse care law. *Lancet*, **i**, 405–412.

Vasey L. A. (1990) DNAs and DNCTs – why do patients fail to begin or to complete a course of physiotherapy treatment. *Physiotherapy*, **76**(9), 575–578.

Wadsworth M., Butterfield M., Harvey R. (1971) *Health and Sickness: The Choice of Treatment*. London: Tavistock Publications.

Walker A. (1995) Patient compliance and the placebo effect. *Physiotherapy*, **81**(3), 120–126.

Weinman J. (1981) *An Outline of Psychology as Applied to Medicine*. Bristol: John Wright.

Williams J. (1989) Illness behaviour to wellness behaviour. *Physiotherapy*, **75**(1), 2–7.

Zola L. (1973) Pathways to the doctor: from person to patient. *Social Science and Medicine*, **7**, 677–689.

9

Stilt Stress
Stephanie Kitchener

Every one of us experiences stress; indeed a certain level of stress is vital if we are to meet day-to-day challenges and cope with life's minor crises. Stress represents an inbuilt homeostatic mechanism enabling us to adapt to our environment, it is necessary to generate motivation and promote development and growth. However, as Wolf and Goodell (1968) point out: 'Sometimes threat evokes reactions of long duration and even of greater magnitude than the threat itself. The resulting protective adaptive reaction when sustained may be more damaging to the individual than the effect of the noxious agent *per se*'. Thus, although the experience and manifestations of stress are perfectly natural and healthy, prolonged or abnormal levels of stress can lead to long-term physical and psychological problems.

The last 40 years or so have seen the publication of an enormous amount of research which has attempted to outline: factors which give rise to stress; physiological, psychological and behavioural responses to stress; coping strategies; and the detrimental effect of sustained stress. Such research has produced a wealth of evidence to suggest causal links between illness, hospitalization and stress. As physiotherapists working with sick people, often within the hospital environment, it is important that we have an understanding of how these links occur, for it has been shown that stress not only interferes with the formation of a good patient–therapist relationship but also hinders effective treatment and rehabilitation following illness and surgery.

Stress and illness

During the course of their working lives physiotherapists will meet patients with an enormous variety of problems. These may range from relatively minor ones such as a sprained ankle, which has a predictable course and is to a large extent self-limiting, to conditions such as multiple sclerosis, spinal cord injury and cancer, where the course may be less certain and long-term disability or death is the final outcome. Physiotherapy education tends to centre around the physiological, physical and functional limitations imposed by illness, with less attention paid to social and psychological consequences of illness. Yet as Weinman (1987) states: 'Any illness occurs within the context of an individual's life and is therefore likely to have effects on psychological and social functioning. For most patients major health problems are perceived as stressful events'.

The link between illness and stress is important to consider because it has major consequences for the patient and his or her family. How the illness is perceived to a large extent determines how the individual will cope with it which in turn will affect participation in treatment and rehabilitation. It is the perception of illness which is the important factor. For example Wellisch (1981) states: 'Cancer perhaps more than any other disease present images of primordial suffering and terror which makes it a uniquely devastating entity, both psychologically and physically. It is not as though other diseases do not kill but this disease ... has long been associated with man's most unspoken and primitive fears, those of boundless suffering'. Yet when one works directly with patients who have a diagnosis of cancer an enormous range of responses are seen.

Factors which have been found to affect illness perception include: the nature of the illness itself and the demands made by it; the social context in which the illness occurs; and individual differences in personality and prior experience of illness. These factors are weighted against the individual's perceived ability to cope in determining how stressful an illness is perceived to be.

The illness itself and the demands made by the illness

The nature of problems associated with different illnesses vary enormously. A sprained ankle may be associated with pain, swelling and loss of movement. But this may have differing consequences for different people. For the office worker it may mean a short time off work, but for the professional ballet dancer it may mean missing the 'all important' opening night and have serious implications for his or her career. The stress these two individuals experience may be very different.

Dewar and Morse (1995) have detailed several problems that people suffering long-term illness find very stressful.

1. Pain particularly when unexplained, unanticipated, disbelieved or intractable.
2. Physical damage and/or altered appearance.
3. The effects of the disease or injury.
4. The effect of treatment including iagenetic problems (problems caused by the treatment itself).
5. Loss of function leading to dependency and loss of dignity.
6. Loss of control over many aspects of life.
7. Isolation.
8. Continuing reality – the unremitting nature of many long-term illnesses, fears about the future.
9. Uncertainty about the diagnosis and prognosis and lack of information.
10. Treatment by carers – being treated like an object and made to feel a burden. Insensitivity and ignorance on the part of carers including their failure to listen.
11. Treatment by others – insensitive comments, sympathy, pity.
12. Disregard from 'significant others'; being made to feel a burden.
13. 'The last straw', for example an incident caused by perceived incompetence or an unexpected setback. This may lead to loss of control by the patient leading to behaviour such as shouting, yelling, swearing, crying, lashing out, fighting and retaliating against carers.

The list is obviously not exhaustive but it does not take much imagination to realize that suffering from a chronic illness or impairment can be very stressful. Physiotherapists should recognize that their reactions and behaviour towards such patients may be a major source of stress.

It is now well recognized that the informal carers of people with long-term illnesses or impairments may suffer severe stress themselves (Nolan and Grant, 1990; 1992). It has also been found that services such as respite care which purport to give carers a break from the stresses of caring can become a source of stress in their own right. For example, Kitchener (1995), in a survey of carers from two respite centres in London, found that 43% of carers found the respite period moderately stressful to very stressful. The reasons given included concerns about the adequacy of care at the respite centre, guilt, demands by the dependent person to be taken home during the respite period, changes in the dependent person's behaviour prior to the respite admission and not having anyone the carers could talk to about emotional problems.

On a more personal note Cooney (1990) speaks openly and frankly about her life as a person with severe rheumatoid arthritis.

> 'Like most people I once plucked my eyebrows and made a cup of coffee when I felt like it, shaved my own legs. Slowly the ability to do these things has been taken from me.
>
> Allowing someone into the yuckier side of your life is hard. Even the most intimate of relationships do not contain the grossly earthy things that are par for the course in ours. I have next to no privacy, my partner knows my every nook and cranny. I am left without a millimetre's worth of mystery. Couples can be close but cutting your own toe nails provides just enough distance for you to regard yourself as separate human beings and appreciate each other as such.
>
> No it's not easy being "cared for". It's not just the messy bits. It's not being able to nick a chocolate biscuit out of the fridge or experiment with makeup or grab just the right scarf to set off your jumper as you rush out of the door. Always you have to ask.
>
> These things may seem nit-picking compared with the more obvious dramatic changes wrought by disability, but taken together they are as momentous as the arrival of the wheelchair or loss of your job. As they are given up a little bit of what outwardly makes you an individual is ended'.

The above quotation emphasizes the importance of looking at situations from the patient's point of view. It has been shown that health professionals often have very little insight into the stresses and problems associated with disability leading to further stress (French, 1994). Failure to understand the patient's point of view can lead to inappropriate goals being set in rehabilitation with frustration to all concerned.

The social context in which the illness occurs

Research has shown that there are marked national and cultural differences in perceptions of and beliefs about the nature and cause of different medical conditions (Helman, 1994). Lay people's perceptions and beliefs about illness can also differ markedly from those of health professionals. Fitzpatrick (1984) reminds us that: 'Illness beliefs shape the response to symptoms by the sufferer and his or her social network. If health care is sought the definition that the lay person brings to bear on his or her illness dictate the kind of help sought and the perception of benefits gained from the treatment'. (For information about lay beliefs about health and illness the reader is referred to Chapter 13.)

A study by White (1982) highlights cultural differences in beliefs. He asked American and Chinese students to list the causes of various problems such as headache, loneliness and loss of appetite. American students tended to cite internal emotional causes whereas Chinese students listed external pressures such as family or the demands of study. A study by Blaxter and Paterson (1982) highlights social class differences. They interviewed mothers from semi-skilled and unskilled social backgrounds in Scotland and found that health tended to be judged in functional terms such as ability to continue to work. They also found that recurrent colds or ear infections in small children were treated as normal occurrences with medical advice seldom being sought.

The amount of social support available to a person has also been found to influence reactions to illness. For example, Spiegal et al. (1989), in a prospective study of women with metastatic breast cancer, found that the survival rate was twice as long in those who received psychosocial support in the form of weekly group therapy with self-hypnosis for pain compared to those who did not.

The importance of social support is now well recognized and hundreds of support groups for patients and their relatives now exist. These include organizations such as: The Stroke Association, The Parkinson's Disease Society, The Motor Neurone Disease Society and The Schizophrenia Society. Many local authorities and individual hospitals run their own support groups in which physiotherapists may be involved. Such groups not only provide social support but are also sources of information, providing a forum in which patients and their carers can meet people with similar problems and experiences. Many groups also act to exert political pressure.

Physiotherapists need to be aware that, for some patients, coming for treatment is a way of gaining social support (Thomas and Parry, 1996). The patient who wants to talk rather than participate in physical rehabilitation is not unusual in physiotherapy departments. Patients, especially those recovering from long-term illness, often come to regard their therapists as friends and confidants. As a result, termination of treatment may be quite traumatic for some patients and needs to be handled sensitively. Termination of treatment also has other implications. It may make the person feel that nothing more can be done (the source of hope is withdrawn) and that he or she has been abandoned. Finishing treatment may be a source of anxiety in that some patients may worry that they will get worse or not be able to cope. For example, Jenkins and Rogers (1995) have found that patients who have suffered heart attacks often experience considerable 'separation anxiety' on transfer from the Coronary Care Unit to a general ward and Christman (1990) found high levels of anxiety in patients with cancer when radiotherapy was terminated. This was attributed to their feelings of uncertainty about tumour recurrence.

The stress caused by long-term illness may vary at different points in the illness. For example, a person who has survived a serious road accident may at first feel relieved and optimistic that he or she has survived. It may only be when the condition becomes stable and the prospect of long-term disability is apparent that stress may arise. Patients with spinal cord injury, amputation and stroke may spend a long time in rehabilitation. In the protected environment of the hospital or rehabilitation centre, where patients mix predominantly with similarly disabled people, they may feel less distressed or unhappy. It may be when they return home that problems become apparent such as social isolation, being the only disabled person around, having to manage alone or being dependent. This may all contribute to a changed perception of the situation and the ability to cope with it. Discharge needs to be handled sensitively and should be well planned. Where possible the person should be offered continued support.

Individual differences and illness perception

A whole host of personality factors have been found to influence illness perception. In a review of the research on reactions to chronic illness, Kline Leidy (1990) lists many personality characteristics which are likely to buffer the impact of stress resulting from chronic physical illness. These include the absence of self-denigration, mastery, high levels of self-esteem, a sense of coherence, self-efficiency, hardness, personal competence and an internal locus of control (a tendency to view oneself as being in control and able to influence the situation). Kline Leidy postulates that pessimism and a low cooperative coping style are associated with increased levels of stress during chronic physical illness. Other personality factors leading to increased stress include high trait anxiety, as measured by Speilberuger's scale, and high levels of neuroticism, as measured by Eysenck's Personality Inventory (Newman, 1984).

Prior experience of illness is another important variable. Witnessing a close friend slowly dying of cancer will obviously have an impact on a person who has just been diagnosed with the condition. Prior experience of hospital can be reassuring or increase a person's level of stress. For example, Friedlander et al. (1982) found, that in a group of patients about to undergo elective surgery, that levels of anxiety were positively correlated with the number of previous admissions to hospital.

Diagnosis and coping

When people are first informed that they have a serious illness they may feel devastated and find it difficult to cope. Sensitive handling and an appreciation of the implication of the knowledge of diagnosis for the individual is vital in helping the person to cope. Kübler-Ross (1969) outlined a series of psychological stages that people go through when they know they are dying, these are, denial and isolation, anger, bargaining, depression and acceptance. The stages follow closely those that people are said to go through when they experience a bereavement. Kübler-Ross argues that during a terminal illness people are grieving for themselves and their loss of life. The model has also been applied to serious illness where the loss may be that of a limb, independence or mobility. The model has been criticized on a number of grounds:

1. Not all people go through all the stages and acceptance may never be reached.
2. People may go backwards and forwards through the stages or get stuck at a particular stage.
3. Some people miss stages out altogether.
4. Oliver (1983) has argued that people who acquire a severe impairment do not necessarily grieve or mourn.

While it is important to bear in mind the criticisms, the model is important because it highlights many of the emotions people are likely to feel during the course of a long or chronic illness. It is important for all health professionals to recognize a patient's emotional state so that constructive help can be provided towards effective and healthy coping. Where an illness is particularly long or protracted or very disabling the process of coming to terms with it may take a long time and patients will fluctuate in their ability to do so. By understanding the nature of stress therapists can provide constructive help as and when it is required. (For further information on death, dying and bereavement, the reader is referred to Chapter 12.)

Hospitalization and stress

Whether patients come to hospital as in-patients or out-patients they are likely to experience stress, not only through lack of knowledge about their condition, but also as a result of the hospital environment itself and the medical procedures they must undergo, including diagnostic tests and surgery. Research investigating stressful aspects of hospitalization has focused on two broad areas: the process of hospitalization, and procedures and surgery carried out in hospitals.

Hospitalization

For most people a visit to the doctor arouses feelings of anxiety. The visit involves a period of uncertainty where the patient is unsure of what to ask, how to behave, or what the outcome will be. As these feelings occur with relatively minor problems it is not difficult to appreciate that admission to hospital can be very stressful. In a variety of studies patients have been asked to rate various aspects of hospital life which they found distressing or worrying. Rapheal (1969), looking at the hospital environment, found that patients most frequently mentioned sanitary arrangements, boredom, noise at night, sleepless nights and the suffering of other patients as most stressful.

Wilson-Barnett (1976) asked 200 patients from two hospitals open questions about 60 aspects of hospital life. The six most distressing aspects were:

1. Using a bedpan.
2. Anticipating a treatment or procedure likely to be painful.
3. Seeing another patient who is very ill.
4. Separation from work.
5. Separation from family members.
6. The actual condition or illness.

Some of these factors, for instance, using a bedpan or seeing someone who is ill may not be regarded as stressful by physiotherapists who, in the course of a day, may see many ill or dying people. Health professionals often develop psychological defence mechanisms over time to help them cope with the anxiety of dealing with seriously ill people (Menzies, 1970; Obholzer and Roberts, 1995). The patient, in contrast, may never have encountered death or serious illness in a fellow human being before. Aspects of hospital life which have been found to give rise to stress have been summarized by Volicer and Bohannon (1975) following a study in the USA, they state, 'Hospitalization as distinct from surgery, is a source of stress and anxiety to most patients in it's own right. The hospital environment is novel to patients and it involves a number of routines and procedures with which they are not familiar. The patients are required to meet and interact with a number of unfamiliar people and frequently have to suffer a loss of privacy. In addition they also lose a considerable degree of independence and have to endure separation from family, friends and work'.

In summarizing the results from various studies, Rachman and Philips (1975) state that five manifestations of stress are commonly seen: fear; increased irritability; loss of interest in the outside world; unhappiness and preoccupation with bodily processes. Such manifestations are not only unpleasant for the patient but are also likely to interfere with communication with hospital staff as well as reducing cooperative behaviour hindering effective and efficient treatment and the speed of recovery.

Surgery and medical procedures

Most people working in the health professions are fit and healthy, few have been admitted to hospital or have experienced routine medical procedures such as ECG, bronchoscopy or barium enema, even fewer have experienced major surgery. This lack of experience makes it difficult to understand the stress and anxiety that many patients go through when they have medical tests and surgery. Reynolds (1978) studied people who had undergone chest X-rays, and found that one-third did not know why the procedure had been carried out. Ninety-three percent received no warning the procedure was to be carried out and 82% were given no information concerning the result. Chest X-rays are a routine procedure before surgery and failure to explain this can lead to patients experiencing considerable stress.

Patients often experience high levels of anxiety which interfere with the process of acquiring, retaining and retrieving information relating to their illness (Ley, 1988). This tends to lead to poor cooperation and delayed recovery. High levels of anxiety also interfere with effective coping and can lead to a vicious circle being set up whereby ineffective coping produces higher levels of anxiety which in turn leads to less effective coping. One of the major issues revealed by this research is that lack of information, or poorly delivered information, correlates positively with stress and anxiety. In the light of such research many hospitals have changed their procedures for giving information. This is a start, but the problems of communicating information adequately is still far from solved (see Ley, 1988).

The research into stress and surgery is vast, with many surgical procedures being studied, ranging from tonsillectomy to cardiac surgery. Many different measures have been used to test preoperative anxiety and postoperative recovery. Measures of anxiety have included: self-rating; adjective check lists; Likert-type scales (5 point scales); the galvanic skin response (measuring sweating of the palms) and blood pressure. Measurements of postoperative recovery have included assessment of subjective mood state (such as anxiety and depression); amount of postoperative analgesia required and length of hospital stay (Newman, 1984). The results are difficult to compare because of the different measures adopted and differing definitions of 'anxiety' and 'recovery' which researchers have used.

Franklin (1974) surveyed 160 male patients who were to undergo surgery and found the most frequently given reasons for worrying were:

1. Not knowing what to expect.
2. The operation and its outcome.
3. The anaesthetic.
4. Concerns about their families.
5. A general dislike of hospitals.

Intuitively it might be expected that the highest levels of anxiety would be reported preoperatively and would decline in the postoperative period, indeed Auerbach (1973) reported that this was the case. However, when Johnson (1980) compared the anxiety scores of patients who had undergone gynaecological and orthopaedic surgery he found the two groups differed. The anxiety levels of the gynaecological patients declined as predicted but they remained high in the orthopaedic patients. Johnson argues that this is because the orthopaedic patient has to wait for some time after the operation before the outcome of it is known. For example, the patient may have to spend some time in a plaster cast and undergo extensive rehabilitation before the final outcome is known. This study highlights the situational context in which surgery takes place.

Other studies have investigated pre- and postoperative anxiety levels. In a rather old study, Janis (1958) divided patients into high, moderate and low level anxiety groups and found that those patients who showed moderate levels of anxiety preoperatively showed the lowest levels of anxiety postoperatively. Patients from the two other groups both suffered high levels of stress postoperatively. Janis concluded that those with low levels of anxiety avoided thinking about the operation and therefore did not prepare themselves for it mentally. In contrast, the group with high levels of anxiety were so anxious that they could neither absorb the information given about the operation nor get relief from reassurance. On the other hand, patients from the moderately stressed group were better informed about their operation and therefore suffered less stress when it was over. Other studies have failed to find the same clear cut relationship between pre-and postoperative anxiety but do report that patients who show high levels of anxiety preoperatively take longer to recover from their surgery (Johnston and Carpenter, 1980). Newman (1984) proposes several explanations for this:

1. Highly anxious patients are more likely to report pain and discomfort and also tend to experience anxiety when confronted by hospital staff and researchers. Thus, to an extent, the difference between them and less anxious patients may be an artefact.
2. Highly anxious patients are less likely to comply with postoperative instructions such as deep breathing and early mobilization.
3. Prolonged anxiety has an inhibitory effect on the immune system which delays healing and leaves the person open to infection.

Egbert *et al.* (1964) compared two groups of patients about to undergo abdominal surgery. The first group received only procedural information (information about what would take place) whereas the second group received sensory information (information about how they were likely to feel during and after the procedure, including how they could reduce pain by relaxation) as well as procedural information. The second group recovered more quickly from their operations, required less analgesia and reported less emotional disturbance postoperatively. Bailey and Clark (1989) suggest that a combination of procedural and sensory information is more effective than procedural information alone because it describes events from the patients' point of view thus allowing them to rehearse their coping strategies and giving them control. When patients are given procedural information alone they are treated as passive recipients rather than the perceiving, appraising and able people they are. For a comprehensive review and evaluation of research in this field see Salmon (1992) and Kincey (1995).

The intensive care unit (ICU)

Imagine yourself to be seriously ill and being treated in an ICU. You are lying on your back with a tube coming out of every orifice. You are ventilated, but are conscious, and have been given drugs to paralyse you. With unceasing regularity a large amount of air is forced into your lungs, but you are unable to speak because of the tube in your mouth. Periodically you are approached by nurses who proceed to do things to you, sometimes they speak to you and tell you what they are doing, sometimes they do not. You have not slept properly since you were admitted to the ICU because of the constant monitoring, the bright lights which are never turned off, the constant 'whirring', 'bleeping' and flashing of the machines, and the intermittent sounds of alarms ringing. Over the past 3 weeks you have seen three of your fellow patients dying and one has had a cardiac arrest. At intervals doctors stand at the bottom of your bed and discuss your progress. And for the last hour (it seems like an eternity) the sharp corner of the sheet has been digging into your leg. Can you doubt that ICUs are unpleasant and stressful places to be in?

Cockran and Ganong (1989) questioned 20 people who had been patients in ICUs about what they found stressful. They used the ICU Environmental Stressor Scale (modified from the Q sort test: Ballard, 1981) which details 42 commonly occurring stressors experienced in ICUs such as having no privacy, not being able to sleep, hearing the buzzers and alarms from the machinery and not having treatments explained. The four items rated as most stressful were:

1. Having tubes in the nose or mouth.
2. Being injected with needles.
3. Being in pain.
4. Not being able to sleep.

Anxiety, fear and depression are commonly experienced by patients in ICU. Bowden (1982) describes these mood states in the following way:

'Anxiety is unpleasant and characterised by feelings of foreboding and bodily discomfort. Physiological symptoms include weakness, dizziness, malaise, insecurity, dread, and a threat of the imminent loss of control. Somatic symptoms include palpitations, dysnoea, chest pain, parapthesia, headache, tremor, fatigue, sweating, dry mouth and frequency of urine. Fear is a response to a recognised external source of danger and the subjective experience ranges from uneasiness to intense dread. Reactive depression is characterised by a range of affective disturbances, from minimal changes to severe misery, gloom and wretchedness. Anxiety is usually present and thinking and action are slowed. Delusional ideas and depersonalisation experiences can arise from mood disorder. Thought can be self-reproachful, hypochondriacal and paranoid, the latter often taking the form of being shamed by others because of moral worthlessness. Sensory deceptions, particularly illusions are not uncommon. Sleep is disturbed and there is loss of appetite. Retardation may progress to stupor'.

While the majority of patients in ICUs experience stress in one form or another a minority of patients show a severe form of stress known as 'ICU syndrome' or 'ICU psychosis'. This is explained by Cookran and Ganong (1989): 'ICU Syndrome (psychosis) is a phenomenon of altered mental functioning which occurs in some patients while in ICU and which resolves after transfer from ICU. Common characteristics of this phenomenon include, confusion, disorientation, hallucinations and delusions. Researchers have found the syndrome to be caused by the stressful ICU environment rather than any physical or psychological factor. The physical symptoms (hyperventilation, tachycardia and anorexia) which accompany ICU psychosis often lead to subsequent impairment of recovery'.

The following factors have been found to contribute to the development of ICU syndrome:

1. Sleep deprivation (Fabijan and Gosselin, 1982).
2. Inability of the patient to communicate (Nastasy, 1985).
3. Sensory deprivation (Jackson, 1979).
4. Physical confinement (Ballard, 1981).
5. Repetitive stimulation – flashing lights on monitors and infusion pumps and the sound of alarms and ventilators (MacKinnon-Kessler, 1983).
6. Noise (Hanwell, 1984).
7. Social isolation (Hester, 1985).

While the ICU environment has been regarded as the main contributing factor, it has been noted that the syndrome tends to develop more readily in patients with impaired cerebral function resulting from metabolic disturbances, procedures such as cardiopulmonary bypass and mitral valve surgery (Hinds, 1987), patients suffering from renal disease, drug and alcohol addiction and those patients who are isolated due to infection (MacKellaig, 1990).

Procedures carried out by physiotherapists working in ICUs are likely to cause particular stress. Treatment often involves positioning and turning patients, disconnecting them from ventilators, manual hyperventilation and suctioning. Stress will be minimized by effective communication – telling the patient what is being done and why, by anticipating and trying to answer patients' questions and above all by empathizing with how they are feeling and remembering they remain thinking and feeling human beings despite the 'high tech' environment they are in.

Work and stress

In a study by Mottram and Flin (1988), of 50 newly qualified physiotherapists in Scotland, 30 said they found their jobs moderately stressful. In a similar study by Schuster et al. (1984), of 160 active members of the American Physical Therapy Association, 84 (53%) said they were currently experiencing symptoms of 'burnout'. A consideration of the relationship between work and stress is important, for not only does it have consequences for the individual physiotherapist but also for his or her patients and the physiotherapy profession as a whole. There is now a good deal of evidence that stress in the caring professions is a major problem giving rise to long-term health problems such as coronary heart disease, alcohol and drug abuse and mental health problems such as anxiety and depression in those experiencing prolonged stress. In a recent study by the Samaritans (Samaritans, 1995) the suicide rate for female physiotherapists aged 20–59 was found to be 2½ times higher than that for the average woman of working age. Female physiotherapists came sixth in the league table for suicide rates among female professionals aged 20–59 with five of the six occupations listed being caring professions. Stress also costs the health service a good deal of money due to absenteeism, decreased efficiency, increased job turnover and loss of individuals from the work force through illness or decisions to terminate employment (Bailey and Clark, 1989; Sutherland and Cooper, 1990). While much of the literature has focused on stress in the nursing profession, it is now recognized that it can be a problem within physiotherapy. The following pages will consider aspects of work which are likely to be perceived as stressful by physiotherapists and the caring professions as a whole. Cooper and Marshall (1978) have outlined five aspects of work that are potential sources of stress:

1. Factors intrinsic to the job itself.
2. Interpersonal relationships at work.
3. Role stress.
4. Organization and structure.
5. Career development.

Factors intrinsic to the job itself

Factors intrinsic to the job itself include the physical conditions under which the person has to work, the task requirements of the job and the workload. Much of the research in this area comes from studies of factories which have looked at the effect of factors such as noise, lighting, temperature and vibration on stress levels and output. Physiotherapists often experience poor working environments; many NHS hospitals are old, run down and have poor facilities. Stress can arise, not only from working in depressing surroundings, but also because poor facilities affect the ability of therapists to provide a good quality of service to patients.

Work overload is another factor that can give rise to stress, but a distinction must be made between quantitative workload (the amount of work one is expected to do) and qualitative workload (the difficulty of the work when matched with one's capabilities). Seventy-one percent of the Scottish physiotherapists in Mottram and Flin's study found being too busy (quantitative overload) stressful. The researchers point out that one reason why being too busy is so stressful is because therapists have to prioritize their case loads and decide which patients to leave untreated. These are decisions that newly qualified physiotherapists lack the confidence and expertise to make. Booth (1988) believes that ethical decision-making is a constant source of stress for nurses. Interestingly, 28% of the Scottish physiotherapists also found having too little to do stressful. Studies of nurses also reveal similar findings with the added stress of always having to appear busy when senior staff are around. (For further details of ethical decision-making, the reader is referred to Chapter 22.)

Physiotherapists are called upon to perform a wide variety of tasks. Some tasks are potentially dangerous if they are carried out in an inappropriate manner or at the wrong time. Physiotherapists also treat patients who are seriously ill or dying. Treatments often have to be carried out in isolation from their colleagues especially when 'on call' or at the weekend. In these situations tasks are likely to be perceived as stressful especially by inexperienced therapists. Defence mechanisms developed over time by senior staff to enable them to cope with stressful situations (Menzies, 1970) may mean that they are unable to acknowledge the stress junior staff experience when carrying out such tasks. Appropriate help and support may not, therefore, be forthcoming.

Interpersonal relationships

Physiotherapists form many interpersonal relationships during the course of their work. These include relationships with patients and their relatives, doctors and other members of the multi-disciplinary team. These relationships may be rewarding but can also be a source of stress. Mottram and Flin (1988) found that newly qualified physiotherapists found the following factors stressful: discussing patients with doctors, nurses and other physiotherapists; thinking staff do not like them; not liking patients; not liking staff; and making decisions with other staff.

A significant source of stress is interdisciplinary conflict within multi-disciplinary teams (Marshall, 1990). Conflicts have been found to occur for several reasons including the struggle for power and autonomy by individuals and individual professions and the fact that individual professions hold different assumptions about what their primary task is with regard to the care and treatment of patients (Stokes, 1995). A frequently occurring conflict arises when a patient is ready for discharge from hospital. The doctor may see early discharge of the patient as his or her primary objective whereas the physiotherapist may want to delay discharge in order to help the patient improve the quality of his or her walking.

Bullying at work is now becoming an increasingly recognized problem (Adams, 1992). The hierarchical structure of the health service and some of the problems related to working in multi-disciplinary teams are often responsible. Bullying can be insidious with one member of the team being singled out. Individuals often feel powerless to complain about such treatment because their self-esteem has been so undermined by the bully, or they feel that no one will challenge the bully because of his or her position in the hierarchy. Such bullying can lead to very high levels of stress and low morale often affecting whole departments.

As discussed earlier social support can reduce stress caused by illness. Social support from colleagues at work is also important in reducing stress, rivalry and competition. Starting work or moving to a new job can be stressful as the therapist may feel isolated until new friends are made and until he or she feels part of the department. A friendly working atmosphere is of great importance to most people.

Role stress

A person's role refers to 'the function a person performs within a particular social context' (Shaw and Constanzo, 1982). Each role has attached to it a set of beliefs, values and behaviours with some space for improvization. Decard and Present (1989) believe that, 'The professional role of the physical therapist is deeply rooted in a commitment to "bettering" the state of the client through a positive and productive therapist relationship'.

Stress is likely to occur when individuals do not feel they are fulfilling their roles. Two major sources of stress have been identified; role conflict and role ambiguity. Role conflict occurs when the demands made of an individual are at odds with his or her perceived role. For example, Wolfe (1981) states that role conflict can occur when the expectation to provide a high quality of care are undermined by an excessive workload and increased documentation and paper work. Role conflict can also occur when a person perceives that he or she has insufficient time or energy to fulfil two or more valued roles to a given standard such as the roles of physiotherapist and mother.

Role ambiguity occurs when an individual is unsure what his or her role entails and how it fits into the wider organization. Stress can also occur when other members of the team or organization do not understand the role and scope of physiotherapy. As a consequence, inappropriate demands may be made of therapists or, alternatively, their advice and skills may not be sought in situations where they feel they have a role to play.

Decard and Present (1989) have looked at the impact of role stress on American physical therapists and have found it is positively correlated with emotional exhaustion, somatic tension, depersonalization and job-related tension. It is negatively correlated with personal accomplishment. In their study the major causes of role stress were perceived to be improper allocation of time, inadequate resources and receipt of incompatible demands. The authors of the study recommend several strategies to minimize role stress:

1. Staff should be involved in the development of departmental and organizational policies.
2. Time stress should be minimized by the introduction of a once-a-month 'office day' for staff to catch up on documentation and continuing education.
3. Staff support groups should be set up to explore potential sources of stress and agreed solutions should be found for each problem.

Organization and structure

Every hospital and physiotherapy department has its own particular set of operational policies, beliefs and customs which give rise to its unique character and atmosphere. For most people when applying for a job, the 'feel' of the hospital and department is an important factor in deciding whether or not they would like to work there. A hospital or department which feels unfriendly, which appears to have lots of unnecessary rules and regulations or has an authoritarian style of management is unlikely to be a good place to work. Sutherland and Cooper (1990) have found that the perceived degree of social support provided by an organization is positively correlated with a sense of belonging and a feeling of loyalty towards it.

Career development

The physiotherapy profession in Britain has a well defined career structure. Newly qualified therapists spend their first couple of years gaining broad general experience with a view to specializing in a particular field as a senior physiotherapist. High grades involve increasingly more management and less clinical work. Climbing the ladder can be fiercely competitive (depending on the speciality) and can lead to some therapists experiencing career stress. Sutherland and Cooper (1990) define four categories of career stress: job insecurity; over promotion; under promotion; and thwarted ambition. In the past most physiotherapists had relatively secure jobs, however recent changes within the NHS including the introduction of job profiling, skill mix, local pay bargaining and performance-related pay has meant that in perceived and real terms, jobs, pay and conditions of work are less secure than they once were. The growth and popularity of alternative sources of treatment, such as osteopathy, acupuncture and chiropractic, may give rise to job insecurity, especially if these practitioners gain licence to practice in the NHS.

Physiotherapists are likely to experience stress if they are over-promoted, as they may lack the skills to do the job well. Under-promotion is likely to give rise to stress if individuals perceive their talents and expertise are not being utilized and that their ambitions are being thwarted. According to Sutherland and Cooper (1990), disruptive behaviour, poor morale and poor quality of interpersonal relationships are associated with the stress of thwarted ambition. Such behaviour is likely to cause problems in the workplace. Under-promotion often occurs in areas where there is only one hospital and where the population is fairly static. In this situation individuals often stay for years in a given post leaving newcomers with little chance of promotion. The system of interviewing for jobs may lead to under- or over-promotion depending on the confidence of the individual at interview. Career stress may be experienced by women who have a break from work while they have children or who move their jobs unwillingly because their partners have gained promotion in a new area.

'Burnout'

Burnout has been defined in many ways. Below are some of these definitions;

1. 'A total loss of purpose, idealism and enthusiasm experienced by the helping professions when conditions at work produce an inability to function because of loss of will' (Squiries and Livesley, 1984).
2. 'To fail, wear out, or become exhausted by making excessive demands on their strength, energy and resources' (Chermiss, 1980).
3. 'Emotional exhaustion and cynicism towards one's work' (Sutherland and Cooper, 1990).
4. The experience of emotional and physical exhaustion together with strong feelings of frustration and failure' (Wolfe, 1981).

Burnout can be viewed as a maladaptive coping strategy which develops through prolonged exposure to stress at work (Schuster et al., 1984). Chronic stress is a major concern because of its links with drug abuse, family problems and work-related problems, including poor performance and loss of concern for patients (Bailey, 1985). Burnout does not have one single cause, it is the result of a variety of excessive demands being placed on an individual at work. Initially the individual shows the common signs of stress such as fatigue, anxiety, moodiness, poor concentration and forgetfulness. However, as the demands continue the individual experiences feelings of frustration and failure and develops the symptoms of burnout – chronic fatigue, job boredom and cynicism, detachment and a denial of feelings, impatience and irritability, depression, disorientation, and forgetfulness, and psychosomatic complaints. The individual experiencing burnout cannot function as an effective therapist.

Squires and Livesley (1984) describe the personality characteristics of individuals who may be more susceptible to burnout. These personality characteristics include idealism, high levels of motivation, a sense of commitment, dedication, apparently tireless energy, inability to say 'no' to work demands, a tendency to perfectionism and a lack of compromise. Most of these characteristics would seem admirable for an individual working within the caring professions. However when faced with poor and ineffective management and scarce resources these individuals are more likely than others to have feelings of frustration and failure if their goals are not achieved.

Burnout develops over a period of time and can occur at any time during a person's career and may even begin before qualifying. Squires and Livesley describe four stages leading to burnout:

1. Enthusiasm – this is the pre-burnout stage when the person possessing the personality characteristics already described enters the profession. These individuals are enthusiastic and hard working and set themselves high standards and many goals. Because of their inability to say 'no' many demands are placed upon them.
2. Stagnation – the person's workload increases because of earlier enthusiasm, but as resources are limited goals are not achieved.
3. Frustration – this occurs when the individual realizes that he or she is not achieving the set goals and because of the lack of resources has no way of doing so. The initial response may be anger and attempts to rectify the situation, for example by trying to get more equipment or staff. But as Squires and Livesley point out 'eventually motivation is decreased and a sense of personal failure allows fatigue to drain any idea of a hopeful future'.
4. Withdrawal – this occurs in an attempt to cope with failure and because of depleted internal resources. The individual withdraws both from his or her job and patients. Finally he or she may break down emotionally and become severely depressed.

Menzies (1970) found that anxiety avoidance was the main coping strategy adopted by nurses under stress which is achieved by avoiding contact with patients, organizing the day around tasks rather than around people and depersonalizing patients.

There have been very few studies which have looked at burnout in physiotherapists. Schuster et al. (1984) surveyed 176 experienced American physical therapists. These researchers found that 53% reported feeling burnout. Four symptoms were found in those reporting burnout, namely: negative attitudes towards others in the workplace; adverse physical and psychological reactions; dissatisfaction with the workplace; and redirection of interest away from the workplace. The occurrence of these symptoms could be predicted by the following eight factors: poor professional preparation; lack of sharing and feedback; organizational dysfunction; excessive demands; perfectionism; overwork; lack of faith in senior colleagues; and low self-esteem. The study makes it clear that the causes of burnout are multi-factorial and usually due to a combination of personality factors and organizational factors.

A later study by Solowij (1992), based on the findings of the Schuster study, found that 35% of experienced Australian physiotherapists reported moderate to high degrees of emotional exhaustion which is a key component of burnout. Scutter and Goold (1995) investigated burnout in Australian physiotherapists with less than 5 years experience. They compared the incidence of three of the symptoms of burnout, namely high levels of emotional exhaustion, high levels of depersonalization and low levels of personal accomplishment, with those in the Solowij study. The results are shown in table 9.1.

Table 9.1   Burnout in experienced and inexperienced physiotherapists

Symptoms of burnout	Experienced therapists (Solowij, 1992)	Inexperienced therapists (Scutter and Goold, 1995)
Emotional exhaustion	12%	60%
Depersonalization	25%	44%
Low personal accomplishment	57%	6%

Scutter and Goold argue that there may be several factors which account for the difference in rates of burnout between the two groups. The experienced groups were more 'professionally mature' and a higher percentage of the experienced therapists were in stable relationships providing social support which helps to mitigate stress.

Preventing burnout

The relationships between workers and those in management is often a major source of stress. Schuster *et al.* (1984) found that lack of professional sharing and feedback from senior colleagues and a lack of faith in them, were significant predictors of stress and burnout. A management style which commands respect, but also allows participation and consultation in decision-making, is probably the most effective in reducing work-related stress.

Squires and Livesley (1984) highlight the importance of good management in the prevention of burnout. Prevention has to begin at the start of a therapist's career. Students entering the physiotherapy profession need to have a clear understanding of the nature of the work they are about to undertake. Clinical tutors and lecturers have a responsibility to ensure that students have a realistic expectation of their role once they are qualified. (For further information on professional socialization and the role of clinical educators, the reader is referred to Chapter 21.)

Managers need to ensure that staff know what standards and goals are expected of them, with joint involvement in the setting of such goals and standards. Managers need to ensure that their staff are given appropriate support and feedback regarding their progress. Effective communication between staff and managers is the key to reducing burnout. Staff should feel valued as people as well as for being part of a team and must feel comfortable about discussing any problems with senior colleagues. At the same time staff need to be aware that managers are under increased pressure within the new NHS and that they themselves may also experience burnout. Mutual support is, therefore, very important. Physiotherapists can protect themselves from burnout by taking a realistic view of their work and, while accepting that dedication and conscientiousness are important, should develop interests in other activities to promote overall personal development.

Conclusion

Patients and physiotherapists are both involved in events which have the potential to be stressful. Physiotherapists need to help patients cope with the stress they are experiencing in order that rehabilitation is maximized, but this is very difficult if their own stress levels are high. An understanding of the nature of stress and what situations and factors may give rise to it are important first steps in learning how to reduce stress both in themselves and their patients. Physiotherapy managers in particular have a responsibility to provide a supportive working environment where physiotherapists and their patients can work happily and effectively. The idea that health professionals do not need support in their professional lives, that their own needs are unimportant and that expressing them is a sign of weakness must no longer remain unchallenged.

References

Adams A. (1992) *Bullying at Work: How to Confront and Overcome it.* London: Virago Press.

Auerback S. M. (1973) Anxiety and adjustment to surgery. *Journal of Counselling and Clinical Psychology*, **40**, 264–271.

Bailey R. (1985) *Coping with Stress in Caring.* London: Blackwell Scientific.

Bailey R., Clark M. (1989) *Stress and Coping in Nursing.* London: Chapman and Hall.

Ballard K. S. (1981) Identification of environmental stressors for patients in a surgical intensive care unit. *Issues in Mental Health Nursing*, **3**, 89–108.

Blaxter M., Patterson E. (1982) *Mothers and Daughters.* London: Heinemann.

Booth K. (1988) Stress and Nursing. *Nursing*, **3**(26), 1017–1020.

Bowden P. (1982) Psychiatric aspects of intensive care. In *Care of the Critically Ill Patient* (Tinker J., Rapplinm N., eds). Berlin: Springer Verlag.

Chermiss C. (1980) *Staff Burnout: Job Stress in the Human Services.* London: Sage Publications.

Christman N. J. (1990) Uncertainty and adjustment during radiotherapy. *Nursing Research*, **39**(1), 17–20.

Cookran J., Ganong L. H. (1989) A comparison of patients' and nurses' perception of intensive care stressors. *Journal of Advanced Nursing*, **14**, 1018–1043.

Cooney K. (1990) The girl can't help it. *The Guardian*, Wednesday January 2nd, p. 28.

Cooper C. L., Marshall J. (1978) *Understanding Executive Stress.* London: Macmillan.

Decard G. C., Present R. M. (1989) Impact of role stress on physical therapist's emotional and physical well-being. *Physical Therapy*, **69**(9), 713–718.

Dewar A. L., Morse J. M. (1995) Unbearable incidents: failure to endure the experience of illness. *Journal of Advanced Nursing*, **22**, 957–964.

Egbert L. D., Batit G. E., Welsh C. E., Bartlett M. K. (1964) Reduction of postoperative pain by encouragement and instruction of patients: a study of patient doctor rapport. *New England Journal of Medicine*, **270**, 823–827.

Fabijan L., Gosselin M. D. (1982) How to recognise sleep deprivation in your ICU patient and what to do about it. *The Canadian Nurse*, 20–23, April.

Fitzpatrick R. (1984) Lay concepts of illness. In *The Experience of Illness* (Fitzpatrick R. *et al.*, eds). London: Tavistock Publications.

Franklin B. L. (1974) *Patient Anxiety on Admission to Hospital.* London: Royal College of Nursing Project.

French S. (1994) (ed.) *On Equal Terms: Working With Disabled People.* Oxford: Butterworth-Heinemann.

Friedlander M. L., Steinhart M. J., Daly S. S., Snyder J. (1982) Demographic cognitive and experimental predictors of presurgical anxiety. *Journal of Psychosomatic Research*, **26**(6), 623–627.

Hansell H. S. (1984) The behavioural effects of noise on man: the patient with 'intensive care unit psychosis'. *Heart and Lung*, **13**, 59–64.

Helman C. (1994) *Culture, Health and Illness* (3rd edn). Oxford: Butterworth-Heinemann.

Hester B. S. (1985) Nursing responsibility in changing visiting restrictions in the intensive care unit. *Heart and Lung*, **14**, 181–186.

Hinds C. J. (1987) *Intensive Care – A Concise Textbook*, London: Baillière Tindall.

Jackson C. (1979) Clinical sensory deprivation: a review of hospitalised eye – surgical patients. In *Sensory Deprivation: Fifteen Years of Research* (Zubek J., ed.). New York: Appleton.

Janis I. L. (1958) *Psychological States Psychosomatic and Behavioural Studies of Surgical Patients*. New York: Wiley.

Jenkins D. A., Rogers G. (1995) Transfer anxiety in patients with myocardial infarction. *British Journal of Nursing*, **4**(21), 1248–1252.

Johnson M. (1980) Anxiety in surgical patients. *Psychological Medicine*, **10**, 145–152.

Johnston M., Carpenter L. (1980) Relationship between pre-operative anxiety and postoperative state. *Psychological Medicine*, **10**, 361–367.

Kincey J. (1995) Surgery. In *Health Psychology: Processes and Applications* (Broone A., Llewelyn S., eds). London: Chapman and Hall.

Kitchener S. J. (1995) *An Exploration of the Emotional Issues Surrounding Respite Care – Carer Perspectives*. Unpublished MSc Thesis, Brunel University College Library, Isleworth, Middlesex.

Kline Leidy N. (1990) A structural model of stress, psychosocial resources and symptomatic experience in chronic physical illness. *Nursing Research*, **39**(4), 230–235.

Kübler-Ross E. (1969) *On Death and Dying*. London; Tavistock Publications.

Ley P. (1988) *Communicating with Patients*. London: Croom Helm.

MacKellaig J. M. (1990) A review of the psychological effects of intensive care on the isolated patient and his family. *Care of the Critically Ill*, **6**(3), 100–102.

MacKinnon-Kessler S. (1983) Maximising your ICU patient's sensory and perceptual environment. *Canadian Nurse*, **79**, 41–49.

Marshall R. (1990) Psychodynamic nature of conflicts within multi-disciplinary groups. *Senior Nurse*, **10**(3), 20–21.

Menzies I. E. P. (1970) *The Functioning of Social Systems as a Defence Against Anxiety*. London: The Tavistock Institute.

Mottram E., Flin R. H. (1988) Stress in newly qualified physiotherapists. *Physiotherapy*, **74**(12), 607–612.

Nastasy E. L. (1985) Identifying environmental stressors for cardiac patients in a surgical intensive care unit. *Proceedings of the 12th Annual Conference of the Association of Critical-Care Nursing*. Newport Beach, Canada.

Newman S. (1984) Anxiety, hospitalization and stress. In *The Experience of Illness* (Fitzpatrick R. *et al.*, eds). London: Tavistock Publications.

Nolan M., Grant G. (1990) Stress is in the eye of the beholder. *Journal of Advanced Nursing*, **15**, 544–555.

Nolan M., Grant G. (1992) *Regular Respite – An Evaluation of a Hospital Rota Bed Scheme for Elderly People*. London: ACE Books.

Norman A. (1987) *Aspects of Ageing: A Discussion Paper*. London: Centre for Policy on Ageing.

Obholzer A., Roberts V. Z. (1995) *The Unconscious at Work: Individual and Organizational Stress in the Human Services*. London: Routledge.

Oliver M. (1983) *Social Work with Disabled People*. London: Macmillan.

Rachman S., Philips C. (1975) *Psychology and Medicine*. London: Temple Smith.

Rapheal W. (1969) *Patients and Their Hospitals: A Survey of Patients View of Life in Hospital*. London: King Edward's Hospital Fund.

Reynolds M. (1978) No news is bad news. *British Medical Journal*, **1**, 1673–1676.

Salmon P. (1992) Psychological factors in surgical stress: implications for management. *Clinical Psychology Review*, **12**, 681–704.

Samaritans (1995) *Behind The Mask*. England: Samaritans.

Schuster N. D., Nelson D. L., Quisling C. (1984) Burnout among physical therapists. *Physical Therapy*, **64**(3), 299–303.

Scutter S. and Goold M. (1995) Burnout in recently qualified physiotherapists in South Australia. *Australian Physiotherapy*, **41**(2), 115–118.

Shaw M. E., Constanzo P. R. (1982) *Theories of Social Psychology*. New York: McGraw Hill.

Sobwijr V. (1992) 'Burnout in physiotherapists in South Australia' (Master's thesis, University of South Australia).

Spiegal D., Bloom J. R., Kraemer H. C., Gottheil E. (1989) Effect of psychosocial treatment on survival of patients with metastatic breast cancer. *Lancet*, **ii**, 888–891.

Squires A., Livesley B. (1984) Beware of burnout. *Physiotherapy*, **70**(6), 236–238.

Stokes J. (1995) The unconscious at work in groups and teams. In *The Unconscious at Work: Individual and Organizational Stress in the Human Services* (Obholzer A., Roberts V. Z., eds). London: Routledge.

Sutherland V. J., Cooper C. (1990) *Understanding Stress: A Psychological Perspective for Health Professionals*. London: Chapman and Hall.

Thomas C., Parry A. (1996) Research on users' views about stroke services: towards an empowerment research paradigm. *Physiotherapy*, **82**(1), 6–12.

Volicer B. J., Bohannon M. W. (1975) A hospital stress rating scale. *Nursing Research*, **24**, 352–359.

Weinman J. (1987) *Psychology as Applied to Medicine*, Bristol: Wright.

Wellisch D. K. (1981) Interventions with the cancer patient. In *Medical Psychology: Contributions to Medicine* (Prokop C. K., Bradley L. A., eds). New York: Academic Press.

White G. M. (1982) The role of cultural explanation in 'somatization' and 'psychologization'. *Social Science and Medicine*, **16**(16), 1319–1530.

Wilson-Barnett J. (1976) Patients' emotional reactions to hospitalisation. An exploratory study. *Journal of Advanced Nursing*, **1**, 351–358.

Wolf F. S., Goodell H. (1968) *Stress and Disease* (2nd edn). Springfield, USA: Charles C. Thomas.

Wolfe G. A. (1981) Burnout of therapists: inevitable or preventable. *Physical Therapy*, **61**, 1046–1050.

10

The psychology and sociology of pain

Sally French

'Dualistic notions that consider pain as either entirely physical or psychological must be abandoned. All pain involves a combination of biological factors, psychological factors (mental, emotional and behavioural) and social–environmental factors.' (Hanson and Gerber, 1990)

The intensity of the pain we experience and the way we respond to it are not merely a function of the degree of physical damage incurred (Sofaer, 1992; Niven and Robinson, 1994). Weinman (1981) believes that, 'Whatever the biological parameters of the symptoms they alone may be insufficient to explain the patient's response'. It is, therefore, very unfair to compare patients who have the same type of pathologies or have undergone similar medical procedures (Sofaer, 1992).

There are individual differences in our perception of pain and the way we respond to it. Engel (1950) referred to this distinction as 'private pain' and 'public pain' and Helman (1994) describes our response to pain as 'pain behaviour'. Philips (1988) and Sofaer (1992) point out that the association between pain experience and pain behaviour is weak, it is possible to be in considerable pain but to hide this from others, or conversely to complain a great deal even though pain is minimal. The intensity of pain is not necessarily strongly associated with the degree of suffering either; people with minimal pain who do not know the cause of it may suffer more than those in severe pain who understand its meaning. Rose *et al.* (1995) states that, 'only the sufferer can assess the severity of pain'.

It would obviously be very helpful if physiotherapists could distinguish pain intensity from pain complaint in their patients, but in practice this is difficult if not impossible to achieve with any degree of accuracy. Pain is a personal and subjective experience and our knowledge of another's suffering is inevitably based on the ways in which he or she responds and our own perception of this, which in turn will be influenced by the social situation. McCaffrey (1983) believes that pain is, 'whatever the patient says it is and exists wherever he says it does'.

Psychological and sociological aspects of pain are, however, often regarded as fringe factors, merely influencing and modifying the 'real' physiological pain. The psychological and social aspects are, however, central to the experience of pain and the behaviour associated with it, as recognized by Melzack and Wall (1988) in their formulation of the pain gate theory. Williams and Erskine (1995) urge us to accept the complexity of pain. They state:

'Most attempts to conceptualise pain have been undermined by dualistic notions of body and mind. It is still hard to find language which integrates rather than separates the physical and the psychological'.

Factors influencing pain perception and pain behaviour

Personality

Research regarding the association between personality traits and pain experience and behaviour, are inconsistent in both laboratory and natural settings (Williams and Erskine, 1995). It has frequently been found, however, that extroverts express pain more freely than introverts even though they appear to be less sensitive to painful stimuli. Griffiths (1980) suggests that this may be because of their greater readiness to accept social disapproval which is likely to be met in British society when emotions are openly displayed. Petrie (1967) found pain tolerance to increase with extroversion, and Eysenck (1961) found that during labour and childbirth introverts felt pain sooner and more intensely than extroverts, yet complained less. They also tended to remember the pain more vividly afterwards. Barsky and Klerman (1983) found considerable individual differences in the degree of attention people pay to normal bodily sensations. Concentrating on the body tends to increase the perception of pain (Klaber Moffett and Richardson, 1995).

Adams et al. (1994a) reviewed the literature regarding personality characteristics in chronic low back pain and carried out an investigation of personality characteristics in patients with chronic low back pain attending physiotherapy out-patient departments (Adams et al., 1994b). They found an increased incidence of depression, anxiety, hypochondriasis and hysteria among patients with low back pain when compared with a control group though they all fell within the normal range. It is unclear whether these characteristics resulted from the pain or whether they predisposed towards it. Little is known about the complex interaction of personality and the experience of pain.

The social context

The social context in which the injury occurs or in which the pain is felt can greatly influence the individual's experience of it and response to it (Hanson and Gerber, 1990). In the Second World War Beecher observed the behaviour of soldiers severely injured in battle. The majority said they were in no pain or very little pain with only one in three complaining enough to warrant the administration of morphine. However, they complained as much as anyone else over routine medical procedures (Beecher, 1959). Beecher also observed civilians with similar injuries to the soldiers; the majority complained of severe pain with most wanting morphine. He explained this in terms of the social context; the soldiers were thankful or even euphoric at still being alive whereas for the civilians the injury was a very depressing and disruptive event (Beecher, 1959). It is also likely that the military role demands greater stoicism than the civilian role.

In a similar way, the pain resulting from injuries sustained in a road traffic accident may well be more severe than the pain following elective surgery, even if the physical injury resulting from the accident is less. In the case of elective surgery the patent will have had the opportunity to prepare him or herself for the event, can look forward to an improved state of health and will probably be thankful that the operation is over; whereas the victim of the road traffic accident is likely to have experienced a sudden, very disturbing and negative event.

If a person's attention is fully occupied he or she may not feel any pain despite considerable injury, as Weinman (1981) explains, 'attention in one sensory source can reduce or abolish awareness of another source'. This can occur in the case of sportsmen and women who continue to play despite considerable injury. Similarly, Rachman and Philips (1978) note that a standard injection which is given following childbirth to aid the expulsion of the placenta is rarely felt. Masochists, on the other hand, tend to label as enjoyable what others would regard as painful, though this too is dependent on the social setting. Another example of how the social context affects pain perception and response is the tolerance people demonstrate towards injuries inflicted as part of various rituals and ceremonies (Mathews and Steptoe, 1988; Melzack and Wall, 1988; Helman, 1994).

Many practitioners, for example Peck (1982), encourage people with chronic symptoms to practise focusing their attention away from the pain and to participate in enjoyable activities, as a way of relieving it. Wynn Parry (1980) reports that people suffering pain following brachial plexus injuries find the most effective way of reducing it is to absorb themselves in their work. Hanson and Gerber (1990) believes that work, recreation, social activity and mental distraction, such as mental imagery, can all relieve pain.

Culture

People seem to have a uniform sensory threshold. Sternbach and Tursky (1965) measured sensory threshold, using electric shock as the stimulus, to American women from four ethnic groups; Italian, Jewish, Irish and Old American. There was no difference in when they first reported feeling the sensation. According to Zborowski (1969), however, cultural background does have an effect on pain perception, that is when people first report feeling pain. Hardy et al. (1952) found that radiant heat, described by Jewish and Italian people as painful, was described as merely warm by Northern Europeans. Zborowski (1952) found that Old Americans had an accepting, stoical attitude towards pain, tending to withdraw when it became intense and preferring to be alone. Conversely Jewish and Italian people were inclined to complain openly and seek support. The underlying attitudes of the latter two groups were, however, different. The Jewish people were most concerned about the cause and the meaning of the pain, whereas the Italian people were concerned about receiving immediate relief. Zola (1966) found attitudinal differences towards symptoms; Italian people were most concerned if the symptoms interfered with their social lives whereas Irish and Anglo-Saxon people were most concerned if they interfered with work.

Interesting though these findings are, care must be taken when interpreting them and acting upon them as there is a serious danger of unfairly stereotyping people according to their cultural or ethnic origins (Sofaer, 1992). It should be remembered that there is more variability within cultural groups than between them. Zborowski (1952) points out that any differences there are tend to disappear over time in cosmopolitan societies and that other factors, such as educational background and occupation, may have an effect on pain behaviour. Pilowski and Spence (1977) suggest that any differences which exist among cultural groups, in regard to their experience and expression of pain, may be due to their immigrant status and the difficulties they experience in adapting to the majority culture. Thus the immediate social situation may influence cultural patterns. In addition, Wolff and Langley (1977) warn of the poor research design of many of these studies. (For further information on people from ethnic minorities and health care, the reader is referred to Chapter 5).

Attitudes and behaviour of health professionals

Health practitioners, including physiotherapists, will have their own notions of appropriate pain behaviour, based on personal and occupational factors. In an American study, Rosengren and DeVault (1976) describe how, in an obstetric hospital, the only place where pain was legitimated, sanctioned and defined as such, was in the delivery room. The expression of pain was deemed inappropriate in any other area, including the labour room. Thus professionals have considerable power to define and manage pain according to their own attitudes and beliefs. It is all too easy to dismiss or become impatient with those who do not fit the stoical British ideal. Helman (1994) states:

'People will receive maximum attention and sympathy if their pain matches the society's view of how people should draw attention to their suffering – whether by an extravagant display of emotion or a quiet change of behaviour'.

Grieve (1987) and Sofaer (1992) warns us not to impose our own stereotypes on patients.

Hough (1987) believes that, 'western culture has a tendency to view the open expression of emotion with some distaste' and Sofaer (1992) states that, 'It sometimes seems that we are more concerned about monitoring patients' expression of pain than the pain itself'. Davitz and Davitz (1981) found that nurses from various cultural groups viewed their patients' pain differently and were also influenced by such factors as the patient's social class, how responsible he or she was judged to be for the condition and the ease or difficulty of diagnosis.

Fagerhaugh and Strauss (1977) found that physiotherapists and nurses tend to assess the severity of patients' low back pain by interpreting their behaviour rather than believing what is said. Saxey (1986) and Sofaer (1992) warn that we should not judge how much pain someone is in by his or her behaviour alone as many people learn to adapt to pain and live relatively normal lives even though it is quite severe. Sofaer (1992) points out that patients may show minimal response to pain because they have devised their own strategies for coping with it. Price (1990) believes that the monitoring of pain should be given as much importance as the monitoring of physiological measures, though Williams and Erskine (1995) state:

'It is not at all unusual for medical and nursing personnel to treat X-rays and other imaging results as "hard" data and the patient's experience as "soft" data. Nor is it unusual for clinicians to feel that they can estimate the pain better than patients themselves on the basis of those data'.

It is all too easy for patients to become negatively stereotyped making it all the more difficult for them to convince others of the pain they are experiencing. Peck (1982) points out that patients may end up being blamed for their pain both by medical staff and their families and are 'left with the burden of having to prove their innocence'.

Baer *et al.* (1970), Lenburg *et al.* (1970) and Johnston *et al.* (1987) found considerable differences in the judgements of various professional groups regarding the degree of pain experienced by real and hypothetical patients. Nurses tend to rate patients' pain higher than either physiotherapists or doctors. Pitts and Healy (1989) found that physiotherapists infer less pain in hypothetical patients than nurses but more pain than doctors. Their ratings were, however, nearer to those of the doctors. These results could not be explained in terms of gender although female doctors did infer more pain than male doctors.

Bendelow (1993) notes the different attitudes towards men and women who experience pain. She found that both men and women tend to believe that women are better able to tolerate pain than men but are 'allowed' to express emotion more than men. Women's pain is also more likely to be perceived as being psychogenic in origin. The research on gender and pain is, however, inconclusive.

Wolff *et al.* (1991) found that a sample of orthopaedic physical therapists in the USA lacked knowledge of pain mechanisms and had poor attitudes towards patients with chronic pain. Ninety-five percent preferred to work with people in acute pain and 75% thought that physiotherapy was not helpful in the treatment of chronic benign pain.

Past experience

As well as the influence of wider cultural factors on pain perception and response, Griffiths (1980) and Sofaer (1992) point out that the individual's unique past history is also of considerable importance. Some families focus great attention on very minor injuries whereas others tend to minimize or ignore quite serious ones. We thus learn how to interpret pain and respond to it by a process of social modelling (Klaber Moffett and Richardson, 1995). There are also differences in the degree and manner to which children are encouraged or discouraged from openly responding to pain. These early experiences may influence our sensitivity to potentially painful stimuli and our pain behaviour throughout life. Sofaer (1992) points out that for some people expressing pain would make them feel ashamed and embarrassed.

Past experience of medical encounters are also important. It is likely that a person who has had a painful experience on one occasion, at the dentist for example, will feel pessimistic and anxious when he or she returns for further treatment. Unsuccessful or painful treatments can lead to lack of trust in the clinician and a loss of confidence that a new treatment will help.

State of mind

People who are anxious are more sensitive to pain than calm people. Kent (1986) found that anxious patients complain more of pain than others and Hill *et al.* (1952a,b) demonstrated that the intensity of pain decreases if anxiety is reduced by giving people control over the situation. The anticipation of pain, and uncertainty regarding its cause, tend to raise anxiety which in turn increases its perceived intensity, thus a vicious circle may operate. Bond (1984) states that, '... pain will be greater for patients who have a tendency to become anxious because pain causes anxiety and, in its turn, anxiety heightens pain'. However, if anxiety is not pain-related it can decrease pain by focusing the person's attention elsewhere (Klaber Moffett and Richardson, 1995).

Many patients experience a reduction in their level of anxiety if they are given information explaining the nature of their illness and the treatment they will receive (Sofaer, 1992; Harding and de C. Williams, 1995; Williams and Erskine, 1995). Many studies indicate that patients are dissatisfied with the degree of information they receive (Ley, 1988), and that giving information is beneficial both in terms of reducing anxiety and speed of recovery. The benefit of giving information to individual patients, however, is difficult to ascertain as a sizeable minority prefer not to know and people differ regarding the amount of information they want. Weinman (1981) believes that their pain tolerance may well be lowered if information is forced upon them or if they are not helped to cope with it. Melzack and Wall (1988) state that knowledge alone may increase anxiety because of the expectation of pain it creates. They suggest that patients must be provided with skills to cope both with their anxiety and with their pain.

If people understand what is causing their pain, for example that chest pain is the result of indigestion rather than heart disease, they are less likely to be anxious about it. Similarly pain is better tolerated, and probably perceived as less intense, if the person believes it is temporary or 'normal'. Examples of 'normal' pain is that caused by exercise, childbirth or menstruation. What is and what is not regarded as a 'normal' symptom, however, varies considerably among different individuals and groups (Helman, 1994).

Anxiety may be relieved and pain reduced by giving patients control (Feuerstein and Beattie, 1995), for example allowing them to terminate a procedure at any time if it becomes uncomfortable. Wright (1987) and Flint (1988) point out that familiarity reduces anxiety, so it is important, if at all possible, that the patient be treated by the same physiotherapist on each visit.

Hall and Stride (1954) found that the appearance of the word 'pain' in a list of instructions increased the subjects' perception of pain, possibly by raising their level of anxiety. The subjects reported a sensation as painful which was not regarded as such when the word was absent from the instructions. This gives rise to a contradiction of significance to physiotherapists; on the one hand it seems that focusing attention on pain – giving information about it pre-operatively, informing people that they are in control of how much pain they receive and so on – decreases their anxiety and perception of pain but, on the other hand, it seems that focusing attention on pain may raise levels of anxiety and pain perception.

Sensitivity to pain is also increased if the person is depressed. This is due to the unpleasant nature of pain, the tendency for it to impose inactivity on the individual, thus reducing enjoyment and leading to a focusing of attention upon it, and the feeling of loss of control (Williams and Erskine, 1995). Peck (1982) points out that guilt, despondency and self-criticism frequently accompany depression, only serving to intensify it. In such a situation the person in pain will tend to perceive it as more intense than he or she would do otherwise, thus a vicious circle may develop.

Mathews and Steptoe (1988) explain that pain can be secondary to depression and can be relieved by antidepressant drugs. They state that emotion and pain, 'appear to be inextricably entangled'. Davison and Neale (1990) point out that depression and anxiety are frequently linked. There is a great danger, however, in assuming that pain is secondary to depression and anxiety. Melzack and Wall (1988) warn that:

> 'The patients with the thick hospital charts are all too often prey to the physician's innuendoes that they are neurotic and that their neuroses are the cause of the pain ... All too often the diagnosis of neurosis as the cause of pain hides our ignorance of many aspects of pain mechanisms'.

Depression may be relieved and pain reduced both by empathizing with the patient and involving him or her in the treatment. People commonly feel in better spirits after engaging in physical activity. Although the mechanism behind this altered mood is not fully understood, exercise is thought to be a way of releasing anxiety as well as improving self-esteem. The trip in the ambulance and the visit to the physiotherapy department may, in themselves, be sufficient to reduce pain by redirecting the patient's attention and improving morale by providing enjoyable companionship. Although physiotherapists may despair of patients who attend 'for social reasons', in reality all patient/therapist encounters are social events and as such have the potential to be highly therapeutic.

There is a danger, however, that repeated contact with health professionals and the constant search for a medical cure may be detrimental to the person with chronic pain. Although many people expect health professionals to cure or alleviate their symptoms, repeated contact with them may actually increase pain by focusing the person's attention upon it, as well as encouraging the idea that a medical cure is possible when this may not be so. Furthermore, Peck (1982) believes that it may sap the person's energy which could be better used to develop realistic coping strategies.

Avoidance behaviour and cognitive processes

The avoidance of physical activity is perfectly rational while pain is acute and while tissues are healing, but this pattern of behaviour sometimes persists and intensifies in those with chronic pain. Philips (1987) believes that this decreases their sense of control over the pain and increases their expectations that exposure to activity will create more pain. Over time the avoidance behaviour intensifies.

Avoidance does not merely concern physical activities but also involves social interaction, hobbies and work. Philips and Jahanshahi (1986) studied people suffering from headaches and found that avoidance was the most common behaviour reported, in particular social withdrawal. There is little evidence that avoidance behaviour reduces chronic pain, and over time avoidance behaviour may become worse even though the symptoms remain static or improve. Philips (1987) believes that this behaviour is a consequence of the patient's beliefs and memories, which are often distorted, rather than a consequence of the pain itself and that these beliefs and memories are in turn reinforced by the avoidance behaviour. This behavioural response is of great significance to the therapist and the patient. The patient believes he or she is controlling the pain by the avoidance behaviour and that the behaviour is a consequence of the pain. The therapist, on the other hand, may view the behaviour as an indication that the patient has developed inadequate and inappropriate coping strategies. Conversely the therapist, for fear that the patient's conditions might recur, may encourage avoïdance behaviour by emphasizing the need to avoid certain activities and to take care.

Understanding how personality, the social context, professional attitudes, state of mind and cultural and family background affect pain perception and behaviour may help to foster empathy and tolerance and improve communication between physiotherapists and their patients. It is now believed that a disease-orientated model is not a suitable perspective for the management of chronic pain.

Because of the highly complex and multi-faceted nature of pain it is essential that the assessment of pain should take into account physical, psychological and social factors (May, 1991; Williams and Erskine, 1995). The McGill Pain Questionnaire has sensory, cognitive and affective components and is often used. Patients may also be asked to keep a diary of their pain and behaviour. Understanding the nature of pain is often highly complex. Pain may, for example, be used (often subconsciously) as a solution to other problems, such as fear of meeting people, and can serve an important role in stabilizing and maintaining relationships. A full discussion of the assessment of pain using a variety of assessment tools is given by Feuerstein and Beattie (1995).

Psychological treatment strategies

Physiotherapists are in a position to incorporate psychological measures into their treatment programmes. Various ways in which this can be achieved have already been discussed, for example, reducing anxiety and depression by giving the patient information and control. It is a mistake to think that the psychological treatment of pain is only indicated if the patient is coping inadequately or if the cause of the pain cannot be found. Pain is as much a psychological as a physiological phenomenon and, therefore, psychological strategies are likely to help the patient control and cope with the pain in many instances.

A good, supportive relationship with the patient is highly therapeutic in itself and the placebo effect, which permeates all treatments is often very powerful (see Chapter 20). In addition to this physiotherapists may use psychological strategies to help their patients, either as the sole treatment technique, or by incorporating them into a programme of physical treatment. The physiotherapist must recognize when the patient needs to be referred to a psychiatrist or clinical psychologist and is likely to work alongside these professionals in some settings, for example in pain clinics. There is considerable overlap between the techniques of various health professionals and alternative practitioners in the treatment of pain. Some of these techniques will now be discussed.

Relaxation

Relaxation may be used to reduce stress, anxiety and depression. Melzack and Wall (1988) state that relaxation reduces activity in the sympathetic and motor nervous systems. The mechanisms of pain reduction may be physiological, for example when the patient succeeds in relaxing tense muscles, or cognitive, for example when the patient manages to direct his or her attention away from the pain. There is considerable evidence that relaxation training brings about pain reduction (Flaberty and Fitzpatrick, 1978; Blanchard et al., 1987; Hellsing and Linton, 1989). Relaxation techniques have been traditionally used by physiotherapists, particularly in relation to antenatal education and respiratory disease. A similar approach is likely to be helpful in the treatment of pain.

Biofeedback

This technique is used if it is thought that the patient's pain is the result of physiological processes such as tense muscles. By giving the patient feedback concerning his or her physiological state the patient may learn to control it (Hanson and Gerber, 1990). The evidence regarding the efficacy of biofeedback in the treatment of pain does, however, conflict. Chapman (1986) reviewed the literature and found no advantage for biofeedback combined with relaxation over relaxation alone. Smith (1987), however, found that the two techniques in combination were more successful than either technique in isolation for reducing headache.

Hypnosis

Hypnotic suggestion has been used for pain relief in many branches of medicine including dentistry, terminal care and obstetrics. Physiotherapists with some additional training may use hypnosis to reduce pain. The patient is put in a trance-like state where he or she is highly suggestible and deeply relaxed. In this state, various ideas can be given to the patient regarding pain, for example that it is not severe or that it will no longer be of any concern. Melzack and Wall (1988) point out that a small proportion of people can undergo surgery while under hypnosis and that many other pain relieving measures, such as drugs, can be reduced when hypnosis is part of the treatment. Melzack and Perry (1980) found that 22% of people who had chronic pain improved with hypnotic treatment compared with 14% who received a placebo. They found that when hypnosis was combined with biofeedback the improvement was considerably greater than when hypnosis alone was given.

Counselling

Many courses now exist on counselling skills for physiotherapists. There are various types of counselling techniques and for further discussion of them the reader is referred to Chapter 19.

In non-directive counselling the therapist creates a warm and empathic relationship and environment whereby the patient can talk and work through his or her problems and difficulties with encouragement but little interruption or direction from the therapist (Burnard, 1992; Swain, 1995). In this way the person in pain may come to the conclusion that the best way to cope is to try to ignore it, or that the pain is being maintained by important secondary gains such as the avoidance of boring or difficult tasks.

In cognitive counselling the therapist takes a more active role, concentrating on the patient's thoughts and feelings in relation to his or her pain and attempting to change them. For example, patients may continually be telling themselves that they cannot cope because of the pain or that they are unattractive to others because of it. These negative messages may be causing anxiety and depression making the pain worse. It is the task of the therapist to help such patients realize that they are responsible for their own thoughts and feelings and to help them develop a more positive outlook by devising a suitable treatment programme (Niven and Robinson, 1994; Williams and Erskine, 1995).

Behaviour modification

This technique is focused on changing pain behaviour rather than pain perception. It is assumed that the person's pain brings about various rewards which he or she wants to maintain, albeit subconsciously, or that the pain behaviour, which was once appropriate, has become maladaptive or debilitating. Whether the patient feels less pain following this treatment is open to question. Behaviour modification is a technique whereby behaviour which is approved of is rewarded while behaviour which is disapproved of is ignored. In this way behaviour is 'shaped'. It may be the case, for example, that the patient has become very isolated because he or she talks of nothing but the pain, so to reduce this behaviour the patient will be rewarded when talking about other matters and ignored when the pain is mentioned. The patient may be fully aware of the aims and objectives of the behaviour modification programme and may even have helped to devise it, conversely it may be covert. Williams and Erskine (1995) state:

> 'Although patients may be sceptical of the extent of change possible through these methods, there is no doubt that selective attention and inattention can bring about rapid change. Behavioural management techniques can be empowering for the patient who can begin to feel in control of him or herself, rather than under the control of the pain'.

Crabbe (1989) claims a 90% success rate when using behaviour modification for the treatment of pain and cites evidence from abroad that maintenance of improvement is of the order of 50%. How it compares with other methods or the placebo, however, is still uncertain.

Harding and de C. Williams (1995) describe a cognitive–behavioural programme for the treatment of pain within a physiotherapy context. The programme includes the setting of realistic goals, the pacing of activities to avoid the 'over-activity/under-activity cycle', education, self-management and the challenging of unhelpful cognitions. Pain is never denied but pain behaviour is not rewarded.

There are important ethical issues with which the physiotherapist should be aware when considering the use of behaviour modification programmes or participating in them, especially if they are covert. (For further discussion of ethical issues in physiotherapy, the reader is referred to Chapter 22.)

Group therapy

According to the patient's temperament, group therapy may have a very positive psychological effect, with the result that pain is reduced or managed more effectively. Human beings are social animals and may be greatly encouraged by working with other people who are experiencing similar difficulties. By seeing others their own suffering may be put into perspective and other group members may act as positive role models. Some people are motivated by competition which the group experience may provide, or may simply feel less anxious and depressed by virtue of enjoyable companionship. Thus the dynamics of the group, for example in back schools or self-help organizations, may have important effects in reducing the person's pain or helping him or her to cope with it.

A combined behaviour modification and group therapy programme has been developed by Williams (1989) for patients with chronic pain who are defined as displaying abnormal pain behaviour and who have not been helped by traditional medical or physiotherapy treatments. Patients take part in a fitness programme in a busy physiotherapy gymnasium. All exercises are directed away from their area of pain. Activity, cheerfulness and effort are praised whereas any demonstration of pain behaviour believed to be abnormal is ignored. Williams claims that most of these carefully selected patients show marked improvement within 3 weeks. She believes that concentrating on physical activity is particularly helpful as most patients strongly resent the suggestion that their pain is 'all in the mind'. No psychotherapy or counselling is given and professionals such as clinical psychologists are not involved. Thus the patient's view of the physiotherapist as someone who is concerned with his or her physical condition, seems to help the programme work. This raises an important ethical issue, however, for clearly the patients are not fully aware of the purpose behind the treatment.

Williams (1989) believes that patients awaiting compensation claims are particularly likely to display abnormal pain behaviour. However, Mendelson (1984) and Melzack *et al.* (1985) found that patients waiting for compensation did not differ psychologically from other patients and Melzack and Wall (1988) point out that pain tends to persist after compensation claims are settled. They warn of the danger of giving people derogatory and inappropriate labels.

Group dynamics can work in a negative as well as a positive direction. For example members may feel obliged to conform to the group norm or some members may succeed in gaining the attention of the physiotherapist while others remain in the background. Not everyone feels happy or confident in a group, or enjoys being treated with other people. Their wishes should be respected, any attempt to force them into a group situation is likely to be counter-productive.

Music

Music brings about physiological and psychological effects and may serve to direct the patient's attention away from the pain. Rozzano and Locsin (1981) found that music of the patient's own choosing aided recovery following surgery and Melzack and Wall (1988) make the point that music and rhythmic drumming often accompany healing ceremonies and probably have a hypnotic effect. Physiotherapists do use music, mostly to stimulate people when exercising in groups, but perhaps the use of music could be extended to help bring about pain relief.

Improving confidence and morale

It is sometimes the case that people reduce their activities, not so much because of the physical limitations of their illness, but because of fear and lack of confidence in their abilities (Feurstein and Beattie, 1995). The person who has recovered from a myocardial infarction, for example, may be afraid to resume even mild physical activity for fear that the chest pain will return. Similarly the person with osteoarthritis may be suffering more from the fear of pain than the pain itself.

Physiotherapists often devise programmes for such people designed to increased their exercise tolerance and reduce their pain by means of carefully graded exercises, along with health education and other treatments when appropriate. Although the programme is usually devised to bring about physiological improvement it is likely that in many cases the improvements seen are equally or more concerned with psychological change. The person who has had a myocardial infarction, for example, will realize that the physiotherapist is not alarmed at the prospect of him or her walking several miles a day, going back to work or riding a bicycle. Thus over a period of time patients undergoing programmes such as these may become confident in their ability to cope with their condition and may eventually define themselves as well rather than ill.

Other techniques

There are many other psychological methods which can be used to help the person in pain. These are not traditionally part of the physiotherapist's work but with the blurring of role boundaries and the growing availability of training, some physiotherapists may become involved. These techniques include psychoanalysis, family therapy, assertiveness training, visual imagery, acupuncture, aromatherapy, homeopathy, reflexology, meditation, various types of massage, diets and faith healing. The precise ways in which each of these therapies work and whether they are purely placebic is a matter of dispute. Much the same can be said, of course, of many of the more orthodox treatments which have been discussed. Many researchers, including Melzack and Wall (1988), have found that combining several methods for the relief of pain leads to greater success than relying on just one. This has important implications for the work of physiotherapists; it is probably unwise to become too devoted to any one technique.

Conclusion

There is no doubt that psychological and social strategies can be used either to reduce the patient's pain or to help him or her cope with it. Such strategies can be combined with each other or with the more familiar physical approaches of physiotherapy practice. To separate psychological from physical treatment is artificial, all of our treatments affect the patient psychologically, however technical they may seem. It is therefore vitally important that physiotherapists understand the nature of pain in all its complexity and treat the patient with this in mind. As Wall (1982) reminds us, 'the simplest of pains is not simple'.

References

Adams N., Ravey J., Bell G. (1994a) Review of personality characteristics in chronic back pain patients. *Physiotherapy*, **80**(8), 511–513.

Adams N., Ravey J., Bell G. (1994b) Investigation of personality characteristics in chronic low back pain patients attending physiotherapy out-patient departments. *Physiotherapy*, **80**(8), 514–519.

Baer E., Davitz L. S., Lieb R. (1970) Inferences of pain and psychological distress in relation to verbal and non-verbal communication. *Nursing Research*, **19**, 388–392.

Barsky A. J., Klerman J. L. (1983) Overview hypochondriasis, bodily complaints and somatic style. *American Journal of Psychiatry*, **140**(3), 273–283.

Beecher H. K. (1959) *Measurement of Subjective Responses*. Oxford: Oxford University Press.

Bendelow G. (1993) Pain: perceptions, emotions and gender. *Sociology of Health and Illness*, **15**(3), 274–294.

Blanchard E. B., Applebaum K. A., Guarnieri P., Morrill B., Dentinger M. P. (1987) Five year prospective follow-up on the treatment of chronic headache with biofeedback and/or relaxation. *Headache*, **27**(1), 580–583.

Bond M. R. (1984) *Pain: Its Nature, Analysis and Treatment* (2nd edn). London: Churchill Livingstone.

Burnard P. (1992) *Counselling: A Guide to Practice in Nursing*. Oxford: Butterworth-Heinemann.

Chapman S. L. (1986) A review and clinical perspective on the use of EMG and thermal biofeedback for chronic headaches. *Pain*, **27**, 1–43.

Crabbe G. (1989) Crossing the pain threshold. *Nursing Times*, **85**(47), 16–17.

Davison G. C., Neale J. M. (1990) *Abnormal Psychology* (5th edn). New York: John Wiley and Sons.

Davitz L. J., Davitz J. R. (1981) *Nurses' Response to Patients' Suffering*. New York: Springer.

Engel G. L. (1950) 'Psychogenic' pain and the pain-prone patient. *American Journal of Medicine*, **26**, 899–909.

Eysenck S. G. B. (1961) Cited in Rachman S. L. and Philips C. (1978) *Psychology and Medicine*. Harmondsworth: Penguin Books.

Fagerhaugh S. Y., Strauss A. (1977) *Politics of Pain Management: Staff–Patient Interaction*. Wokingham: Addison-Wesley.

Feuerstein M., Beattie P. (1995) Behavioural factors affecting pain and disability in low back pain: mechanisms and assessment. *Physical Therapy*, **75**(4), 267–280.

Flaberty G., Fitzpatrick J. (1978) Relaxation techniques to increase comfort levels of post-operative patients. *Nursing Research*, **27**, 352–355.

Flint C. (1988) Know your midwife. *Nursing Times*, **84**(38), 28–32.

Grieve G. P. (1987) Psychological aspects of benign spinal pain. *Physiotherapy*, **73**(9), 499–501.

Griffiths D. (1980) *Psychology and Medicine*. London: Macmillan Press.

Hall K. R. L., Stride E. (1954) The varying response to pain in psychiatric disorders: a study in abnormal psychology. *British Journal of Medical Psychology*, **27**, 48–60.

Hanson R. W., Gerber K. E. (1990) *Coping with Chronic Pain: A Guide to Self-Management*. London: The Guildford Press.

Harding V., de C. Williams A. C. (1995) Extending physiotherapy skills using a psychological approach: cognitive–behavioural management of chronic pain. *Physiotherapy*, **81**(11), 681–688.

Hardy J. D., Wolff H. G., Goodell H. (1952) *Pain Sensations and Reactions*. New York: Williams and Wilkins.

Helman C. G. (1994) *Culture, Health and Illness* (3rd edn). Bristol: John Wright.

Hellsing A., Linton S. (1989) Chronic headache treatment in an occupational setting: a pilot study. *Physiotherapy Practice*, **5**(1), 3–8.

Hill H. E., Kornetsky C. H., Flanary H. G., Wikler A. (1952a) Effects of anxiety and morphine on discrimination of intensities of painful stimuli. *Journal of Clinical Investigations*, **31**, 473–479.

Hill H. E., Kornetsky C. H., Flanary H. G., Wikler A. (1952b) Studies of anxiety associated with anticipation of pain. *Archives of Neurological Psychiatry*, **67**, 612–617.

Hough A. (1987) Communication in health care. *Physiotherapy*, **73**(2), 56–59.

Johnston M., Bromley I., Boothroyd-Brooks M., Dobbs W., Illson A., Ridout K. (1987) Behavioural assessment of physically disabled patients: agreement between rehabilitation therapists and nurses. *International Journal of Rehabilitation Research*, **10**(5), 205–213.

Kent G. (1986) Effect of pre-appointment inquiries on dental patients' post-appointment ratings of pain. *British Journal of Medical Psychology*, **59**, 97–100.

Klaber Moffett J. A., Richardson P. H. (1995) The influence of psychological variables on the development and perception of musculoskeletal pain. *Physiotherapy Theory and Practice*, **11**(1), 3–12.

Lenburg C. B., Glass H. P., Davitz L. J. (1970) Inferences of pain and psychological distress in relation to the stage of illness and occupation of the perceiver. *Nursing Research*, **19**, 392–398.

Ley P. (1988) *Communicating with Patients*. London: Croom Helm.

McCaffrey M. (1983) *Nursing the Patient in Pain* (2nd edn). London: Harper and Row.

Mathews A., Steptoe A. (1988) *Essential Psychology for Medical Practice*. London: Churchill Livingstone.

May B. (1991) Pain. In *The Psychology of Health: An Introduction* (Pitts M., Phillips K., eds). London: Routledge.

Melzack R., Perry C. (1980) Psychological control of pain. Cited in Melzack R., Wall P. (1988) *The Challenge of Pain*. Harmondsworth: Penguin Books.

Melzack R., Katz J., Jeans M. E. (1985) The role of compensation in chronic pain: analysis using a new method of scoring the McGill Pain Questionnaire. *Pain*, **23**, 101–102.

Mendelson G. (1984) Compensation pain complaints and psychological disturbance. *Pain*, **20**, 169–177.

Niven N., Robinson J. (1994) *The Psychology of Nursing Care*. London: Macmillan.

Peck C. (1982) *Controlling Chronic Pain*. London: Fontana.

Petrie A. A. (1967) *Individuality in Pain and Suffering*. Chicago: University of Chicago Press.

Philips H. C. (1987) Avoidance behaviour and its role in sustaining chronic pain. *Behaviour Research and Therapy*, **25**(4), 273–279.

Philips H. C. (1988) Changing chronic pain experience. *Pain*, **32**, 165–172.

Philips H. C., Jahanshahi M. (1986) The components of pain behaviour report. *Behaviour Research and Therapy*, **24**, 9117–9125.

Pilowski T., Spence N. (1977) Ethnicity and illness behaviour. *Psychological Medicine*, **7**, 447–452.

Pitts M., Healy S. (1989) Factors influencing the inferences of pain made by three health professions. *Physiotherapy Practice*, **5**(2), 65–69.

Price S. (1990) Pain: its experience, assessment and management in children. *Nursing Times*, **86**(9), 942–945.

Rachman S. J., Philips C. (1978) *Psychology and Medicine*. Harmondsworth: Penguin Books.

Rose M. J., Slade D. P., Reilly J. P., Dewey M. (1995) A comparative analysis of psychological and physical models of low back pain experience. *Physiotherapy*, **81**(12), 710–716.

Rosengren W. R., DeVault S. (1976) The sociology of time and space in an obstetrics hospital. In *Basic Readings in Medical Sociology* (Tuckett D., Kaufert J. M., eds). London: Tavistock Publications.

Rozzano G. R. A. C., Locsin A. C. (1981) The effect of music on the pain of selected post-operative patients. *Journal of Advanced Nursing*, **6**, 19–25.

Saxey S. (1986) Nurses' response to post-op pain. *Nursing Times*, **3**, 377–381.

Smith W. B. (1987) Biofeedback and relaxation training: the effect on headache and associated symptoms. *Headache*, **27**(9), 511–514.

Sofaer B. (1992) *Pain: A Handbook for Nurses* (2nd edn). London: Chapman and Hall.

Sternbach R. A., Tursky B. (1965) Ethnic differences among housewives in psychophysical and skin potential responses to electrical shock. *Psychophysiology*, **1**, 241–246.

Swain J. (1995) *The Use of Counselling Skills: A Guide for Therapists*. Oxford: Butterworth-Heinemann.

Wall P. (1982) The introduction. In *Controlling Chronic Pain* (Peck C., ed.). London: Fontana.

Weinman J. (1981) *An Outline of Psychology as Applied to Medicine*. Bristol: John Wright.

Williams A. C. C., Erskine A. (1995) Chronic pain. In *Health Psychology: processes and applications* (2nd edn) (Broome A., Llewelyn S., eds). London: Chapman and Hall.

Williams J. (1989) Illness behaviour to wellness behaviour. *Physiotherapy*, **75**(1), 2–7.

Wolff B. B., Langley S. (1977) Cultural factors and the response to pain. In *Culture, Disease and Healing: Studies in Medical Anthropology* (Landy D., ed.). New York: Macmillan.

Wolff M. S., Michel T. S., Krebs D. E., Watts N. T. (1991) Chronic Pain – assessment of orthopedic physical therapists' knowledge and attitudes. *Physical Therapist*, **71**(3), 209–214.

Wright S. (1987) Patient-centred practice. *Nursing Times*, **83**(38), 24–27.

Wynn Parry C. B. (1980) Pain in avulsion lesions of the brachial plexus. *Pain*, **9**, 41–53.

Zborowski M. (1952) Cultural components in responses to pain. *Journal of Social Issues*, **8**, 16–30.

Zborowski M. (1969) *People in Pain*. San Francisco: Jossey Bass.

Zola I. K. (1966) Culture and symptoms: an analysis of patients' presenting complaints. *American Sociological Review*, **31**, 615–638.

Psychological principles applied to sports injuries

Richard J. Butler

Introduction

Sporting performance might be typically construed as a fusion of an individual's physical attributes, technical competence and psychological skills. Whilst today this might be proclaimed as axiomatic, such a sentiment has not always been the case. Until quite recently there was but a tacit acknowledgement of the important part psychology plays in influencing a performance. Preparation for performance was bereft of psychological input yet the abiding rhetoric for failure was fashioned in terms of psychological detriment. Athletes tend to rationalize errors and below par performances in terms of depleted confidence, lapses of concentration or faulty strategy, whilst coaches typically accord the athlete's failure with choking under pressure, lacking motivation or abject failure to follow instructions. The dilemma of enlisting psychology as a worthy, if retrospective, account of performance, yet disregarding its potency in assisting the athlete to prepare for competition is now being addressed.

With success in sporting endeavour demanding ever greater sophistication of training methods, the astute coach is now engaged in a study of how best to harness and consolidate appropriate psychological approaches and techniques. The natural by-product is an invitation to the psychological community to play a part and offer its constellation of skills and ideas to sporting scrutiny.

Orlick and Partington (1988), in a comparative study of Olympic competitors, discovered the only factor which significantly distinguished those who performed well at the Games from those who underperformed was indeed the degree to which they had prepared psychologically. Many of the athletes who had employed psychological techniques in their training were able to exceed their personal bests despite the pressurized setting of the Olympic stage.

From a more qualitative and individualistic perspective the important role played by psychology is captured in the following comments, all of which adopt a theme of proportion. Ion Tiriac described tennis as, '80% head and 20% legs', Duncan Goodhew enthused that swimming is '95% of the time psychological', Jim Wolhford suggested, '90% of baseball is half mental', and the golfer Mark James said, 'Putting is 70% technique, 30% mental'. The psychological characteristics of successful performers has been examined quite extensively. Both Highlen and Bennett (1979) and Mahoney and Avener (1977) identified a proficiency to control anxiety, a high level of confidence, an adeptness to focus on the present and the applied use of imagery as seminal psychological factors.

More recent investigations have sought not necessarily to understand the characteristics of an athlete, but alternatively, have attempted to analyse the composition of exceptional performances. Garfield and Bennett (1984) and Gould *et al.* (1992a,b) have extrapolated physical relaxation, no fear of failure, confidence, freedom from distraction, being highly energized and a preparation for competition which includes the use of visualization, as common themes indicative of such performances.

Traditionally, the sports psychologist's role has involved facilitating such attributes with a desired attempt to raise the athlete's performance level and once raised, to formulate ways of securing consistently superior performances. Often referred to as mental skills training, this might be considered a narrow portrayal of psychology. The focus, much like the coach encouraging the acquisition and development of a technique, is instructional. Relaxation, confidence building, visualization and focusing become the cornerstones of a psychology programme.

A broader vista however invites a diverse and sundry range of influences for psychology. Syer (1989), for example, developed a notion that all sports specific skills – physical, technical and psychological – could be enhanced by the application of psychological techniques. Butler (1995) has drawn attention to other critical variables in determining performance, such as mental toughness and strategy, which may be enhanced and strengthened through the employment of psychological techniques. Further tasks for the psychologist, particularly at the elite level, involve generating a means of coping with pressure (Anshel, 1994), dealing with slumps in form (Prapavessis and Grove, 1995), developing appropriate attributions for performance (Van Raalte, 1994) and enhancing team spirit and communication (Slater and Sewell, 1994). There are additionally many instances when athletes and coaches are faced with difficulties, of both a sporting and personal nature, where problem solving skills, counselling and clinical interventions prove helpful. Finally, and apposite in this context, is the role psychology has to play when an athlete is injured.

Whilst many psychologists initially adopted a role of 'expert' in educating athletes and coaches in psychological approaches, a more recent model favoured by an increasing number of psychologists is the one of 'equal expertise', whereby athlete, coach and psychologist are each considered expert in his or her field (Butler, 1995; Terry, 1996). The athlete arrives with a broad understanding of his or her strengths, weaknesses, recent progress, aspirations and so forth; the coach understands the schemata of demands and pressures of competition and the strategies needed for success; the psychologist has a grasp of the processes which might be invoked to improve performance. Employing the virtuosity of each improves the chances of success. Not only does the athlete heed what the coach and psychologist suggest, but imperatively the coach and psychologist discover the athlete's distinctive ways. Butler developed a process called 'Performance Profiling' which facilitates an understanding of the athlete, and enables the coach and/or psychologist to generate training strategies appropriate to the athlete's needs (Butler and Hardy, 1992; Butler *et al.*, 1993; Butler, 1995). The model of equal expertise can be justly adapted to encompass all members of the sports science team working with the athlete and coach – nutritionist, exercise physiologist or biomechanic. The governing philosophy brings the athlete's needs into relief, expanding an understanding of the athlete which can be taken into account and embodied in the design of a training programme, a process which increases the athlete's commitment to the programme. The delicate balance of designing a training plan thus hinges on valid contributions and ultimately a sense of appropriate ownership.

The injured athlete

As far as the athlete remains free from injury this network, or relationship with the coach and sport scientist operates well. However, injury generally triggers a more anomalous, and much less intensive relationship with the coach. With a team, or group of individuals to manage, a coach is inexorably more inclined to maintain a focus on their training schedule, than become 'distracted' by the fervent needs of those who are injured or out of action. That is not to imply the coach becomes insensitive to the injured athlete's dilemma, but in reality the commitment, and in many respects, the duty of the coach is directed towards those preparing for competition.

Metaphorically the injured athlete thus steps, or limps, into an unknown arena. An arena in which the physiotherapist becomes, in many respects, the foremost contact for the athlete. Not only will the physiotherapist deal with the injury but also learn to treat and support the athlete as an individual. Cockerill (1992) reflects on a comparative acceleration of recovery where physiotherapists show interest in athletes as people rather than exclusively attend to their injuries. Just as the coach is pivotal in the training schedule, the physiotherapist is central to the recovery schedule. Also, just as it is palpably obvious that the effective coach employs psychological techniques, through tuition or intuition, then it is equally clear the effective physiotherapist does likewise. Indeed, both Gordon *et al.* (1991) and Pearson and Jones (1992) stress how the close relationship between physiotherapist and athlete places the physiotherapist in an ideal position to apply psychological principles.

Applying the 'equal expertise' model with the injured athlete is also intrinsically valid. Effective recovery demands an understanding of the athlete's predicament – the impact of the injury, his or her commitment to return to action, the effects of exclusion from the team and so forth. The medical fraternity apply diagnostic techniques to further an understanding of the degree of injury, whilst the physiotherapists plan and instigate a rehabilitation programme based on their expansive knowledge of the most effective course of action. The psychologist's input might best be construed as providing a broad understanding of the emotional consequences of injury and the application of psychological techniques to promote rapid recovery from injury.

Wiese and Weiss (1987) elaborated this role by suggesting a credible input for the sports psychologist might include:

1. An awareness of the cause of injury, leading to an appreciation of the potential risk factors, culminating ideally in preventative measures to alleviate the physical and psychological suffering.

2. An understanding of the impact of injury for the athlete.
3. The generation of psychological methods to assist the rehabilitation process, taking into account notions about the favourable time for a return to competition.

Causative factors in injury

A corpus of knowledge concerning the likely antecedents of injury is steadily accumulating. Familiarity with factors which increase the risk of injury encourages a greater sense of awareness amongst both athletes and coaches, and further implies a requirement to monitor those aspects carefully during a training programme. A range of risk factors includes:

1. The demands of the sport – some sports, especially contact events unequivocally increase the risk of injury. However, even in sports such as figure skating, synchronized swimming and gymnastics, where physical attractiveness is perceived by the athlete to play a key part in success, the prevalence of eating disorders is high, with a consequent increased vulnerability to problems such as stress fractures (Lloyd *et al.*, 1986).
2. The increased pressures to succeed – to maintain a level of success many athletes push themselves to the limit, and are expected to continue to do so at ever greater frequency as the rate of competition increases. An expectation that immoderate effort is expended in order to achieve results, encourages athletes to take risks which potentially increases the likelihood of injury. To maintain a place on the team, a professional ranking, retain a sponsor or avoid being considered unreliable, an athlete may struggle to play through pain and injury, reluctant to report any injury, thus increasing the possibility of a more chronic injury arising (Tajet-Foxell and Rose, 1995).
3. The athlete's capacity to cope with stress – a concept of 'injury proneness' has regularly been mooted to explain why some individuals seem to suffer a recurrence of injury. There is, however, little empirical evidence to support such a thesis which aligns the problem with the personality of the athlete (Lamb, 1986; Williams *et al.*, 1986). Nevertheless there is evidence accumulating which supports the notion that an increase in life events may precede injury. A life event is typically defined as a situation, such as moving house, becoming married, or losing a job, which necessitates the individual having to make changes or adaptations to his or her life style. Many such situations create stress for the individual, and indeed the 'life event' theory is fundamentally based on an assumption that such events are inherently stressful. It may not, however, be the magnitude of the life event itself which is crucial, but the athlete's perception of how severely it disrupts daily functioning, and additionally how adept the athlete is in coping with such events. Interestingly Williams *et al.* (1986) found that minor or day-to-day 'hassles' can predict the occurrence of injury equally as well as major life stresses. Kerr and Fowler (1988) suggest life events may prove distracting for athletes, thus leading to vacillations in focusing on the essential performance requirements. Alternatively, or compoundingly, a further intervening factor,

suggested by Kerr and Fowler (1988) could be fatigue, both physical and psychological, which contributes to the individual's susceptibility to injury.

4. Pain – the climate of modern sport desires, perhaps even demands, that athletes play or compete with pain. The maxim 'no pain, no gain' stoically prevails. Heil (1993) suggests playing with pain is often encouraged whereas playing with injury is generally discouraged. However, the distinction between the two can become indistinct especially where athletes interpret pain positively and re-label the experience as exertion. Heil (1993) has attempted to formulate a discrimination between pain which is harmless – dull, not persisting after activity and not associated with swelling – from pain which could have long-term detrimental consequences – sharp, localized, persists after exercise and is accompanied by swelling – which should be regarded as a sign for discontinuing exercise.

5. Fear of re-injury – the daunting thought of having to cope again with injury leads some athletes to 'overprotect' or become acutely sensitive to the previously injured area. This in turn may create increased muscular tension, and a distracted focus leading to poorer performance and increased vulnerability to further injury, a scenario undoubtedly familiar for those athletes who fail to achieve the zenith of previous performances despite a full return to physical fitness.

6. Returning to competition too early – some athletes increase the risk of further injury or delay the recovery process by their eagerness to return prematurely to training.

Monitoring physical and psychological states

Whilst clearly not all injuries are predictable, an understanding of those factors which increase the risk of injury suggests a way forward in terms of preventing injury. Many psychologists argue that an athlete's vulnerability to injury is manifest in his or her physical and emotional state. Thus an athlete at risk of injury because of a pressure to succeed or recent life events, for example, will exhibit physical and/or emotional signs. Inviting the athlete to monitor his or her physical and emotional state fairly regularly during training can prove remarkably helpful in this context. This is also consistent with Kerr and Fowler's (1988) suggestion that day-to-day, repeated measures of the athlete's state is likely to be the most sensitive way of capturing the degree of stress the athlete is experiencing. It is also in accord with Rotella and Heyman's (1986) notion that the coach and support services should be constantly monitoring the athlete's state in order to identify who might be at risk of injury.

Many psychologists have elected to use the Profile of Mood Scales (POMS), an adjective checklist designed to tap transient emotional states (McNair *et al.*, 1971), to monitor the athlete during turbulent personal times, intensive training schedules or the build up to a major competition (Morgan *et al.*, 1987; Terry, 1996). Abbreviated versions of POMS (Grove and Prapavessis, 1992) and visually constructed displays of emotional state (Butler, 1995) offer feasible and practical means of monitoring the athlete's emotional reactions and phases.

Kerr and Fowler (1988) suggest when an athlete shows a dramatic change in his or her emotional state, there is a need to:

1. reduce training intensity;
2. emphasize the perfecting of basic skills;
3. vary the training techniques;
4. employ exercises which reduce the stress experienced by the athlete such as relaxation, massage, sauna and swimming;
5. provide the athlete with an opportunity to explore the causes of stress and possible options or solutions he or she might employ.

The impact of injury

Most athletes experience injury, especially serious injury, as traumatic. The abrupt halt to activity initiates a series of challenges. The higher the level of competition, because of the wider implications of being out of action, the more distressing an injury is likely to be. Some theorists have postulated that the grief response – as described when people experience loss – adequately generalizes to the scenario athletes undergo when they become injured (Gordon, 1986; Oglesby, 1988). However, Smith *et al.*, (1990) argue that athletes do not enter the grief cycle, but rather experience a range of emotional states simultaneously. The impact of an injury can be condensed and understood in terms of anxiety, threat and hostility.

Anxiety may be conceptualized as the individual's difficulty in predicting the events with which he or she is faced (Bannister and Fransella, 1986). The injured athlete is confronted with a series of questions, the answers to which are unknown. It is the inability to predict which creates the feeling of anxiety. Chan and Grossman (1988) found injured runners were more likely to report anxiety than uninjured contemporaries. Thus instead of adopting the usual committed, focused and goal-directed approach to training and competition, injury forces a major shift of thinking. Important issues are suddenly and inextricably unable to be addressed in the same 'professional' manner. Typical issues for the injured athlete to grapple with include:

1. the seriousness of the injury;
2. the extent of lay off;
3. the lost opportunities;
4. the loss of a place on the team;
5. the loss of financial security and sponsor's interest.

Threat has been defined as an awareness of an imminent change in the individual's construing of self (Bannister and Fransella, 1986). Athletes frequently project their identity as closely enmeshed in their sport. They find it difficult to see themselves as anything but a competitor. It is difficult to contemplate how they will function or construe themselves as someone not participating in their event. Boris Becker recently described tennis as defining his individuality, without which he would fail to be unique, an inclination which served to maintain his interest in the sport and search for continual improvement. As Heil (1993) reflects, because athletes are so dependent on their physical skills and because their identities are so wrapped up in their sport, injury is enormously threatening. Wacquant (1995) provides a further evocative example from the field of boxing in stating that, 'because it demands and effects a far reaching restructuring of the self as well as an integral colonisation of one's lifeworld, boxing is what they *are*: it defines at once their innermost identity, their practical attachments and everyday doings'.

Having constructed a well elaborated sense of self as an active and participating athlete, a change in self-construing is threatened when an injury occurs. The athlete can no longer validate notions of him or herself as an active sportsperson, but has to make a re-construction in self-concept. Lost are the opportunities for elaborating the self as active, competitive, and in control. Unable to put him or herself to the test, with ambitions thwarted, the injured athlete is faced with a dramatic revision of the sense of self.

McGowan *et al.* (1994) empirically demonstrated the loss in self-worth following injury, during a prospective study of American football players. Interestingly, 16 of the 29 players studied during the season long study, were injured severely enough to prevent them competing. Chan and Grossman (1988) also found a loss of self-esteem, measured by the Rosenberg Self Esteem Inventory, in a group of runners prevented from running for 2 weeks as a result of injury.

Hostility might be seen as the continued effort to seek evidence in favour of a prediction which has already been ruled out (Bannister and Fransella, 1986). This surfaces immediately as disbelief (Weiss and Troxel, 1986) or a playing down of the problem and may subsequently result in a denial of the seriousness or extent of the injury. If the athlete agrees to physiotherapy, he or she may subtly seek to undermine treatment, in order to maintain a view of self as not injured. Thus, as Gordon *et al.* (1991) suggest, an indicator of denial or non-acceptance of injury is a reluctance to change a life style to accommodate the injury. The athlete strives to continue as if not injured. Manifestations of this include playing through the pain and injury and attempting to return to competition before being fully physically fit, Smith *et al.* (1990) provide an interesting interpretation of denial in suggesting that some athletes may prefer the physical discomfort of continued participation in the presence of an injury, rather than experience the prospect of 'emotional discomfort' which may accompany the cessation of exercise. If, and when, the athlete finally acknowledges an injury and its implications, frustration and anger surface (Quackenbush and Crossman, 1994). Smith *et al.* (1990) found anger especially noticeable in younger, seriously injured athletes, and suggest it is directed at self, team mates, the coach, equipment, opponents, referees and physicians.

Support

Eldridge (1983) highlights the lack of support many athletes encounter in coming to terms with the emotional trauma of injury and how few opportunities they have to reconcile the turmoil of sudden loss of such a significant part of their life. The provision of what has been called 'social support' has been described as one of the central tenets of rehabilitation (Heil, 1993; Brewer *et al.*, 1994), enabling the athlete to protect him or herself from a perception of social isolation which seems invariably to occur alongside injury. Both adherence to treatment (Levy, 1983; Fisher *et al.*, 1988) and favourable progress in rehabilitation (Gordon *et al.*, 1991; Wiese *et al.* 1991) are facilitated by effective social support.

Structuring social support for the athlete will invariably involve a number of people. The role of the physiotherapist is especially crucial given the extended contact an athlete is likely to have through the course of injury. A particular dilemma for the athlete is realized in voicing how he or she feels given that the athlete is ordinarily expected, in order to perform well, to have developed a flawless means of controlling his or her emotional state. The independent role of the physiotherapist is invaluable in providing the support of encouragement, protection, allegiance and understanding. So too are other members of the team – coach, team mates, physician, psychologist – in addition to 'outside' support from family, spouse and friends.

An often unresolved quandary for many injured athletes is reflected in the choice of maintaining solace and contact with the team, but which invariably breeds frustration at watching former team mates from the sidelines. Oglesby (1988) suggested that athletes might maintain a relationship with the team and coach to lessen the feeling of loneliness and alienation. Wiese and Weiss (1987) indicate a range of participatory roles including assisting in keeping scores, times and statistics, helping the coach officiate and providing feedback and encouragement to team members.

Social support can invariably take a range of forms:

1. Explanation of how the injury will heal and specific information about rehabilitation methods will ease the athlete's uncertainty and anxiety. Heil (1993) remarks on the significance of such education in assisting athletes to recover quickly and effectively. One goal must be to ensure athletes are not left with unanswered questions or an inadequate understanding of the injury. Heil (1993), Weiss and Troxell (1986) and Wiese and Weiss (1987) have provided a comprehensive list of areas to cover in educating athletes about injury. This incorporates basic anatomy of the injured area, changes causes by the injury, a description of rehabilitation methods and the reasons for such interventions, the anticipated timetable for rehabilitation, what to expect in terms of pain, mobility and recovery, possibility of treatment plateaux or setbacks, rationale for limits on daily activity, injury as a source of stress itself and long-term maintenance and care of the healing injury.
2. Reassurance provides a means of helping athletes to cope with anxiety. Providing clear information on the nature of the injury and the expected outcome, along with a description of the athlete's role in recovery is essential in this process (Smith *et al.*, 1990). Perceiving injury as something of an 'occupational hazard' can be helpful in encouraging athletes to construe the situation as a challenge.
3. Counselling offers the athlete an opportunity of expressing his or her concerns privately, detached from those individuals who have a vested interest in the athlete's return to athletic activity (Smith *et al.*,

1990; Brewer *et al.*, 1994). Eldrige (1983) provides a schema for under-standing the meaning injury has for an athlete. This involves addressing the significance sporting activity plays in the athlete's life; the impact injury has on self-esteem, dependency, body image, perceived competence and achievement of goals; an exploration of current life stresses; and identification of personal strengths and competencies which can play a part in developing appropriate and positive coping strategies.

4. Peer modelling involves setting up a liaison between the injured athlete and another athlete who has previously incurred a similar injury and who has made a successful recovery (Weiss and Troxell, 1986). Such a relationship can provide support through an empathic understanding coupled with a model for the injured athlete of how to overcome the predicament of inactivity.

Following injury an athlete may start to spend an inordinate amount of time at physiotherapy. This may reflect the need an athlete has for both the intense physiotherapeutic contact, but also for psychological support. Alternatively, the contact may serve to reinforce the athlete's notion of him or herself as injured, which in turn may be a protective mechanism in serving to rationalize not being selected for the team, being substituted, being dropped into the second team or having not performed up to expectation.

Psychological methods to assist rehabilitation

Heil (1993) notes that the impact of an injury is the net effect of the stress and emotional consequences of the injury itself coupled with the athlete's coping resources. As Heil (1993) again astutely observes, in contrast to the non-athlete, the athlete is uniquely challenged by injury, and particularly well prepared to cope with it, by virtue of an expertise in seeking challenges, mental toughness and goal setting skills. Athletes are further characterized by their need to feel they are doing something. Advice to rest is therefore not something an athlete readily welcomes or will adhere to. What differentiates athletes who seemingly cope successfully with injury from athletes who become enmeshed in the trauma of injury may be summarized as follows:

1. They put the injury into perspective by seeking to understand the impact and anticipated recovery, accepting restrictions the injury places on them and acknowledging that injury is part of an athletic career (Gordon *et al.*, 1991).
2. They adopt an attitude of taking control, devoting time and effort to what can be done rather than bemoaning their luck and their lot. Taking an active involved stance to injury might involve the following:
   - undertaking exercises to maintain both the strength of uninjured limbs and the general aerobic conditioning of the athlete (Smith *et al.* 1990).
   - working on aspects of performance which might, whilst actively engaged in training, have been neglected, such as developing a

greater tactical awareness, improvement or fine tuning of a technical skill, the incorporation of psychological skills such as visualization or planning, and an increased understanding of the role nutrition might play in improving performance.
- undertake a programme of study related to their sport (Weiss and Troxell, 1986), involving perhaps reading books or watching films and videos of competitions to develop an in-depth assessment of strategy, history and influential factors.
- develop adjuncts which might assist in the athlete's performance when fully recovered, such as collecting and editing a video of the athlete's best performances to incorporate into a programme of confidence building.

3. Interventions of a psychological nature have been advocated to improve the psychological state of the injured athlete, increase the athlete's commitment to rehabilitation and facilitate the physical rehabilitation of injured athletes (Weiss and Troxell, 1986; Smith *et al.*, 1990; Fisher *et al.*, 1993; Rotella and Heyman, 1993). They should always be integrated into the physical rehabilitation programme, so that psychological interventions are not construed as extra or additional (Brewer *et al.*, 1994). The most common interventions include:
   - Goal setting. Gould (1986) and Weiss and Troxel (1986) suggest the athlete's commitment to rehabilitation and inherent sense of achievement will be enhanced where goals, specific and measurable, and owned by the athlete are established. Simplified by Wiese and Weiss (1987) into 'Who? Will do what? By when?' goals help form direction, provide a positive climate for intervention and set challengeable yet realistic targets. Once set, the athlete requires strategies for accomplishing the goals, and the physiotherapist's role here is crucial, in designing the necessary techniques. Additionally, the enthusiastic athlete may be encouraged to record progress through diaries, graphs or contracts.
   - Visualization. Usually accompanied by relaxation, the athlete may initially be assisted in coping with the stress and anxiety associated with the injury, in addition to the pain (Rotella and Heyman, 1986). Heil (1993) has tabled a range of images such as ultrasound creating a 'healing glow' which athletes may incorporate to help in the healing process. Formulating an image of the self returning to competitive participation and visualizing the execution of difficult skills have further been advocated as useful for the injured athlete (Gordon, 1986; Weiss and Troxel, 1986; Wiese and Weiss, 1987).
   - Cognitive restructuring. There is a tendency amongst injured athletes to dwell on the drama of tragedy, to construct avenues of negative thinking about themselves and a future return to sport. Central to any programme of physical rehabilitation must be a theme of developing a positive approach to the rehabilitation tasks and a realistic anticipatory schemata of the future. Rotella and Heyman (1986) and Weiss and Troxell (1986) describe some technical approaches to enable athletes to alter the way they construe themselves and injury, involving an identification of the causative

stress and their reaction to it, the development of more effective coping strategies, and the implementation of such positive approaches.

Despite the increasing employment of psychological interventions in rehabilitation, Brewer *et al.* (1994) correctly suggest, such interventions have yet to be empirically tested with the injured athlete. It might be assumed that only those methods which are perceived as credible and acceptable to the injured athlete will prove beneficial or effective (Ievleva and Orlick, 1991). Brewer *et al.* (1994) did find that psychological interventions were on the whole considered in a favourable light.

Integration of psychological approaches with physiotherapy input would seem the way forward. The psychologist's role, whilst always in collaboration with the physiotherapist, would appear to increase where circumstances lead to particular problems of adjustment. Such times might include:

1. The timing of the injury. The impact of injury tends to be more severe if it happens close to or during a major competition, or late in the season (Gordon *et al.*, 1991).
2. The severity of the injury, perhaps leading to retirement issues.
3. The chronic nature of the injury, caused by the athlete underplaying or ignoring the severity of the injury and playing on through it.
4. The emotional impact, particularly when severe, might invite referral to clinical psychology services.
5. The perception of the injury, especially where the athlete 'over-generalizes' to the extent of believing his or her life style is under threat, or where an attribution of being out of control, leaves the athlete feeling impotent to influence the rehabilitation process.
6. Where the athlete expresses a fear of future injury.
7. Where the athlete's incapacity is profoundly linked with psychological aetiology, such as pathological weight control behaviours (Parker *et al.*, 1994), bulimia or psychosomatic complains.

Conclusion

Heil (1993) has developed a set of principles which richly encapsulate the psychological stance with the injured athlete:

1. Preventing and coping with injury is, like playing sport well, something the athlete must actively address if success is to be forthcoming.
2. Rehabilitation from injury relies on much the same skills as employed in sport performance.
3. Effective return to play depends not only on physical function, but also on psychological status.
4. The athlete who has physically recovered from injury but remains psychologically unprepared to compete is not fully recovered.
5. Treatment effectiveness is enhanced when the athlete feels confident with the treatment providers.
6. The athlete remains actively involved in decision-making and the role required in rehabilitation.

7. Treatment effectiveness is improved when the athlete senses an alliance between those professionals responsible for delivering the care and rehabilitation.

The role of the physiotherapist in facilitating athletes' recovery from injury is, without question, pivotal. An intuitive understanding of psychological principles often underpins the treatment approaches adopted by physiotherapists. This chapter has emphasized the important role physiotherapists have in the psychological care of injured athletes. It has also sought to explore the breadth of psychological influences involved in sports injury, taking as a particular focus, the requirement to understand each individual's unique perspective on injury. An acknowledgement of the 'expertness' of the athlete generally facilitates a confidence in the physiotherapist which tends to increase the effectiveness of a chosen intervention. Inviting physiotherapists to develop their psychological know-how should further strengthen their crucial role in assisting athletes to recover from what is increasingly being seen as an occupational hazard – injury.

Acknowledgements

I am grateful to the Sports Council through the SSSP project with amateur boxing for their support of my applied psychological work. I am also indebted to Britt Tajet-Foxell, Emma Hiley and Gillian Roberts for their comments and suggestions during the various stages of writing the chapter.

References

Anshel M. H. (1994) A test of the COPE model on motor performance and affect. *Perceptual and Motor Skills*, **78**, 1016–1018.

Bannister D., Fransella F. (1986) *Inquiring Man: The Psychology of Personal Constructs*. Beckenham: Croom Helm.

Brewer B. W., Jeffers K. E., Petitpas A. J., Van Raalte J. L. (1994) Perceptions of psychological interventions in the context of sport injury rehabilitation. *Sport Psychologist*, **8**, 176–188.

Butler R. J. (1995) *Sports Psychology in Action*. Oxford: Butterworth-Heinemann.

Butler R. J., Hardy L. (1992) The Performance Profile: theory and application. *Sport Psychologist*, **6**, 27–46.

Butler R. J., Smith M., Irwin I. (1993) The Performance Profile in practice. *Journal of Applied Sport Psychology*, **5**, 48–63.

Chan G. S., Grossman, H. Y. (1988) Psychological effects of running loss on consistent runners. *Perceptual and Motor Skills*, **66**, 875–883.

Cockerill, I. M. (1992) Psychological aspects of sports injuries and overtraining. In *Physiotherapy: A Psychosocial Approach* (French S., ed.). Oxford: Butterworth-Heinemann.

Eldridge W. D. (1983) The importance of psychotherapy for athletic related orthopedic injuries among adults. *International Journal of Sport Psychology*, **14**, 203–211.

Fisher A. C., Domm M. A., Wuest D. A. (1988) Adherence to sports-injury rehabilitation programs. *Physician and Sportsmedicine*, **16**, 47–52.

Fisher A. C., Mullins S. A., Frye P. A. (1993) Athletic trainers' attitudes and judgements of injured athletes' rehabilitation adherence. *Journal of Athletic Training*, **28**, 43–47.

Garfield C. A., Bennett H. Z. (1984) *Peak Performance: Mental Training Techniques of the World's Greatest Athletes*. Los Angeles: Tarcher.

Gordon S. (1986) Sport psychology and the injured athlete: A cognitive–behavioural approach to injury response and injury rehabilitation. *Science*

Periodical on Research and Technology in Sport. Ottowa: Coaching Association of Canada.

Gordon S., Milios D., Grove J. R. (1991) Psychological aspects of the recovery process from sport injury: the perspective of sport physiotherapists. *Australian Journal of Science and Medicine in Sport*, **6**, 53–60.

Gould D. (1986) Goal setting for peak performance. In *Applied Sport Psychology: Personal Growth to Peak Performance* (Williams J., ed.). Palo Alto, CA: Mayfield.

Gould D., Eklund R. C., Jackson S. A. (1992a) 1988 US Olympic wrestling excellence: I. Mental preparation, precompetitive cognition and affect. *Sport Psychologist*, **6**, 358–382.

Gould D., Eklund R. C., Jackson S. A. (1992b) 1988 US Olympic wrestling excellence: II. Thoughts and affect occurring during competition. *Sport Psychologist*, **6**, 383–402.

Grove R. J., Prapavessis H. (1992) Preliminary evidence for the reliability and validity of an abbreviated Profile of Mood States. *International Journal of Sport Psychology*, **23**, 93–109.

Heil J. (1993) *Psychology of Sport Injury*. Champaign, Ill: Human Kinetics.

Highlen P. S., Bennett B. B. (1979) Psychological characteristics of successful and non-successful elite wrestlers: an exploratory study. *Journal of Sport Psychology*, **1**, 123–137.

Ievleva L., Orlick T. (1991) Mental links to enhanced healing: an exploratory study. *Sport Psychologist*, **5**, 25–40.

Kerr G., Fowler B. (1988) The relationship between psychological factors and sports injuries. *Sports Medicine*, **6**, 127–134.

Lamb M. (1986) Self concept and injury frequency among female college field hockey players. *Athletic Training*, **21**, 220–224.

Levy R. L. (1983) Social support and compliance: a selective review and critique of treatment integrity and outcome measurement. *Social Science and Medicine*, **17**, 1329–1338.

Lloyd T., Trianthafyllou S. T., Baker E. R. *et al.* (1986) Women athletes with menstrual irregularity have increased musculoskeletal injuries. *Medicine and Science in Sports and Exercise*, **18**, 374–379.

McGowan R. W., Peirce E. F., Williams M., Eastman N. W. (1994) Athletic injury and self diminution. *Journal of Sports Medicine and Physical Fitness*, **34**, 299–304.

McNair D., Lorr M., Droppleman L. (1971) *Manual for the Profile of Mood States*. San Diego, CA: Educational and Industrial Testing Service.

Mahoney M. J., Avener M. (1977) Psychology of the elite athlete: an exploratory study. *Cognitive Therapy and Research*, **1**, 135–142.

Morgan W. P., Brown D. R., Raglin J. S., O'Connor P. J., Ellickson K. A. (1987) Psychological monitoring of overtraining and staleness. *British Journal of Sports Medicine*, **21**, 107–114.

Oglesby C. (1988) Coaches can help the injured cope. *American Coach*, March/April, 10.

Orlick T., Partington J. (1988) Mental links to excellence. *Sport Psychologist*, **2**, 105–130.

Parker R. M., Lambert M. J., Burlingame G. M. (1994) Psychological features of female runners presenting with pathological weight control behaviours. *Journal of Sport and Exercise Psychology*, **16**, 119–134.

Pearson L., Jones G. (1992) Emotional effects of sports injuries: implications for physiotherapists. *Physiotherapy*, **78**, 762–770.

Prapavessis H., Grove J. R. (1995) Ending batting slumps in baseball: a qualitative investigation. *Australian Journal of Science and Medicine in Sport*, **27**, 14–19.

Quakenbush N., Crossman J. (1994) Injured athletes: a study of emotional responses. *Journal of Sport Behaviour*, **17**, 178–187.

Rotella R. J., Heyman S. R. (1986) Stress, injury and the psychological rehabilitation of athletes. In *Applied Sport Psychology: Personal Growth to Peak Performance* (Williams J. M., ed.). Mountain View, CA: Mayfield.

Slater M. R., Sewell D. F. (1994) An examination of the cohesion–performance relationship in university hockey teams. *Journal of Sports Sciences*, **12**, 423–431.

Smith A. M., Scott S. G., Wiese D. M. (1990) The psychological effects of sports injuries: coping. *Sports Medicine*, **9**, 352–369.

Syer J. (1989) *Team Spirit*. London: Simon & Schuster.

Tajet-Foxell B., Rose F. D. (1995) Pain and pain tolerance in professional ballet dancers. *British Journal of Sports Medicine*, **29**, 31–34.

Terry P. (1996) The application of mood profiling with elite performers. In *Sport Psychology in Performance* (Butler R. J., ed.). Oxford: Butterworth-Heinemann.

Van Raalte J. L. (1994) Sport performance attributions: a special case of self serving. *Australian Journal of Science and Medicine in Sport*, **26**, 45–48.

Wacquant L. J. D. (1995) Through the fighter's eyes: boxing as a moral and sensual world. In *Boxing and Medicine* (Cantu R. C., ed.). Champaign, ILL: Human Kinetics.

Weiss M. R., Troxell, R. K. (1986) Psychology of the injured athlete. *Athletic Training*, **21**, 104–109.

Wiese D. M., Weiss M. R. (1987) Psychological rehabilitation and physical injury: implications for the sport medicine team. *Sport Psychologist*, **1**, 318–330.

Wiese D. M., Weiss M. R., Yukelson D. P. (1991) Sport psychology in the training room: a survey of athletic trainers. *Sport Psychologist*, **5**, 15–24.

Williams J. M., Tonymon P., Wadsworth W. A. (1986) Relationship of life stress to injury in intercollegiate volleyball. *Journal of Human Stress*, **12**, 38–43.

12

Death, dying and bereavement
Mary F. McAteer

Physiotherapy is a dynamic profession where there has been an increasing need to justify the treatments based on clinical reasoning and published work. The age of high technology, outcomes measures and audit has dawned. Physiotherapy aspires to be highly academic but is, perhaps, becoming insufficiently intuitive. Hollenbery (1994) is concerned that the current approach may lead to a lack of sensitivity to the real needs of patients.

Thanatology, the study of death and its related phenomena and rituals, is a vast resource which may be used by practising physiotherapists. It embraces academic literature, fiction, poetry, philosophy and theology. The medical literature on death and dying tends to be inaccessible to the general public, though the profession of nursing and the academic disciplines of psychology and sociology have made some attempts to disseminate their knowledge to the wider public readership. While it is obvious that a more cohesive approach to the understanding of death, dying and bereavement would be beneficial, a proper understanding must always embrace the vast range of human experiences. Death cannot be the sole preserve of any one profession or group of carers (Dickenson and Johnson, 1993). This brief exploration of such a vast subject area must serve only as an introduction to thanatology for physiotherapists who want to embrace this field of study. It concentrates on death, dying and bereavement in the developed world.

Death and dying are of universal concern (Feifel, 1990). Many physiotherapists encounter death in their professional lives on an almost daily basis since approximately 70% of all deaths occur in public sector facilities of one sort or another. Purtillo (1972) recognized that the family of a patient may also wish to discuss death-related topics with the physiotherapist. The purpose of this chapter is not to help the physiotherapist to become a bereavement counsellor, but to enable him or her to care, to communicate and to help which is the essence of all counselling processes. Counselling skills are at the heart of all human relationships, and human relationships are important in the work of all formal and informal carers and helpers (Swain, 1995).

The historical perspective

Death in the last years of the twentieth century is shaped by the secularist and consumerist society in which we live. Euphemistic language describes how the deceased has 'passed away' or 'gone home', rarely stating the fact that he or she has died. The various arts and sciences of the undertaker ensure that many people look better in death than they did in life. In many graveyards coffins are not interred in the ground in the presence of mourners but are placed on grass-like mats to be committed to the earth only when the mourners have left the cemetery. Behaviours such as these serve to illustrate the vain attempts that people employ to help deny the reality of death. Historically death and dying were dramatic but natural events which took place in the family arena. Death was common in all age groups before the discovery of antibiotics. Many people lived within multi-generational family units dependent upon the resources available within that unit. With this type of inter-generational life style, birth and death were viewed as natural aspects of the life cycle. This family structure has largely disappeared in modern, industrialized and urbanized communities and death no longer impinges so frequently on people's lives.

Before this century many people died in the prime of life leaving spouses, children and other dependents. Death-bed, funeral and mourning rituals helped the survivors deal with their loss. Religion was a potent force. Declining religious practices in many countries, coupled with the fact that most deaths now occur in the elderly population has meant that many rituals have been abandoned in some cases because there are few, if any, survivors. Walter (1993) contends, however, that the poor have always been buried without much ritual and are probably dispatched with more respect in today's welfare state than in any other epoch. Two women, outstanding in their work to lift the taboo on death have been Dame Cicely Saunders, founder of the British hospice movement, and Dr Elizabeth Kübler-Ross who tirelessly promoted openness with dying patients by talking about their illnesses and feelings.

It is inevitable that physiotherapists are coming into contact with more older people as the age profile of the population increases. Many patients referred for physiotherapy will be in the palliative or terminal phases of treatment, while others will have been bereaved themselves. As a requirement of humane care, the physiotherapist will be expected to cope with grief states of varying types and intensities. The ability to cope with issues surrounding death and dying will be influenced by personal beliefs and philosophies as much as by education and training programmes. Purtillo (1972), writing about the physiotherapist as part of the death-denying society, searched through 12 years of publications of *Physical Therapy* (an American journal) to find only two articles written on the subject, neither of which were written by a physiotherapist. The paucity of articles in this journal, as well as the British journal *Physiotherapy*, is similar to the present day. The dearth of literature is indicative of how the area of death, dying and bereavement has been neglected by physiotherapists.

Terminal illness

A common perception that people have is that cancer and terminal illness are synonymous, and while this is often the case it is not necessarily so. Physiotherapists are involved in the management of a wide variety of terminal conditions which may be vascular, neurological or respiratory in origin without necessarily being cancerous. AIDS has greatly increased in prevalence since it was documented in the USA in the 1970s. This disease has brought with it the possibility of millions of untimely deaths in contrast to the current situation where deaths occur mostly among elderly people. Kübler-Ross (1987) suggests that it is AIDS which affords society the ultimate challenge to either cherish and help those affected by it, or to abandon them.

Health professionals in general have a common core of values centred around the promotion of health, the restoration of health to sick and injured people and the prolonging of life, insofar as that is reasonable. Even the notion of what is reasonable is no longer as obvious as it once seemed to be with 'end-of-life' issues being debated by doctors, nurses, lawyers and the general public in many countries. It is perhaps just a matter of time before physiotherapists formally join this complex debate.

Perhaps the most quoted work in the area of death and dying is the seminal work of Elizabeth Kübler-Ross, *On Death and Dying* (1969) where she focused on the feelings of patients with cancer who were fully informed of their diagnoses. She identified stages through which terminally ill people frequently pass. These stages comprise the following: denial and isolation; anger; bargaining; depression and acceptance. This work, while it has been a cornerstone in palliative care, has had some adverse criticism because of its simplistic presentation. Kübler-Ross did not claim that every dying person passes through all stages, but the use of the word 'stages' implies a linear sequence. Saunders (1978) supports the classification and suggests that it describes a process of realization whereby the person eventually recognizes the inevitability of his or her own death.

Reactions to impending death

Most of Kübler-Ross's 200 subjects exhibited denial as their first reaction on hearing of their diagnosis. They believed there had been a mistake, that the X-rays had got mixed up. Frequently second opinions were sought in the vain hope that a more optimistic diagnosis could be given. Denial may take other forms such as the dying person referring to a large tumour as a 'wound'. Lamerton (1973) found that the first thing people did with bad news was to deny it. Many people in their daily lives cope with bad news or unpleasant events in this way, so it is not surprising that they adopt this strategy when faced with a life-threatening diagnosis. Hinton (1972) believes that people who are dying should not be denied the comfort of make-believe or consoling daydreams. Kübler-Ross strongly contends that denial is a healthy way of dealing with uncomfortable and distressing situations. It acts as a buffer which allows people time to mobilize other, less radical defences. Veatch (1976) not only supports this view, but suggests that denying a terminal illness is what many people do to maintain their sanity.

Staff members who do not recognize denial or understand its function, may be intolerant or judgemental and may tend to leave patients alone and isolated with their grief. Empathic health professionals will not shatter the coping mechanisms of patients. Physiotherapists who are willing to spend time with their patients, to sit, to talk or to listen, will instill a feeling of confidence in them that there is someone who cares and is available. It is in such a person that a dying patient is likely to confide. Few patients will deny their mortality without wavering; most people will, in time, come to some level of acceptance. Kübler-Ross compares the prospect of impending death to looking at a bright sun insofar as one can look directly at it for short periods before being forced to look away. When denial is no longer easy to maintain, by reason of persistent ill health, anger, rage, envy and resentment may surface. Anger is easy to understand in the person who may never see the fruits of his or her life's work, the happy years of retirement and leisure which have been anticipated for years, or the growth of children and grandchildren. They may feel anger about the loss of life itself and this may be vented on family members or hospital staff. It is not uncommon for anger to be directed at God by a person who feels that terminal illness would be more appropriately visited on someone else – some old or worthless person who is perceived as making no worthwhile contribution to society. There may also be feelings of jealousy towards the healthy people around the terminally ill person.

Angry patients are almost impossible to please. They tend to be very demanding of attention and at the same time they complain that they are bothered by staff and cannot rest. Visits by loved ones to the hospital can be very strained and uncomfortable when the visitor is overwhelmed by grief and may be made to feel guilty by the patient to the extent that further visits are avoided. Saunders (1978) has shown that formerly loving relationships have broken down because of the anger evoked by severe physical and mental distress. However, not all terminally ill people are distressed by their diagnoses. Hinton (1972) found that to feel needed and to have a sense of belonging is profoundly important to many people and the recognition that their loved ones can manage without them can give rise to considerable anger. Staff and loved ones who understand this will realize that the anger is not directed at them personally, even though they are the targets. An attitude of understanding and patience and a willingness to share the unhappiness will show the patient that he or she is still a cherished human being.

Bargaining, as practised by demanding children, is a tactic adopted by dying people. Many terminally ill people make bargains with God which only the pastor may hear about. Bargains may take the form of a promise to give money or service to the poor or to the church in return for a cure or a remission. Kübler-Ross found that many patients promised to donate their bodies to medical research if the doctors could cure them. Various forms of bargaining may be seen among terminally ill people, all of which are attempts to postpone the dreaded day. Glaser and Strauss (1965) recognized bargaining, coaxing, persuasion and hinting as some of the ways in which dying patients negotiated in order to achieve their aims.

Depression in terminally ill people has been a controversial subject. Many people when told of their diagnosis are not feeling ill and in such circumstances denial and anger are readily explicable. Glaser and Strauss (1965) believe that when a person is told that he or she is terminally ill the response is one of depression after which the person may choose to accept or reject the prognosis. In Kübler-Ross's classification of the stages of dying (1969), depression arises when the person's health declines, when the body is thinner, weaker and more debilitated. The depression may be compounded by other losses such as the loss of a breast, a limb, income, or social status and the prospect of loss of life itself. Lamerton (1973) points out that some people worry about unfinished business from the past, or the anticipated suffering and bereavement of others.

Hinton (1972) believes that bereavement is the commonest emotional upset in terminally ill people. The sadness, apathy and misery experienced tends to be under-rated by health professionals, including physiotherapists, who may believe that such emotions are evoked entirely by the person's poor physical condition. This is an erroneous assumption since other people who have the prospect of recovery do not exhibit the same degree of misery. It is certainly not helpful to tell the dying person, 'It could be worse', for clearly it could not. Depression is normal and fully understandable in terminally ill people and Saunders (1978) believes that it is not helpful to label them with psychiatric diagnoses.

Everyone knows that life ends in death, yet many people have a private belief that death cannot touch them. Someone who has had a sudden illness of short duration may not have even contemplated his or her own demise. Those who have a terminal illness of protracted course are likely to come to some level of acceptance in time and are more fortunate, in some respects, than those with short-term terminal illness as they have had the opportunity to confront and deal with the gamut of emotions which terminal illness evokes. The person may eventually become resigned and accepting of the inevitable. Attitudes to death and expressions of grief are variable, but, almost always, they are influenced by a person's cultural background (Valk Lawson, 1990). Essentially, people die as they live. Halper (1979) talks about the now fashionable dogma that dying people should accept death, but for many people this is totally out of character with the broad pattern of their lives and may not be an appropriate coping mechanism. The empathic physiotherapist may recognize a quieter state of mind where the patient begins to question the purpose of continuing treatment, no longer interests him or herself in reading or watching television and spends more time sleeping. The physiotherapist must be ready to discuss the continuation of treatment with the patient and the physician. The patient's wishes are paramount and must always be respected, but sometimes an explanation will show him or her that physiotherapeutic procedures, such as passive movements and chest clearance, are performed for comfort rather than for cure. The patient's queries regarding the purpose of treatment may indicate a readiness to die and there may be a need for reassurance that the care team will not give up if the patient feels he or she is benefiting from the treatment.

The preparation for death

In facing death people are confronted with mixed and sometimes conflicting emotions, many of them centred on the nature and purpose of life itself. People move in and out of belief and disbelief concerning their mortality. Kübler-Ross (1969) found that denial, anger, bargaining, depression and acceptance lasted for varying periods of time or existed alongside each other from time to time. One feeling that tends to persist throughout a terminal illness is hope. Hope is not incompatible with acceptance and there is a growing body of literature to support the view that patients tend to show the greatest confidence in medical personnel who offer them hope, whether it is realistic or not, and that patients who maintain hope are the ones who tend to outlive the physician's expectations for them (Siegel, 1988). Halper (1979) questioned the ability to be both resigned and hopeful simultaneously and thought that acceptance was fundamentally incompatible with hope. Saunders (1978), however, found that hope and truth concerning terminal illness were not mutually exclusive insofar as informed patients were better able to fight for life, with knowledge and understanding of the real battlefield.

Purtillo (1972) points out that terminal illness gives rise to many fears of which the physiotherapist should be aware. Communication about matters of life and death is often fraught with difficulties caused by the fear it evokes in the dying person, his or her family and the care-givers themselves. This often results in the communication being ineffective. Fear is a natural reaction to danger and it is easy to see why it occurs in a person whose life is threatened. What is less generally recognized is the extent to which the expression of fear often becomes blocked, distorted or fragmented in people with incurable disease (Saunders, 1978). Many dying people admit to feeling anxious, but, according to Saunders (1978), few of them can identify the cause of their anxiety. Some may experience fear on behalf of someone else, for example, a spouse or a child who is affected by their illness, but they will frequently deny feeling any fear themselves. The effect of this situation may be that the dying person restricts his or her communication to trivialities and pointedly ignores the opportunities given by carers to talk about the illness. In contrast, Hinton (1972) found that most dying people were only too willing to communicate with anyone who was prepared to listen.

It is not always easy to recognize the main source of a dying person's fears, for as well as pain, there are many dangers, real and imagined, with which terminally ill people must cope. Halper (1979) speaks about the fear that the doctor will give up on them too soon, that the nurse will not come quickly enough with the medication, that the aide will not come in time with the bedpan. Qvarnstrom (1979) discussed fears such as loss of identity, loss of vital functions, loss of the body, loss of self-control, loss of relatives and the fear of what will happen when death has occurred.

The moment of death after a terminal illness is invariably peaceful. Hinton (1972) states:

'The moment of death is not often a crisis of distress for the dying person. For most the suffering is over a while before they die. Already some of the living functions have failed and consciousness goes early. Before the last moments of life there comes a quieter phase of surrender, the body appears to abdicate peacefully, no longer attempting to survive. Life then slips away so that few are aware of the final advent of their own death'.

The hospice concept of living until death has ensured that pain can be managed in almost every instance. Many physiotherapists have had the experience of witnessing a patient's death while quietly performing passive moments or other palliative measures. Many young physiotherapists may not have experienced death among their own relatives and friends and may, quite naturally, have apprehensions about encountering it for the first time in the professional situation. Quietly holding a person's hand may be the last service a physiotherapist can give to a patient, a final act of kindness for which no thanks can be given.

Mount (1979) reports on an International Work Group on Death, Dying and Bereavement which first met in 1974 to propose standards of care for terminally ill people. At that time the needs of dying people were described in the following way:

1. To be relieved of pain and other distressing symptoms;
2. To be in an environment of care where the patient's demands can be met without him or her suffering the fear of being a burden and where his or her individuality and integrity as a person can be maintained;
3. To have time and opportunity to voice his or her fears and to come to terms with the illness.

From the literature it seems that pain relief is of greatest concern to the dying person (Lamerton, 1973). Hanratty (1989) describes four main types of pain in terminal illness.

1. Physical pain.
2. Mental pain (e.g. anxiety, depression).
3. Social pain (e.g. isolation, embarrassment).
4. Spiritual pain (e.g. desolation).

Physiotherapists have sometimes felt themselves unqualified to evaluate the psychological effects of pain. Swann (1989) believes, however, that they have the requisite skills, or can acquire them, to treat not only the physical symptoms but to help alleviate the associated psychological manifestations of pain. (For a full discussion of the psychology and sociology of pain, the reader is referred to Chapter 10.)

Physiotherapy and terminal care

Terminally ill people develop physical impairment directly from the disease process or secondarily, especially in cancers, from surgery, chemotherapy and radiotherapy. With recent advances in diagnostic procedures, many therapies for cancer are now highly effective. The fact that people are living longer has led to an increase in the demand for rehabilitation services. Rehabilitation is not a matter of physical treatment alone, but rather is a consideration of the whole person; body, mind and spirit.

The concept of the physiotherapist treating the whole person is not new. Downie (1971) stressed the need for physiotherapists to be adaptable, to transcend their traditional role and to interest themselves in everything that involved total patient care. This means making time to listen, to talk, to empathize and to understand what is happening to a person who is facing death. The patient must be accepted and respected as he or she is. Knowledge of the thanatology literature is, of itself, not a recipe for helping dying patients. There is always the danger that a health professional may look for the reactions and emotions which are described in the literature, in an attempt to categorize the patient. Karl (1987) believes that such attempts show insensitivity to the needs of dying people and give the impression of turning their personal grief into a mechanical process.

Good terminal care may be defined as rehabilitation of dying people and is exemplified in the modern hospice (Twycross, 1981). For maximum efficiency, rehabilitation is delivered by means of a team approach. The physiotherapist in such a team needs to know the range and extent of services offered by other team members. Professional education may make it difficult for people to exchange roles or to accept the blurring of professional boundaries. Flexibility and mutual support of colleagues is essential if optimum care is to be given.

Terminal and palliative care require that all the professionals looking after the patient are responsive, not to the disease, but to the needs of the person (McAteer, 1990). Needs are as variable as the people who manifest them and physical requirements vary with the disease itself. Most recipients of palliative care are suffering from cancerous diseases, but increasing numbers of people with AIDS and motor neurone disease are in need of high quality care. There is no dichotomy between palliative/terminal care and rehabilitation when rehabilitation is viewed as the process whereby a patient is treated to ensure maximum function in a given set of circumstances and in accordance with the person's own wishes. Rehabilitation needs can be met at each stage of the disease process.

Below are some guiding principles which will assist the planning of physiotherapy programmes for terminally ill people:

1. The unique nature of each person must be recognized with respect to temporal, social, psychological and spiritual needs.
2. Health professionals must coordinate their response to the patient's needs.
3. Care of the patient must include the family, friends and any other significant person.
4. Physiotherapy goals must be reasonable and attainable.
5. Treatment must be determined by constant assessment and the wishes of each individual patient.

There are no specific techniques of physiotherapy that are employed for dying patients. Educational programmes for physiotherapy students teach not only the basic skills of electrotherapy, kinesiology and manipulative procedures, but employ an analytical approach which enables students to apply, synthesize and analyse various modalities for a given clinical problem. Palliative care involves the easing and controlling of symptoms in a patient with an incurable disease. In making decisions about treatment it is important to avoid inappropriate procedures which might prolong a poor quality of life and cause distress. Decisions must be made with the close involvement of the patient, his or her loved ones and the whole care team. Choices and plans must be feasible for the carers and realistic in terms of the resources available within the community (Oliver, 1993).

Physiotherapists spend relatively long periods of time with their patients carrying out treatments and so they are likely to hear a lot about how patients are feeling, not only in terms of physical well being, but with respect to needs, fears, anxieties, joys or woes. Hargreaves (1987) believes that touching, when it occurs as part of the therapeutic process, can indicate encouragement, support and caring. There are few people, healthy or otherwise, who do not feel better having had a massage from a physiotherapist. For the dying patient it can be a potent message that he or she is a valued human being.

Most physiotherapy services for dying patients will be given in the setting of the hospital, nursing home or hospice. Dying in public sector institutions is a phenomenon of the late twentieth century. Throughout history people tended to die at home. Most people, if asked, would choose to die at home, provided the essential care were available (Hanratty, 1989). Hanratty found that people making this choice associated their home with safety, comfort and love – elements which they felt would mitigate against the suffering of their last illness. A comfortable and home-like ambience is achieved in many hospices throughout Britain and Ireland. There are also growing numbers of home-care hospice teams which bring the range of hospice services into the patient's home. Many clinicians of various disciplines appear to be working towards a philosophical concept of hospice in any location where there are dying patients rather than the notion of a hospice as a building.

Physiotherapists who gain insights into the various affective states associated with terminal illness will develop a richer understanding of the person whose life is fading away. This understanding will edify and illuminate terminal care.

Bereavement

Bereavement essentially means the loss of someone with whom the survivor has had a close association. Responses to death will be variable, depending on the closeness of the relationship, the manner of death and whether it was sudden or expected. When a person has died after a protracted illness the loved ones will have had time to anticipate and to prepare for the death. Such anticipatory grief was recognized by Worden (1983) to have the effect of loosening the emotional ties with the dying person to such an extent that when the moment of death arrived there was no great outpouring of grief. Immediate reactions to death are culturally determined and vary considerably as do the religious practices associated with the death rituals. For Buddhists, Muslims, Sikhs, Hindus, Jews and Christians, there are definitive tasks to be completed soon after death. The physiotherapist who has looked after the patient in life will be well rewarded by familiarizing him or herself with these requirements, in order to dignify the person in death as in life. Grief is the expression of, and reaction to, loss and its intensity will be related to the nature of the attachment to the person who has died. A person who is mourning has usually been bereaved by death, but people may also mourn a wide variety of losses, such as loss of limb, loss of body image, loss of independence and loss of mobility. Bereavement by death has been used as a conceptual framework for understanding losses in many areas of physiotherapy practice (McAteer, 1989).

Uncomplicated grief

Grief has been the subject of much investigation in the twentieth century. Early work suggested a pathological or psychiatric basis but now grief is seen as a normal response to loss. A terrible fire in the Cocoanut Grove Nightclub, Massachusetts, in the Autumn of 1942, led to a classic study by Eric Lindemann (1944). He studied a large sample of the people who were bereaved by the 500 deaths which resulted from the fire. Lindemann is considered to be the father of the modern study of grief since his publication of the characteristics of normal, acute grief. These are:

1. Somatic distress.
2. Preoccupation with the image of the deceased.
3. Guilt.
4. Hostile reactions.
5. Loss of patterns of conduct, manifested by restlessness, lack of daily routine and an inability to sit still.
6. Appearance of traits of the deceased in the bereaved.

When a death is unexpected, shock and disbelief are the common responses. Shock is experienced even in cases where death was expected. Shock, disbelief and denial are particularly intense when a young person dies suddenly, as for example, in a motor-cycle accident. Frequently the response is 'there must be some mistake', or, 'Is there another person of the same name?'. These reactions closely resemble the typical response to the diagnosis of terminal illness.

Anger is a common and confusing emotion experienced by bereaved people. Many accident and emergency staff have borne the brunt of this anger. Widows, most of them former loving wives, become angry at their dead husbands and these feelings may persist throughout the first year of bereavement (Murray-Parkes, 1975). Widows may be angry that they are left without sufficient funds, adequate insurance or other less tangible goods. Worden (1983) believes that anger is at the root of many of the problems of the grieving process. Anger is often directed at friends or family and it may be rationalized by blaming someone else for the death. In some cases the hospital authorities or the doctor-in-charge is targeted for blame and in some circumstances this may proceed to litigation.

When the shock wears away the reality of the loss becomes apparent. Sadness fills the bereaved person's waking hours, crying and tearfulness are common. This state of anguish, sadness and despair is described by Karl (1987) as a coping phase. The bereaved person goes about his or her daily business feeling tired, aimless, confused, indecisive, apathetic and lacking in confidence. Crying is a variable feature since sadness is not always manifested by tears. Many bereaved people describe how they wake up in the morning feeling for a brief moment that the death of their loved one was all a dream, but reality quickly shatters this moment.

The feeling of guilt is also common among bereaved people and is widely reported in the literature (Lindemann, 1944; Worden, 1983; Walsh 1995). Families may feel guilty that they did not get a second opinion, a private hospital or a special nurse. Some may feel that they should have dissuaded the patient from allowing an operation to take place. Parents whose children die are highly vulnerable to feelings of guilt which often focus on the fact that they could not ease the child's distress or prevent the death (Worden, 1983). Other people feel guilty about the sense of relief they feel after the death of a loved one, even though they may have nursed him or her over a long period of time. Yearning and pining for the dead person is normal and persists throughout the mourning period. When it diminishes in intensity it usually indicates that mourning is coming to a healthy termination.

Mourning a loss is considered an essential part of the restoration process (Imara, 1983). The term 'recovery' poses a difficulty, however, insofar as the person who is lost is not recovered. Mourning, or the adaptation to loss, is described in almost all the literature as 'grief work'. Worden (1983) identifies the main tasks of mourning as follows:

1. To accept the reality of the loss.
2. To experience the pain of grief.
3. To adjust to an environment in which the deceased is missing.
4. To withdraw emotional energy from the deceased person and invest it in other relationships.

To accept the reality of a loss may be a difficult task. Some practices of denial may help to mitigate against the loss and may be useful in the short term. Denial of the facts may involve a slight distortion or a more serious delusion. Seeing the body is the first recognition of the reality of what has happened. Absence of a body, in an air crash or a drowning, for example, leads to what may be a complicated or prolonged grief (Van der Hart, 1988). Parents who have been dissuaded from seeing the body of their child killed in a mutilating accident, frequently have difficulty with this first task of mourning and invariably regret not having said the 'last goodbye' (Jones, 1988).

Funeral rituals help to confirm the reality of death, especially if they take place some days after death has occurred. Keeping the bedroom of a dead person exactly as he or she had left it creates a type of shrine and is, in reality, a denial of the death. Queen Victoria derived comfort from having her dead husband's clothes left out each day as though he were alive. If such practices are carried out for too long the bereaved person may never get past the first stage of mourning without some professional counselling intervention. It appears that to suppress the pain of grief is to store up mental or physical dysfunction in the future (Zisook and de

Vaul, 1976). Drugs which suppress these sad emotions are not considered suitable for most people since taking them merely prolongs or postpones the period of mourning. The funeral rituals have a valuable role to play in facilitating the outpouring of grief, but not all bereaved people will feel such pain.

For those who are bereaved the environment is totally different without the deceased person. Living without a loved one has many connotations. Murray-Parkes (1975) points out that the death of a spouse may be viewed as the loss of a breadwinner, a sexual partner, a babysitter, an accountant, or all of these. The death of a child before that of his parents seems to go against the natural order of things and is particularly difficult to accept. In ancient Greece, Aristotle recognized this as the unbearable loss. Responses to bereavement are as variable as the people concerned and while some people are not able to cope with the practical or emotional demands of their changed situation, others go on to achieve new dimensions of personal growth.

The final task of mourning is to achieve an emotional detachment from the deceased which will enable the bereaved person to enter into new and meaningful relationships. This is possible when the other tasks of mourning have been dealt with and should not be viewed as disloyalty to the dead person. The tasks of mourning take varying periods of time, ranging from months to years, but in some respects it can be said that mourning never ceases. Society supports bereaved people in various ways, but there are many situations where the mourner is more secretive and is, therefore, not so amenable to the concern and understanding of others. These situations include:

1. Those grieving unborn babies lost through miscarriage, abortion or stillbirth.
2. Those grieving for very young children.
3. Those grieving for pets.
4. Those grieving for a homosexual partner or lover.
5. Those grieving for a divorced or separated partner.
6. Those grieving for a deceased person with whom they had a secret relationship. (Walsh, 1995).

Worden (1983) identified some major determinants which can influence the type, intensity and duration of grief. These determinants are:

1. Who the person was. It is almost axiomatic that the intensity of grief is determined by the intensity of love. Grief for a spouse, for example, is usually totally different to the grief for a grandparent.
2. The mode of death. Traditionally, deaths have been categorized under four headings; natural, accidental, suicidal and homicidal. All the feelings and responses already discussed here may be experienced by bereaved people, whatever the type of death, but there may be extreme anger at a homicidal death and certainly suicide brings many complex feelings to the bereaved people.
3. Mental health. The bereaved person's mental health and history of

dealing with past losses are relevant. People with a history of depressive illness usually fare rather poorly in coping with their grief.

4. Ability to cope. The ability of the bereaved person to cope with anxiety and stress is an important consideration. When a key attachment figure provides a secure base, the bereaved person is more likely to establish comforting and reliable relationships and to manage bereavement without experiencing extended or atypical grief (Sable, 1989).

5. Cultural factors. Ethnic and religious sub-cultures provide rituals for most life events including death, funeral rites and mourning. It is frequently assumed that Irish Catholics and Orthodox Jews grieve well because of their extensive funeral arrangements. However, the effects of the participation in such 'rites of passage' have yet to be established.

Caplan (1990) summarizes the ability to cope with loss when he recognizes that competence in this area incorporates both constitutional and acquired elements.

Health in bereavement

Some people express their pain of bereavement emotionally in the expression of feelings, while others 'somatize' the pain of grief, that is their bodies express it (Walsh, 1995). Most people experience both emotional and physiological manifestations. Lindemann (1944) showed that various types of somatic distress were evident in normal grief. Many people interpret the features of grief as being 'sick' and, consequently, they seek medical help. When doctors write prescriptions for these 'ills', they confirm the bereaved person in his or her 'sick role'. Not only does this help to suppress the normal physiological and psychological manifestations of grief, but it leaves people open to medical, psychiatric and even surgical mismanagement.

Physical symptoms associated with grief are many and varied. Lindemann (1944) lists tightness of the throat, shortness of breath, digestive symptoms, nausea and loss of strength. Murray-Parkes (1975) mentions headaches, dry mouth, a lump in the throat and aching limbs, and Worden (1983) talks of hollowness in the stomach, breathlessness, lack of energy and over-sensitivity to noise. This can be experienced either as difficulty in going to sleep or waking up after only a short period of sleep. Sleep disorders can sometimes symbolize certain fears such as fear of dreaming, fear of being in bed alone or fear of not awakening. A patient of Worden's conquered her night-time fears by taking her dog to bed with her for the first year of her bereavement. The rhythm of her dog's breathing was a source of comfort and reassurance to her.

Appetite for food was shown by Murray-Parkes (1970) to be severely depressed during the first month after bereavement, resulting in loss of weight. This may be accounted for by the hollow feeling in the stomach, nause or dry mouth.

The pain of grief has been described as the 'broken heart', not just in poetry and song, but by Murray-Parkes (1985). The classic broken heart on the death of a spouse reflects the puzzling association between bereavement and the death of the survivor from heart disease. There is a significant increase in death rates from heart disease in men in the first year after the death of their wives, although not all types of bereavement are equally dangerous for the heart. The death of a spouse has long been recognized as one of life's most stressful experiences (Schleifer *et al.*, 1983) and, clearly, few survivors of conjugal loss can be entirely healthy in the first year of the bereavement. The effect of conjugal loss may be so profound as to result in future illness, demonstrating the adverse effect of separation on biological homeostasis (Oberfield, 1984).

The first study to demonstrate a connection between bereavement and the immune system was carried out by Bartrop *et al.* (1977). Schleifer *et al.* (1983) showed that lymphocyte responses were significantly suppressed in the first 2 months of bereavement following the death of a spouse. These findings may account for the increased morbidity and mortality associated with bereavement, although it is equally possible that lymphocyte function may be affected by changes in nutrition, exercise levels, sleep patterns and drug use. Lymphocyte functions in bereaved spouses could also be influenced by centrally mediated stress effects. Psychosocial processes, such as stressful life experiences, may be associated with changes in central nervous system activity. Research is currently exploring the links between bereavement and a wide range of physical and psychosomatic disorders, such as cancer, arthritis and allergies.

Jacobs and Douglas (1979) see grief as a mediating process between a significant loss and possible illness; there now seems to be little doubt that the expression of grief in mourning is essential for health. Tears may have a potential healing value. Stress causes chemical imbalances in the body and some researchers believe that tears remove toxic substances and help to redress the balance. Frey (1980) suggests that the chemical content of tears caused by emotional stress is different from that of tears shed as a result of eye irritation. Subjectively, tears relieve emotional stress, but this is a perception not yet fully understood. Research is needed to establish if it is harmful to suppress tears.

Bereavement and physiotherapy

The implications for physiotherapists treating bereaved people are considerable. Patients who have recently been bereaved may suffer from any or all of the physical manifestations of grief which have been considered in this chapter. Wortman and Silver (1989) point out that the loss of a loved one removes a major source of social support which, in itself, can account for some of the pathogenic effects of bereavement. It would be of considerable help to the physiotherapist to know, as part of each routine interview and assessment, if his or her patient has recently been bereaved, and if so who had died. Many symptoms, for example, vague joint and muscle pains, can be attributed to acute grief. The physiotherapist, with even a limited knowledge of the grief process, can be of considerable help to patients by being a good listener or non-directive counsellor. According to Sim (1990), the physiotherapist who wants to create and enhance health in others needs a more ambitious and wide-ranging definition of health than the mere removal of illness and disease. Becoming responsive to any need that the patient may have is what gives breadth and movement to the accountability aspect of professional responsibility (Purtillo, 1986). The physiotherapist who understands the grief and mourning process will convey to bereaved, but otherwise healthy, patients that while they may have physical signs and symptoms, these do not constitute sickness and should not be medicalized.

There are a number of ways in which the physiotherapist can provide practical help in promoting the health of bereaved people.

1. If sleep is difficult, rest is possible without recourse to a drug-induced sleep. Most physiotherapists have a range of relaxation techniques to offer, or they may suggest some commercially produced audio/video tapes.
2. Sensible exercise may promote relaxation. Walking is considered to be one of the safest ways to maintain cardiovascular fitness. It may also enhance the immune system and alleviate depression.
3. The bereaved person should ensure that three meals, consisting of wholesome foods, are consumed daily.
4. A check-up with the general practitioner is a good idea for bereaved people. The patient should not be labelled a 'hypochondriac' if there are physical signs and symptoms of emotional distress. These are real problems and should be regarded as such.
5. The physiotherapist should recognize when the patient would benefit from referral to a bereavement counselling service. Bereavement following particular types of death, such as stillbirth, homicide and suicide, are usually catered for by specialist counsellors or other helping agencies.
6. Reaching out to empathize with another human being will always help to dispel loneliness and isolation.

Professional carers are not immune from grief themselves. Physiotherapists may mourn the loss of a patient for whom they have cared and may feel anger, guilt and remorse when such a loss occurs. They, too, need the help, understanding and support which sensitive colleagues can provide.

Conclusion

Working with dying and bereaved people is neither depressing nor unrewarding. Death and dying are everyday realities. Fowler (1989) believes that in some respects health professionals are guilty of cultivating an expectation of a painless life without suffering. Life is painful and full of sorrow for many people, but death need not be so. Working with fellow human beings who are facing death has many rewards for physiotherapists not least of which is the very significant personal growth and development they are certain to experience.

References

Bartrop, R. W., Lazarus L., Luckhurst E. *et al.* (1977) Depressed lymphocyte function after bereavement. *Lancet*, **i**, 834–836.
Caplan G. (1990) Stress and mental health. *Community Mental Health Journal*, **26**(1), 27–48.

Dickenson D., Johnson M. (1993) *Death, Dying and Bereavement*. London: Sage Publications.

Downie P. A. (1971) The physiotherapist and the patient with cancer. *Physiotherapy*, **57**(3), 117–125.

Feifel H. (1990) Psychology and death. *American Psychologist*, **45**(4), 337–343.

Fowler M. D. M. (1989) Weal and woe: on the loss of lament. *Heart and Lung*, **18**(6), 640–641.

Frey W. H. (1980) Not-so-idle tears. *Psychology Today*, **13**, 91–92.

Glaser B. G., Strauss A. L. (1965) *Awareness of Dying*. Chicago: Aldine Publishing.

Halper T. (1979) On Death, dying and terminality. *Journal of Health Politics, Policy and Law*, Spring, 11–29.

Hanratty J. F. (1989) *Palliative Care of the Terminally Ill*. Oxford: Radcliffe Medical Press.

Hargraves S. (1987) The relevance of non-verbal skills in physiotherapy. *Physiotherapy*, **73**(12), 685–688.

Hinton J. (1972) *Dying*. Harmondsworth: Penguin Books.

Hollenbery S. (1994) Looking to the future: an alternative view. *Physiotherapy*, **80**(A), 103A–104A.

Imara M. (1983) Growing through grief. In *Hospice Care: Principles and Practice* (Corr C. A., Corr D. M., eds). New York: Faber and Faber.

Jacobs S., Douglas L. (1979) Grief: a mediating process between a loss and illness. *Comprehensive Psychiatry*, **20**(2), 165–176.

Jones J. H. (1988) The importance of children's funerals in the mourning process. *Bereavement Care*, **7**(3), 34–37.

Karl G. T. (1987) A new look at grief. *Journal of Advanced Nursing*, **12**, 641–645.

Kübler-Ross E. (1969) *On Death and Dying*. London: Tavistock Publications.

Kübler-Ross E. (1987) *AIDS: The Ultimate Challenge*. New York: Macmillan Publishing Company.

Lamerton R. (1973) *Care of the Dying*. London: Priory Press.

Lindemann E. (1944) Symptomatology and management of acute grief. *American Journal of Psychiatry*, **101**, 141–148.

McAteer M. F. (1989) Some aspects of grief in physiotherapy. *Physiotherapy*, **75**(1), 55–58.

McAteer M. F. (1990) Reactions to terminal illness. *Physiotherapy*, **1**, 9–12.

Mount B. M. (1979) International group issue proposal for standards for care of the terminally ill. *Canadian Medical Association Journal*, **120**, 1280–1283.

Murray-Parkes C. (1970) The first year of bereavement. *Psychiatry*, **33**, 443–467.

Murray-Parkes C. (1975) *Bereavement*. Harmondsworth: Penguin Books.

Murray-Parkes C. (1985) Bereavement. *British Journal of Psychiatry*, **146**, 11–17.

Oberfield R. (1984) Terminal illness: death and bereavement – towards an understanding of its nature. *Perspectives in Biology and Medicine*, **28**, 140–155.

Oliver D. (1993) Ethical issues in palliative care – an overview. *Palliative Medicine*, **7**, 15–20.

Purtillo R. B. (1972) Don't mention it: the physical therapist in a death denying society. *Physical Therapy*, **52**(10), 1031–1035.

Purtillo R. B. (1986) Professional responsibility in physiotherapy. *Physiotherapy*, **72**(12), 579–583.

Qvarnström U. (1979) Patients' reactions to impending death. *International Nursing Review*, 26 April, 117–119.

Sable P. (1989) Attachment, anxiety and loss of a husband. *American Journal of Orthopsychiatry*, **59**(4), 550–556.

Saunders C. M. (1978) *The Management of Terminal Disease*. London: Arnold.

Schleifer S. J., Keller S. E., Camerino M. *et al.* (1983) Suppression of lymphocyte stimulation following bereavement. *Journal of the American Medical Association*, **250**(3), 374–377.

Siegel B. S. (1988) *Love, Medicine and Miracles*. Essex: Arrow books.

Sim J. (1990) The concept of health. *Physiotherapy*, **76**(7), 423–428.

Swain J. (1995) *The Use of Counselling Skills*. Oxford: Butterworth-Heinemann.

Swann P. (1989) Stress management for pain control. *Physiotherapy*, **75**(5), 295–298.

Twycross R. C. (1981) Rehabilitation in terminal cancer patients. *International Rehabilitation Medicine*, **3**(3), 135–144.

Valk Lawson L. (1990) Culturally sensitive support for grieving parents. *American Journal of Maternal Child Nursing*, **15**, 76–79.

Van der Hart O. (1988) An imaginary leave-taking ritual in mourning therapy. *International Journal of Clinical and Experimental Hypnosis*, **36**(2), 63–69.

Veatch R. M. (1976) *Death, Dying and the Biological Revolution*. New Haven: Yale University Press.

Walsh M. P. (1995) *Living After a Death*. Dublin: Columba Press.

Walter T. (1993) Modern death: taboo or not taboo. In *Death, Dying and Bereavement* (Dickenson D., Johnson M., eds). London: Sage Publications.

Worden J. W. (1983) *Grief Counselling and Grief Therapy*. London: Tavistock Publications.

Wortman C. B., Wilver R. C. (1989) The myths of coping with loss. *Journal of Consulting and Clinical Psychology*, **57**(3), 349–357.

Zisook S., de Vaul R. (1976) Grief-related facsimile illness. *International Journal of Psychiatry in Medicine*, **7**(4), 329–336.

13 Lay beliefs about health and illness

Michael Calnan

This chapter examines lay perspectives and knowledge about health and illness mainly from a sociological point of view. Lay knowledge about health and illness is an important area to examine for a number of reasons. Firstly, sufferers, and those who make up their social networks, call upon it to make sense of signs and symptoms and other health problems. While lay knowledge may be influenced, in terms of its structure and substance, by scientific knowledge given by professionals and/or through the media, it is nonetheless different from professional, scientific knowledge. Secondly, lay health knowledge is important because it may influence health-related behaviour and other behaviour. Lay knowledge may, for example, influence decisions concerning patterns of food consumption, decisions to self-medicate, to go to the doctor or to do nothing. Finally, lay perspectives on health and health care are important as they can be used, along with assessments of medical effectiveness and economic efficiency, to evaluate health care programmes.

These are three practical illustrations of the need to examine lay beliefs about health and illness. The approach to the subject has changed over the last decade or so, but before recent research is outlined the more traditional perspective will be briefly discussed.

The traditional perspective

This perspective is well represented in what has been popularly termed the Health Belief Model. The model was extended by Janz and Becker (1984) and is used to predict compliance with official health recommended actions such as screening, immunization, diet, exercise, personal habits and entering or continuing treatment programmes. Thus it covers not only the uptake of health services but also compliance with recommended health action, for example that given in health education campaigns. The model consists of a number of dimensions of health beliefs which comprise the concept 'readiness to undertake recommended compliance behaviour'. These dimensions include motivation, value of illness threat reduction and probability that compliant behaviour will reduce the threat of illness. In addition it is suggested that demographic, structural, attitudinal and interactional factors can modify and enable action. The approach can be described as the 'ballistic' approach, since the image of the proto-patient is one of a missile ready to be hurled towards the health services. The view is that these different dimensions of health beliefs work in concert to produce a decision to act or not. (For further information on patient compliance, the reader is referred to Chapter 8.)

An alternative construct or framework which is also rooted in learning theory, is the health locus of control. The general principles behind the health locus of control are that people who feel they control their own health are likely to engage in healthy behaviour and to act in accordance with the recommendations of official health agencies, whereas those who feel powerless to control their own health, will be less likely to do so. Since its original inception the general construct of the health locus of control has been modified (Wallston and De Vellis 1978) and the favoured concept is now that of the multi-dimensional health locus of control. This construct consists of three distinct dimensions of belief about health: the internal; the powerful other (e.g. the doctor or physiotherapist); and chance. People who score high on the internal scale are more likely to believe that health is the result of their own behaviour, while those who score high on the other dimensions believe either that health depends on the power of health workers, or on chance, fate or luck.

While both these approaches have been popular, there are some fundamental problems which occur at both the conceptual and empirical level. At the empirical level studies have shown that both models have limited explanatory value. For example, a study by Calnan (1989), using data from two large scale community surveys (n = 4224), examined the relationship between multi-dimensional health locus of control and exercise, cigarette smoking and alcohol use. The results showed that none of these relationships were more than modest in strength even within different social and economic contexts. Obviously this analysis did not exhaust all health behaviours, for example dietary practice was not included.

Similarly, in studies examining the predictive power of the health belief model, the evidence suggests only a modest relationship between the belief dimension and behaviour (Langlie, 1977). Calnan and Rutter (1986) examined the predictive power of the health belief model for explaining changes in the practice of breast self-examination. Three groups of women were investigated – 278 who accepted an invitation to attend self-examination classes and were taught the techniques in detail, 262 who declined the invitation and 594 controls to whom no classes were offered. Beliefs and self-reported behaviour were measured shortly before the classes took place and again a year later. The results suggested that beliefs do predict behaviour; both perceived susceptibility and perceived benefits/barriers made significant contributions to the belief behaviour equations and the relationships were generally highly statistically significant.

To that extent the model was supported. However, the evidence also suggested that the relationship between the behaviour and the dimensions of health which the model stresses was not a strong or a simple one. Two pieces of evidence in particular deserve attention. First, only a small proportion of the variance was explained in the analyses, which is a common finding in studies using the health belief model. The figure was never higher than 25% and was generally much lower. It was also noticeable that the greatest amount of variance was explained in the control group, where the smallest amount of behaviour change was found. The second piece of evidence was that a supplementary analysis of the data showed that prior behaviour was a stronger predictor of subsequent behaviour than were beliefs. When prior behaviour was introduced into the analysis, the proportion of variance explained was increased markedly – as much as 48% in one case. In summary, this empirical evidence suggests that the health belief dimensions identified in the health belief model and the health locus of control have limited explanatory value.

It is important that physiotherapists gain insight into patients' beliefs about health and illness as this may affect their behaviour. For example, a patient who believes he or she has control over his or her illness may be more inclined to work hard to recover than one who believes in the curative powers of the physiotherapist. Eachus (1990) states: 'Patients who do not believe that they are, at least in part, responsible for and can influence their own health, are likely to prove particularly frustrating. This will be particularly true for those conditions which require the active participation of the patient during the course of treatment'.

Eachus (1990) measured the health locus of control of physiotherapy students and compared it with that of the general public. He found that the students' beliefs were basically very similar to those of the general public, with very little change occurring over the course of their professional education. The physiotherapy students were slightly less inclined to believe that illness was the result of chance factors or that they could influence its course. A rather larger difference was seen with regard to powerful others with the physiotherapy students having less belief in their power to control illness. Eachus states: '... it might be expected that the public attribute greater power to physiotherapists than student physiotherapists do themselves'.

In addition to the weaknesses at the empirical level there are also problems at the conceptual level. Some of the conceptual weaknesses of the health belief model have been discussed elsewhere (Calnan, 1987). The concept of perceived vulnerability to illness in general, or to a particular disease, is central to the health belief model (Janz and Becker, 1984). This concept appears to be derived from epidemiological models which, using probability theory as their basis, identify the range of factors that might influence a population's or an individual's vulnerability to disease in general or to a specific disease. The concept has been shifted to the area of health behaviour where it is argued that certain levels of vulnerability are associated with a greater likelihood of compliance with officially recommended health actions. This approach has been accepted and adopted by those who are involved in designing health education campaigns where one of the major objectives is to educate the individual into an awareness of how 'at risk' he or she is to certain diseases.

One of the conceptual problems of the health belief model, however, pertains to the concept of perceived vulnerability to illness. Calnan and Johnson (1985) explored the concept through an ethnographic study and found that it tended to embrace a wide range of beliefs and feelings.

Respondents very rarely said with certainty that they felt vulnerable to a specific illness unless there was some concrete justification for doing so, such as the presence of signs and symptoms. A clear distinction was also made between worries about diseases such as cancer, and actually thinking that they would or might develop them. The possibility of getting a disease was more frequently mentioned by respondents, although this was not based on a probability model of disease causation, but rather reflected a lack of good evidence, such as previous experience of the illness in question. For some people even thinking about the possibility of getting a disease was viewed as a sign of 'neurosis'.

The models of disease causation which predominated appeared to derive from the medical model in that the respondents tended to use criteria that characterized disease as a fundamentally biological phenomenon with a specific aetiology. Little emphasis was placed on behavioural elements, and social and economic factors were completely ignored. Hereditary explanations were commonly used by both groups but usually as collaborating evidence in the interpretation of the significance of symptoms. According to these data, perception of vulnerability has little to do with health and more to do with the experience of illness and how it occurs.

A similar criticism could be applied to the health locus of control in that it focuses solely on the medical definition of health, i.e. health as the absence of illness and dependence on medical professionals to manage health problems. Yet evidence from ethnographic research has shown that lay conceptions of health include many dimensions such as health as being strong, health as being fit and active and health as the absence of illness (Calnan, 1987). Thus the instrument is probably tapping people's beliefs about illness rather than their beliefs about health. It may therefore be more valuable for explaining the use of curative or preventative services, which are more concerned with the early detection of disease, and predicting behavioural change in those suffering illness, than for maintaining good health or predicting the behaviour of the 'healthy'.

Ethnographic perspective

One of the assumptions which is inherent in the models described in the previous section is that the public shares the same values and interests as the medical profession, accepts the authority of the profession and has faith in medical knowledge and medical expertise. In this context the lay person is depicted as passive and uncritical. In contrast, the ethnographic perspective suggests that the provider and the consumer may have different and even conflicting perspectives. The image of the lay person in this approach is one who is active and critical, who manages his or her own health requirements and is discriminating in his or her use of medical knowledge, advice and expertise. The doctor is seen by the potential patient as one source of advice within a network of consultants. There is a shift away from an emphasis on explaining behaviour in terms of medical rationality, towards attempting to understand the lay person's actions in terms of his or her own logic, knowledge and beliefs. The ethnographic approach involves a shift away from such questions as, 'Why do people fail to follow officially recommended advice and practices?', to 'Why do people comply?', and to much broader questions such as, 'What is health and what is illness?'.

Lay concepts of health

Previous approaches such as the health belief model seem to assume that as a whole the general public's definitions of health are congruent with official medical definitions. The assumption is surprising given that there is little consensus among professional groups about how health should be defined. Official definitions highlight both the positive aspects, i.e. feelings of well-being, and the negative, disease-orientated aspects, i.e. the absence of disease. These and other definitions are also found in lay representations of health. Evidence from the Health and Life Style survey, comprising about 9000 men and women, showed that three different concepts of health were prevalent (Blaxter, 1990). The first was positive fitness, that is having strength and energy and an efficient or athletic body. This concept was most prevalent among men, young people and the better educated. The second concept was a social or functional one associated with the requirements of living, it was most common among old people. The final concept was 'not being ill' which was found equally in all social groups, although more often among women than men. This has implications for the physiotherapist as his or her patient's definitions of health and illness will differ one from another and may be out of line with that of the physiotherapist.

Explanations for the presence of these different dimensions of health in lay concepts have emphasized the power and influence of scientific medicine which uses the medical model of health (the absence of disease) in combination with the influence of more traditional values such as the importance of work. However, perhaps one of the most interesting explanations comes from Crawford (1984), who elicited ideas about health and illness from 60 mainly white, middle class adults living in Chicago. He found that there were contradictions in people's definitions of health. On the one hand health was seen in terms of control and discipline and the importance of maintaining a healthy body for work, and on the other it was seen as a 'release' where being healthy was concerned with seeking pleasure and satisfying desires. Crawford explains these contradictions in terms of the demands made upon Americans by capitalist society. The stress on health as discipline is congruent with the ethics of present day employment, with ideas of a disciplined workforce, holding down jobs and producing goods and services, but at the same time industry requires market outlets for its goods, hence all the advertising which encourages self-indulgence and 'release'. Other studies have also shown evidence of these complementary discourses of 'control' and 'release'. (Backett, 1992; Davison *et al.*, 1991; Lupton and Chapman, 1995). Backett (1992) found that informants emphasized the importance of exerting discipline in one's life in the interests of good health and an attractive (i.e. slim) appearance, it was also deemed necessary to be able to 'let go' and to enjoy life, including eating the 'wrong' types of food, for a 'little bit of what you fancy does you good'. Food sometimes served as a source of 'release', like alcohol, for alleviating tensions.

These studies have suggested that the public holds concepts of health which contain a range of different, sometimes contradictory elements. But when are these concepts used in practice and how far are concerns about health a priority for the majority of people in their daily lives?

This particular issue was examined in a recent study by Calnan and Williams (1991) where they attempted to identify how salient health was in people's daily lives. A novel methodology, at least in this area of research was adopted in that informants were asked to describe, in detail, a day in their life (spontaneous discourse) and this was followed by more specific questions (probed discourse) about health and 'life style'. The evidence from the study showed that irrespective of socioeconomic circumstances, matters of health rarely surfaced in people's descriptions of their daily lives. Neither did a concern with health in the context of behaviour. Moreover, the emphasis placed within the first part of the interview upon spontaneous discourse left open the possibility that alternative forms of health-related behaviour may emerge. However, this did not prove to be the case, and it was only at the level of probed discourse that discussions of health matters seemed to emerge.

One interpretation of this evidence, and the most likely, is that health is not a priority for most people in the course of their daily lives and only surfaces when 'health problems emerge or when trouble looms large'. Thus, general discussion of health-related matters only seemed to surface spontaneously within respondents' accounts when they, or their families, suffered actual health problems. This is well illustrated in the following accounts:

> 'As I think I said ... I'm diabetic, so I have to do my injections in the morning and in the evening ... Make a cup of tea, had some cod liver oil for me aches and pains ... a teaspoonful a day. It seems to have stopped me joints aching and burning.'

This highlights the taken-for-granted nature of health in routine daily life and the manner in which, paradoxically, it is only spoken about in its absence. For example, as one man remarked when asked to define health:

> 'Its very difficult to say what you define as "fit" and "well" if what you have you take for granted. I mean, if you take a man who, for argument sake, has suffered with rheumatism, then you appreciate that you are presumably better off and fitter. It is very difficult to describe, something that I suppose you take for granted.'

Moreover, as other studies have shown (Cornwell, 1984), respondents may have different bodies of knowledge which they use in different contexts. This might be explained by the framework suggested by Young (1981) who argues that health and illness should be seen in the context of process and practice rather than in abstract terms. In this analysis of the nature of medical knowledge, Young makes a distinction between respondents' representational knowledge ('knowledge of something') and their practical knowledge ('knowledge produced in response to something'). Thus, when respondents are asked, 'what is health?', they produce a wide range of concepts. This might be seen as abstract or representational knowledge that was clearly present in the prompted questions on health and behaviour. However, in everyday life such concepts are rarely adopted and more functional concepts such as the absence of incapacitating signs and symptoms are utilized. Calnan and Williams (1991) found that the only exception to this was in relation to exercise where, among middle class men and women, there was an emphasis on 'well-being' and 'relaxation' and physical exercise was used as a resource to achieve that end. A further, related explanation for the absence of discussion of matters of health in peoples' descriptions of their lives, is that decisions about current everyday activities have been taken for granted and have become routine.

Other studies show how social and economic factors may shape health beliefs. For example, studies such as that by Cornwell (1984) show how ideas about health are grounded in everyday life, and in turn, structured by social and economic circumstances. Cornwell, in her ethnographic study in East London, found that the set of moral and philosophical assumptions which underlay beliefs about work almost replicated those which underlay beliefs about health and illness.

Health maintenance

Some logical connection between concepts of health and beliefs about health maintenance is evident in that a dimension of health which is very prevalent in lay concepts of health is that of being fit and active and strong. This is at least logically connected with lay ideas about health maintenance, as evidence has shown that diet and exercise are the most popular means of maintaining health (Blaxter, 1990; Calnan, 1990). Calnan (1989) found that respondents' ideas about health included, 'Well balanced diet and plenty of exercise' and 'To eat properly and exercise and walk instead of going by taxi'. Regular exercise is clearly logically linked with health as fitness and health as activity, whereas food and diet can be viewed as 'fuel' for maintaining levels of energy and providing the resources necessary to keep active and fit in order to perform daily tasks.

Studies of food and health beliefs have shown interesting differences between social groups. For example, Calnan (1990) compared working class women and middle class women and showed that in contrast to the middle class women's emphasis on a balanced diet and 'everything in moderation', the working class women were more concerned about meals being substantial and filling. This was particularly evident when the two groups discussed notions such as a 'balanced diet'. There was also some similarities between the two groups. For example both agreed that good diets should be based on 'fresh' food and vegetables. The following was a typical response: 'I would say all fresh food is good and processed food I don't believe in. I mean those ready made meals I don't believe in. I don't believe in fish fingers or frozen things – you never know what's happened to them. It's all right going into Safeways and getting them off the shelf, but where have they been before that? Fresh goods are more nutritious. Well they have not been preserved and I don't know I suppose it's the fact I can see what I'm buying and also to me it tastes better'.

A similar emphasis was placed on 'fresh' food in a previous study by Calnan (1987). It appears that the women in these studies operate with ideas about diet which are products of periods where there was a shortage of food, such as during the war years and the depression when fresh food was in short supply and when items, such as fresh fruit, were regarded as a symbol of prosperity. With a group of younger women, however, Calnan (1990) found that concerns about fresh food were a product of more contemporary ideas. The data indicated a dislike of artificially packaged food and a preference for 'natural' food. Food additives were high on the agenda of this generation of women as potential sources of ill health.

While there appears to be some evidence of a logical connection between concepts of health and beliefs about health maintenance, how far do these concerns about health influence patterns of health-related behaviour? The study by Calnan and Williams (1991), which examined 'life style' behaviours, found that it was only in relation to food consumption that there was evidence from spontaneous discourse that concerns about health might have an influence. It was also evident that health concerns may be more influential on patterns of food consumption in the middle class households. Other studies have also suggested that food choice may be shaped by health knowledge although there may be class differences in this relationship. For example, Calnan and Cant (1990) examined influences on food purchase, food preparation and cooking and the serving and consumption of meals in middle class and working class households. They found that concerns about health were important in guiding food purchase although there were class differences. For example, working class women tended to talk about the influence of concerns about health on food purchase when it appeared to be associated with the occurrence of particular family problems. These problems were divided into diagnosed medical problems associated with diet and those where women believed that certain foods affected family members' health. The latter category is more clearly exemplified in the beliefs of several women that additives, especially in orange juice, contributed to hyperactivity in their children:

> 'I buy orange juice without additives or preservatives because I find he gets very high. Especially the orange juice that stains round the mouth'.

The middle class women on the other hand, tended to report a category that the authors describe as 'health knowledge' which included ideas from books, general knowledge, and the medical press.

> 'I'm a believer in whole foods ... it's the thing, you read and hear, regarding for instance the cancers and the colitis, that medically speaking it seems that if you have the right amount of fibre, this is going to be far better for you ... I think to me that seems to be enough evidence that we need these foods. I used to buy white bread and now I only buy brown ... its just that you see all this on television, its better for you, all the roughage and that, also we used to have butter and I now have Gold because that's low fat and we have skimmed milk now'.

However, in addition to health concerns, there were other more powerful influences on food purchase associated with the internal structure of the family such as gender roles and the division of labour in the households. The responsibility for, and management of, food purchase fell primarily on the shoulders of women whose food purchases were influenced by the preferences, needs and requirements of more powerful family members. For example, Charles and Kerr (1986) found that the purchase of various foods were ranked hierarchically in terms of the social status of family members and that the distribution of food in the family reflected the relative power and status of each member. Similarly, Graham (1987) found that lone mothers no longer had to adapt to the food preferences of their male partners whereas when they had partners the women's preferences were 'eclipsed and reshaped to conform to the choice of their partner'.

The relationship between social position, health benefits and health-related behaviour is also illustrated in Graham's studies (1989) on tobacco use among families living in poverty. These studies emphasize the direct impact of the material circumstances in which people live and work on health-related behaviour. She found that spending money on tobacco is strongly related to particular forms of inequality and specifically with caring for children in poverty. In a qualitative investigation of women bringing up children living in poverty Graham showed how, in some families, smoking was associated with breaks from care when they rested and 'refuelled'. She also found that cigarettes were smoked during breaks in care when the demands of the children became too much with which to cope. When women were forced to cut back on luxury goods for themselves, such as shoes, hair cuts etc., cigarettes could be the only 'luxury' purchase they made for themselves. Thus smoking reflects the social isolation and stress of caring for children in poverty. In these circumstances the social benefits of habits such as smoking outweigh the known costs and even if some of these women would like to give up smoking, changing their health habits is difficult given the lack of resources such as time, energy and finance (Graham, 1993). (For further information on inequalities in health, the reader is referred to Chapter 2.)

Illness and its management

The public's conceptions of health and its maintenance also provide a general framework for making sense of the signs and symptoms of illness. Studies have shown that sufferers and their families, when faced with a disturbance in body functioning, ask a series of questions which include, 'What is happening?', 'Why is it happening to me?' and 'Why is it happening now?'. Sufferers examine their own theories of causality of disease in an attempt to answer some of these questions. These theories will be considered later but before this the focus will turn to the meaning of illness.

What is illness

'Disease is something an organ has; illness is something a man has' (Helman, 1981).

Disease and illness are distinct and the relationship between the two is not simple. Diseases may be discovered, for example through screening, but the person concerned may not be experiencing any change in bodily functioning. Conversely, a person may have signs and symptoms in the absence of a disease process.

How do lay people perceive illness? Not all problematic signs and symptoms lead the sufferer to define himself or herself as ill and in many cases 'health' problems are normalized and accommodated and people continue with their everyday routine tasks. Locker (1979) has argued that actions such as staying in bed, not going to work and going to see the doctor characterize people who are ill. He believes that illness is essentially a moral category where those labelled as ill are usually absolved of responsibility for action because the major causes of illness are believed to be outside their control, i.e. illness is viewed in terms of biological disorder.

Herzlich (1973), in her study of a sample of middle class French people, found that respondents conceived of illness as inactivity and discussed their reactions to illness in terms of their response to inactivity. The significance of inactivity for lay people is well illustrated by a respondent of Calnan and Johnson (1983) when discussing the possible impact on her life of having breast cancer:

> 'That's the funny thing about it because I don't think they fear pain or mutilation. Even I can't understand that. Everyone's got some fear of death but then we all know that we can die by so many other means, so it can't be just death. Perhaps it's the thought of being incapable and somebody having to look after you and not having your own mind, or being able to carry on with your life. I think that's probably my fear, all of a sudden perhaps being up in a bedroom with nobody to talk to except those who are very close popping in to say hello'.

This respondent identifies the more negative and destructive influences of inactivity and views illness as a destroyer. It illustrates one of the three types of responses to illness inactivity that Herzlich (1973) identified. People who respond to illness in this way might be less likely to seek medical care because of a refusal to acknowledge the problem. This might describe women referred to as 'deniers' by researchers investigating people with breast cancer, who delay medical consultation. Reluctance to seek medical care might also arise if it is thought to be of limited value. For example one of Calnan and Johnson's (1983) respondents states in relation to breast cancer, 'Well, I mean they can't really cure it can they … in spite of what they tell you?'. Radley (1989), in his study of chronic heart disease, gives similar evidence where illness is minimized through increased engagement in everyday activities and limited communication about signs and symptoms.

The other two types of response to illness identified by Herzlich (1973), are described as 'illness as an occupation' and 'illness as a liberator'. Those who explained illness in terms of an occupation emphasized the need to fight and control it. When defined in this way the respondent might do anything possible to manage the illness including seeking medical care. The group who saw illness as a liberator described illness or inactivity as a source of freedom from their everyday commitments. In these cases there was also a likelihood of consultation with the medical profession. The way people respond to illness has obvious implications for physiotherapists. For example a patient who feels liberated by his or her illness is likely to behave very differently from a patient who fights to control it. Eachus (1990) is of the opinion that if the physiotherapist has different views to those of his or her patient concerning the appropriate response to illness, there is likely to be conflict between them. He believes there is, on occasions, some justification for attempting to change the patient's beliefs. He states: 'The patient who can be encouraged to take active responsibility for his health is likely to benefit in terms of more rapid and successful recovery, as well as feelings of increased participation and satisfaction with the treatment process'.

Other studies have focused on the social processes involved in illness behaviour and help-seeking behaviour. The first cognitive stage involved in this process is the initial identification that something is wrong and an attempt to apply, if possible, a diagnostic label to the problematic experience. Helman (1981) has pointed out that each individual has a unique relationship with his or her body and thus his or her own personal models about what is abnormal and what is not. What is more difficult for the sufferer and significant others (e.g. relatives and friends), however, is applying a general label to the problematic experience. For example, there seems to be considerable variation and uncertainty about what a breast lump (possibly an early sign of breast cancer) might look like. One woman in a study by Calnan and Johnson (1983) stated: 'One of my friends who had breast cancer was in her fifties and she just told me one day that she had a lump in her breast and at that time I did not know that it was more dangerous to have little lumps than a large lump, yet the first friend of mine told me she had a lump like a pigeon's egg. So I just don't know. It is one of those subjects that one tends not to go into carefully'.

Some resolved the uncertainty by adopting a policy of 'If in doubt go to the doctor'. For example one woman stated, 'I think that if I found a lump, whatever size, I would go to the doctor and say, "Look I've found this little lump" '. The policy of going to the doctor with any sign or symptom does, however, have its costs as a respondent clearly stated: 'Well I had a small pimple on the nipple on the left side so I went alone – one has to make an appointment at our doctor … I telephoned to make the appointment for the following day, went along to the doctor and there was no pimple. I felt such a fool. He said to me "No there's nothing the matter" '.

This respondent was particularly concerned about wasting her general practitioner's time with what she considered to be a minor ailment and it illustrates the difficult position patients find themselves in. On the one hand they are uncertain about whether their signs and symptoms are serious and would like to go to the doctor to ease their minds, but on the other hand they do not want to be seen as 'bad' patients by their general practitioners or the type of people who over-utilize the service. For example one respondent stated, with reference to the early diagnosis of breast cancer, 'Oh, I would not think my doctor had time for that sort of thing. He would go mad if I bothered him with nothing'.

This leads to the second cognitive stage in the illness behaviour process which involves decisions about what to do about the health problem. The sufferer and significant others, have the options, at least in theory, of ignoring the problem, waiting and seeing what develops, or deciding to do something about it which might involve self-treatment or seeking outside help.

The number of empirical studies which have examined decision rules that people use to decide what to do about health problems is small. However, Cowie (1976), in a study of cardiac patients examined the ways in which signs and symptoms were evaluated and how patients responded to them. He found that their responses were coloured by the context in which pain was experienced. Perception of the need for urgent medical attention was more likely to occur when the pain was sudden, acute and unexpected. However, 16 of the 23 patients initially applied a common sense lay diagnostic category. Some identified the pain as a bout of indigestion and others related it to a recurrence of other minor illnesses they had recently had.

This process of normalization was upset by their failure to understand the physical experiences in terms of the interpretive framework available to them and by changes in the quality and duration of the signs and symptoms. Cowie (1974) reports that this sometimes happened when lay others, such as spouses, evaluated something as wrong when the sufferers were not behaving in accordance with their spouses' conceptions of how they normally behaved. Thus, decisions to seek medical care tended to occur when sufferers and significant others could no longer account for signs and symptoms within their framework of everyday knowledge. (For further information on pain, the reader is referred to Chapter 10.)

Clearly, uncertainty about what is wrong is a significant influence on people's decisions to seek medical care. However, in relation to cancer, uncertainty can have an inhibiting effect. For example, a woman in a study by Calnan and Johnson (1983) stated that sometimes she was hesitant or nervous about seeking medical help. She explained when this occurred: 'If I have got something pretty foreign to me and I cannot sort of create a self-diagnosis, I automatically think the worst. I feel that this is what everybody does … For instance, should I have a lump appear on me I would automatically think it must be cancer because I had a friend who was about 3 months younger than I was – she just suddenly died of cancer – and it hit me – and I thought that …'

In these circumstances some women may consult their doctors because they feel they should and because they want to know what is wrong. However, others might prefer to stay ignorant because they believe that nothing can be done about it anyway. Robinson (1974) has suggested that sufferers, although aware of the salience of their signs and symptoms, still tolerate and accommodate them on the grounds that the social, psychological or economic costs of accepting the illness, in terms of the dependent sick role and seeking medical care, far out-weigh the benefits.

Making sense of signs and symptoms

Lay theories about disease causation are important for interpreting and making sense of signs and symptoms. The available evidence suggests that people hold specific theories about a range of diseases, although there is a mode of thought or logic common to these theories. For example, heart disease and depression are viewed as products of an imbalance between the individual and the environment. A logic of degeneration is inherent in lay theories about diseases such as arthritis, and a logic of invasion in others such as AIDS. Calnan (1987) found that cancer was the disease with which people found the most difficult identifying a clear logic of causality because it is shrouded in mystery. One respondent said: 'I really have no idea but it's just sort of a nasty bogey that is tucked away in the back of the cupboard. I have no idea – my husband's brother he died of cancer when he was twenty eight'.

People's theories about the causality of illness also have implications for feelings of control and responsibility. For example the following quotations concerning heart attacks and AIDS, taken from a study by Calnan (1991), suggest that some diseases are viewed as punishments which people bring upon themselves, whereas others are thought to be outside their control.

> 'Heart attacks, some people have defective hearts, some people cause their hearts to be defective through smoking. I suppose you could say they deserve it in a way, but in the case of a smoker it's self-induced, obviously the person who was born with a defective heart can do little about it.
>
> 'Well, if you are daft enough to use a dirty needle, and stick it in your arm you get what you are asking for. If you are sleeping around with the wrong people or indeed anybody, and you know you don't have the right precautions, you're asking for what you get. That's a very broad view, but there's always the unlucky one who gets you know ...'.

Thus for some diseases some degree of responsibility is imputed, although as Pill and Scott (1982) point out, the majority of people feel that illnesses are caused by factors outside their control such as hereditary or environmental factors (Davison *et al.* 1991).

Evidence from empirical research suggests that people's theories about disease causation not only contain ideas about the typical circumstances likely to produce an illness but also stereotypes or images of those types of people who are particularly vulnerable to specific diseases. For example, West (1976) showed how parents with children with epilepsy sometimes doubted the clinical diagnosis as their child's identity did not match up with what they considered to be a typical epileptic. The type of person thought most likely to develop coronary heart disease was described in a study by Calnan (1991) as the anxious and nervous type. This stereotype was similar in some ways to that used by people to characterize those who are particularly vulnerable to breast cancer. A respondent in a study by Calnan and Johnson (1983) said: 'Well, these two women I know who have had breast cancer, they are both highly nervous people. When I say nervous I do not mean that they are frightened of their own shadows but they are both very thin. They are both wiry people, probably people who tend to live on their nerves'.

This image of the thin and nervous person being particularly vulnerable to cancer is compatible with how Sontag (1979) has portrayed the vulnerable person, who she describes as internally repressed. Thus, the lay person, when assessing vulnerability, or the meaning of symptoms, asks him or herself if the circumstances are compatible with his theory about the causation of the disease and whether he or she is the type of person who is likely to get it.

Chronic illness

For some the experience of illness is short term, for others such as those who suffer from chronic illness it is, by definition, a long-term and perhaps permanent event. Bury (1982) identifies two forms of meaning with regard to chronic illness. The first involves the consequences of the illness for the individual in terms of disruption to daily life. In this case advice about the management of symptoms may be sought from a range of different networks. Also, in the early period of a medical condition, management by individuals may be tentative and uncertain as they attempt to control and perhaps minimize the effects of signs and symptoms.

Second, the meaning of chronic illness, may be seen in terms of its social significance i.e. the image of the disease and how individuals think it is seen by others. Meanings surrounding illness often change as they interact with different stages of the life course. Robinson (1988), for example, shows that patients with multiple sclerosis report being at risk of having their symptoms misunderstood as signs of mental illness, malingering or even being drunk by those who do not understand.

There is also the important issue of how sufferers and their families cope with chronic illness long term. Various factors may explain variations in coping such as the impact of social position or gender. Kelleher (1988) shows that women who have diabetes are more likely to normalize and deny their condition than men as they are more likely to suffer anxiety in the management of their condition. (For further information about illness behaviour, the reader is referred to Chapter 8.).

Conclusion

The aim of this chapter has been to illustrate lay perspectives on health and its maintenance and on illness and its management, by drawing on different kinds of empirical material. The material clearly illustrates that lay people have their own complex models of health and illness which they use to make sense of health problems and other health-related matters. This health knowledge influences their decision to seek professional help and affects their response to professional treatment and their reaction to illness and disability. Sim (1990) believes that physiotherapists should attempt to understand and respect the lay beliefs of their patients. He states: 'Lay theories of health and illness should be assessed as to their usefulness. If they are functional in aiding people to make sense of, or come to terms with, their health experience, then they are valid. Their 'rightness' or 'wrongness' is largely an irrelevance'.

References

Backett K. (1992) Taboos and excuses: lay health moralities in middle class families. *Sociology of Health and Illness*, **14**, 255–274.

Blaxter M. (1990) *Health and Lifestyles*. London: Routledge.

Bury M. (1982) Chronic illness as biographical disruption. *Sociology of Health and Illness*. **4**, 167–182.

Bury M. (1991) The sociology of chronic illness: a review of research and prospects. *Sociology of Health and Illness*. **13**(40), 451–468.

Calnan M. (1987) *Health and Illness: The Lay Perspective*. London: Tavistock.

Calnan M. (1989) Control over health and patterns of health related behaviour. *Social Science and Medicine*, **2**, 131–136.

Calnan M. (1990) Food and health. In *Readings in Medical Sociology* (Cunningham-Burley S., McKeganey N., eds). London: Tavistock.

Calnan M. (1991) *Preventing Coronary Heart Disease: Prospects, Politics and Policies*. London: Routledge.

Calnan M., Cant S. (1990) The social organisation of food consumption. *International Journal of Sociology and Social Policy*, **10**(2), 53–79.

Calnan M., Johnson B. (1983) Understanding non-compliance with cancer education campaigns. In *Public Education about Cancer* (Hobbs P., ed.). Geneva: IUAC, pp. 49–64.

Calnan M., Johnson B. (1985) Health, health risks and inequalities. *Sociology of Health and Illness*, **7**(1), 55–75.

Calnan M., Rutter D. (1986) Do health beliefs predict health behaviours. *Social Science and Medicine*, **22**, 673–678.

Calnan M., Williams S. (1991) Style of life and the salience of health. *Sociology of Health and Illness*, **13**, 506–529.

Charles N., Kerr M. (1986) Servers and providers: distribution of food within the family. *Sociological Rview*, **34**(1), 115–157.

Cornwell J. (1984) *Hard-Earned Lives: Accounts of Health and Illness from East London*. London: Tavistock.

Cowie B. (1976) The cardiac patient's perceptions of a heart attack. *Social Science and Medicine*, **10**, 87–96.

Crawford R. (1984) A cultural account of health-control, release and the social body. In *Issues in the Political Economy of Health* (McKinlay J., ed.). London: Tavistock.

Davison C., Davey Smith G., Frankel J. (1992) Lay epidemiology and the prevention paradox. *Sociology of Health and Illness*, **13**, 1–19.

Eachus P. (1990) Health locus of control in student physiotherapists. *Physiotherapy*, **76**(7), 366–370.

Graham H. (1987) Being poor. In: *Give and Take in Families; Studies of resource distribution* (Brannen J. and Wilson G. eds). London: Allen and Unwin.

Graham H. (1989) Women and smoking in the UK: the implications for health promotion. *Health Promotion*, **3**, 371–381.

Graham H. (1993) *Hardship and Health in Women's Lives*. London: Harvester Wheatsheaf.

Helman C. (1981) Disease versus illness in general practice. *Journal of the Royal College of General Practitioners*, **31**, 548–552.

Herzlich C. (1973) *Health and Illness*. London: Academic Press.

Janz N., Becker H. (1984) The health belief model: a decade later. *Health Education Quarterly*, **11**, 1–47.

Kelleher D. (1988) *Diabetes*. London: Tavistock.

Langlie J. (1977) Interrelationships among preventive behaviour. *Public Health Report*, **94**, 216–220.

Locker D. (1979) *Symptoms and Illness*. London: Tavistock.

Lupton D., Chapman S. (1995) A healthy lifestyle might be the death of you. *Sociology of Health and Illness*, **17**(4), 458–476.

Pill R., Stott N. (1982) Concepts of illness causation's and responsibility. *Social Science and Medicine*, **16**, 43–52.

Radley A. (1989) Style, discourse and constraint in adjustment to chronic illness. *Sociology of Health and Illness*, **11**, 231–252.

Robinson D. (1974) *The Process of Becoming Ill.* London: Routledge and Kegan Paul.

Robinson I. (1988) *Multiple Sclerosis.* London: Routledge.

Sim J. (1990) The concept of health. *Physiotherapy*, **76**(7), 423–428.

Sontag S. (1979) *Illness as a Metaphor.* London: Allan Lane.

Wallston H., De Vellis D. (1978) Development of the multidimensional health locus of control. *Health Education Monograph*, **6**, 160–170.

West P. (1976) The physician and the management of childhood epilepsy. In *Studies in Everyday Life* (Wadsworth M., Robinson D., eds). London: Martin Robertson.

Young A. (1991) When rational men fall sick – *Culture, Medicine and Psychiatry.* **5**: 317–335.

14

Age-related cognitive change: working with elderly people

Janet M. Simpson

Most old people, at least those under 80 years of age, are living in the community and having as good a time as the rest of us (Hunt, 1978). Those of them who required physiotherapy usually present with a single health problem such as low back pain, a fracture, a chest infection and, apart from the date of birth on their referral form, and perhaps a few more wrinkles and grey hairs, there is nothing much about these people to suggest that they are very different from people 10 or even 15 years younger, and on the whole they are not (Hunt, 1978). These clients are to be distinguished from very old people, who have been fortunate in reaching their eighth or ninth decade of life but at the same time have been unlucky enough to have accumulated several health problems. These very old people are usually under the care of a specialist in old age medicine (Young, 1989) and they are regular users of physiotherapy services (Simpson *et al.*, 1993).

In this chapter I shall focus on changes in cognitive processes (to do with the acquisition and use of knowledge) that occur with ageing. Awareness of these changes helps therapists to understand their elderly clients and enables them to gain their clients' co-operation in rehabilitation.

First I shall show that ageing is not just a straightforward, chronological process but, among other factors, is increasingly related to health. I shall then summarize current thinking on changes in cognitive performance before going on to draw implications for working with elderly people. But first a note about terminology. There is considerable fluidity in this respect in cognitive psychology. Several words have similar meanings and tend to be used interchangeably although they are not really synonymous: psychological, mental, cognitive, intellectual; also performance, ability, skill. The references I shall cite are either key studies or papers or they are useful reviews or text books for readers who wish to explore the subject of age related cognitive change further.

Processes of ageing

Old age itself is not a disease and chronological age is merely an index of the passing time. But the more time that has passed the wider is our experience and the more different we become from one another. Also, the older we are the more likely we are to have acquired an array of pathologies. Thus various factors both intrinsic and extrinsic to the person contribute to the ageing process. Several useful models of ageing have been proposed (see Stuart-Hamilton, 1994, Chapter 1; Hayslip and Panek, 1993, Chapters 1 and 2). For our purposes I will describe the simple distinction between *primary* and *secondary* ageing made by Busse (1969).

Primary ageing encompasses those changes that we can all expect to take place to some extent as we grow older. In terms of onset and duration these changes show a fairly strong relationship to chronological age and are largely, but not exclusively, biologically determined. They occur in highly similar ways for all individuals in a given culture.

Secondary ageing refers to those processes which do not affect everybody to the same extent and are usually attributable to injury and other health problems. They do not occur in the same way to all individuals.

This distinction implies that old people, even in one culture at one point in historical time are very variable. Because each person's life experiences are different, the longer we live the more different from each other we become. It is much more difficult to visualize the typical 80-year-old person that it is to conjure up a picture of the typical 4-year-old child. There are also going to be differences between age groups at any one point in time which may be attributable to the effects of ageing itself but also to differences in the context in which generations of people have grown up (cohort effects). National policy on education or health care, the occurrence of wars, food shortages and disease epidemics for example, as well as cultural norms regarding appropriate age-related behaviour may all influence the way in which a person develops. Below I shall show how between-cohort variability can have critical implications for researchers seeking to understand the way people change with age. In general then, therapists would be unwise to assume that all old people are experiencing the same amount of change in intellectual performance. Deterioration will be less noticeable, if at all, among old people who have had the benefit of good education, are healthy and living stimulating lives and there will always be some old people who function at higher levels than some young people.

Health status and mental performance

Organic diseases of the brain such as Alzheimer's disease or multiple strokes directly impair mental functioning. I shall not cover the particular psychological changes associated with these conditions but therapists working with sufferers and with severely depressed people require specialist knowledge and communication skills (Holden and Woods, 1995; Kunanac and Simpson, 1995; Pomeroy, 1995).

However, even subclinical ill health is now recognized to affect mental performance, even slightly raised blood pressure is related to poorer performance on a variety of psychological tests (Elias *et al.*, 1990). Moreover among generally healthy people there is still a relationship between level of fitness and mental ability. Among a group of 60–90 year olds who rated their own general physical health as above average for their own age group, the better they reported their health on a detailed questionnaire, the better, in general, was their intelligence test performance (Perlmutter and Nyquist, 1990). Mental speed, as measured by the time taken to process verbal material correlated modestly with self-reported fitness among normal, healthy adults aged between 55 and 86 years (Hultsch *et al.*, 1993). Birren and Fisher (1995) review the growing body of evidence indicating a positive association between aerobic fitness and cognitive functioning.

Most of these studies are, however, correlational and so the causal direction of the relationship cannot be established with certainty. It is just possible, as Perlmutter and Nyquist (1990) point out, that in their study poorer intellectual functioning might have led to poorer self-perceptions of health, especially mental health, rather than the other way round. Also, whatever is causing people to have raised blood pressure may also be causing their mental performance to deteriorate rather than the raised blood pressure itself being the direct causal agent.

Changes in intellectual abilities

Intelligence is defined as the general ability to think, solve problems and learn new tasks. Rather than a single unified construct it is regarded as a system of abilities, probably a hierarchy, which changes in different ways with ageing.

A commonly used intelligence test is the Wechsler Adult Intelligence Scale (WAIS). The full scale consists of 11 sub tests, a person's score on each of them is added up to yield his or her final score. WAIS data from cross-sectional studies, in which data are collected at the same period in time from groups of people of different ages, suggests that peoples' intellectual abilities peak in the mid-twenties and decline steadily after that (see Figure 14.1). But between-cohort variability poses a problem for cross-sectional studies as the effects of primary ageing may be confounded with cohort effects. For example early studies showed how the WAIS curve could be mapped onto a histogram of the number of years each cohort had, on average, spent in school (Birren and Morrison, 1961). Old people who participated in these studies had also had less opportunity for schooling than the younger cohorts; thus age was confounded with amount of education.

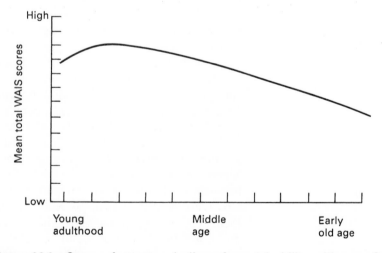

Figure 14.1 Curve of average decline of mental ability with age. Cross-sectional data.

Not all the WAIS sub-tests, however, show the same pattern of rapid decline starting in early adulthood. One group of sub-tests, designated verbal, are not performed under time limits. They draw on stored wisdom and are related to educational achievement. The subject must recall miscellaneous information for example, or explain the meaning of words and of familiar facts. In contrast, another group, called performance measures, have time limits on their completion and tap abilities which are relatively unaffected by educational attainments but which require mental speed. For example, the testee is timed while arranging a set of pictures into a logical sequence, or while recoding a set of digits as abstract symbols (Hayslip and Panek, 1993, Chapter 6, describe the WAIS and other intelligence tests in more detail, see also Stuart-Hamilton, 1994, Chapter 2).

Figure 14.2 illustrates the shape of the curves that emerge when results for the verbal and performance WAIS sub-tests are plotted separately. Older people's decrement in total test scores is seen to be due for the most part to their inefficiency, compared with younger people, on the performance sub-tests. This finding is very robust: it has been demonstrated for different races, for different social classes and for men as well as women. Furthermore, a similar pattern of results appears in data gathered with other types of intelligence test.

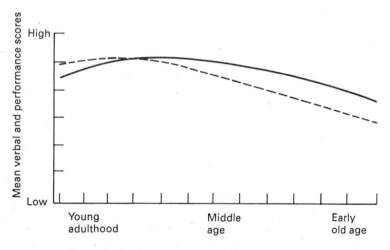

Figure 14.2 Comparative decline of verbal and performance sub-tests on WAIS with age. Cross-sectional data. ——— verbal; – – – performance.

Between-cohort differences, i.e. generational differences, tend to exaggerate the apparent intellectual deterioration in old age. Longitudinal studies, which record age changes in the same individuals over time, show less decline in test performance. They also suggest it starts later in life than cross-sectional studies imply. But problems of distortion are also associated with this type of investigation – it may under-estimate change. People who score rather poorly on intelligence tests when first recruited to a study appear to be more likely to drop-out for one reason or another than those who score better (Siegler and Botwinick, 1979). Hence the people available to be tested later in the study tend to be the cleverer ones in the original sample.

To overcome these difficulties, sophisticated study designs have been developed which combine elements of both cross-sectional and longitudinal studies (Hayslip and Panek, 1993, Chapter 2). Research conducted in this way confirms that various intellectual abilities change at different rates (Schaie, 1990). The peak of overall intellectual capacity, which sets limits on performance in the absence of any effect due to poor health, lack of education or absence of motivation, is probably reached in the 20s coinciding with biological maturity. After that people gradually become less proficient at tasks such as reasoning, problem solving and integrating new information especially if performing under time pressure. However, noticeable decline in these skills may not become apparent until the 50s or 60s or even later. Our knowledge and experience-related abilities show little or no decline although they may plateau later in life. Schaie (1990) emphasizes inter-individual variability. In the Seattle longitudinal studies, the incidence of significant decrement was quite limited until age 60 and even by age 81 it was apparent in only 30–40% of participants. Very few individuals showed global decline in all mental abilities and about 50% of people in their 80s maintained their level of previous functioning in most of them. Beyond that, however, most people did show evidence of global decline.

Ageing and mental speed

It is tempting to attribute all the slowing in performance apparent as we age to peripheral factors involved in the time required to sense the stimulus and to make the response. That is, to changes in sense organs, in speed of muscle contraction, in range of joint movement. Research suggests however, that slowing is due to changes at the CNS-level leading to slowing in the central mechanisms responsible for interpreting incoming stimuli and for deciding on the appropriate response to make (Salthouse, 1985; Welford, 1985; Cerella, 1990; Craik and Jennings, 1992; Birren and Fisher, 1995).

Changes in sensory mechanisms probably mean that the strength of signals from the sensory receptors to the brain is diminished. As we grow older we have more difficulty in bringing objects we see into focus, we become more susceptible to glare, require more time to adapt to the dark and our visual acuity decreases so that less detail can be appreciated. We also experience some loss of hearing especially for high frequency sounds as well as alterations in other senses (see Stuart-Hamilton, 1994, Chapter 1; Hayslip and Panek, 1993, Chapter 4). But evidence comparing simple reaction time (SRT) and choice reaction time (CRT) tasks suggest that neither sensory changes nor changes in movement time to make responses contribute greatly to slower performance.

In an SRT task subjects must respond as quickly as possible, usually by pressing a button or raising a finger from a button, to the onset of a signal such as a light or sound. The actual amount of movement required is minimal. In CRT tasks the movement required to respond is similar but rapid thinking is necessary to decide which response to make. For example there may be several different light signals, some needing a button to be pressed with the left index finger when they flash on and others needing a button to be pressed with the right index finger when they flash on or a response being required to a high but not a low tone.

As the decisions to be made become more complex, the more mental operations will be required to select an appropriate response. An age–complexity interaction in response time has been found, the more complex the decision, the more time older adults need to respond. This finding suggests that much of the age-related slowing in performance is due to slower thinking time. Other contributory factors have been proposed especially motivational factors such as increased difficulty in ignoring irrelevant information and emphasizing accuracy at the expense of speed. However, evidence from the Baltimore longitudinal study is inconsistent with the latter. Fozard *et al.* (1994) report simultaneous increases in both response time (RT), response variance, and errors (pressing the wrong button in response to the target auditory stimulus).

One explanation at a higher level is based on the concept of signal to noise ratios (Welford, 1985). Whether or not a person detects a stimulus, such as an auditory or visual signal, depends on the strength of the stimulus itself relative to the amount of conflicting, irrelevant, background 'noise' that is also impinging on his or her sense organs. Thus the likelihood of a stimulus or signal being successfully detected depends on the signal to noise ratio. For example, it is more difficult to hear someone over a poor, crackly telephone line than over a clear crackle-free line. It is also more difficult to hear a caller who mumbles quietly than one who speaks clearly and it is very difficult indeed to understand a mumbler over an unclear line and with a car-engine being revved in the background.

As we have noted above, changes in the sense organs may result in weaker signals entering the central nervous system in old age. Welford (1985) hypothesizes that these weak signals may then have to compete against increasing levels of neural noise in the CNS itself. Neural noise may arise as a result of age changes in neurones and their connections. So the person may have to allow more and more signals to accumulate before the nature of the signal can be registered and interpreted.

For a satisfactory theory of age-related changes, a hierarchy of explanations must be sought such that changes at the physiological, cognitive and intelligent behaviour levels link together (Birren and Fisher, 1995). On the one hand it is widely accepted that slower information processing can account for all cognitive and intelligence-related changes and that slowing is linked to biological variables, possibly white matter changes. On the other hand there are two theories of slowing: the generalized and the process specific. According to Cerella's (1990) 'accumulated loss hypothesis' slowing is due to more and more breaks in the neural network which makes up the CNS. These breaks simply mean that nerve impulses are often diverted and hence need more time to reach their destinations. Thus each component process in a complex task is slowed and these losses accumulate. Slowing of a highly complex task should be proportional to that of a less complex task. Alternatively the rate of slowing may be specific to a particular task. These two theories are not incompatible and both may be incorporated in a hierarchical model. At the neuronal level slowing may be general but this may be mediated by higher level components such that it appears as performance differences between tasks. The neural noise theory may fit into this scheme.

Nevertheless, old people's slowness in decision-making may not be particularly apparent in everyday life. Also, as Rabbitt (1986) makes clear, not all old people deteriorate and some remain very proficient until very late in life. He tested 998 people aged 18 to 92 on various reaction time tasks. Of the people aged between 75 and 85 years, 10% performed as fast and as accurately as the best subjects aged 30–50 years.

Mental speed, learning and memory

Decrease in information processing speed can explain much of our age-related loss of memory efficiency. Of course, we can still learn new information and new skills in old age, a foreign language, for example or how to operate a video-player or a word-processor, but we tend to need more time to do so.

Five processes have been identified in the chain of mechanisms by which material is learnt and then recalled (Welford, 1985):

1. Material is perceived and comprehended.
2. It is held for a few seconds in short-term memory (STM) until it is either lost or passes to the third stage of processing. These items are in conscious awareness and are lost rapidly if not processed further.
3. Registration in long-term memory (LTM) occurs, i.e. the material is encoded into a durable memory trace.
4. The coded material is stored in long-term memory until required.
5. It is recovered from long-term storage.

This model shows that memory itself is conceptualized as a number of processes, which in practice are closely linked, rather than a single 'box' in the head. Elderly people seem to have problems with some memory processes more than with others.

Perception and comprehension: Several processes are involved when we perceive and comprehend the material to be learnt. I have already described how changes due to age in our peripheral sensory mechanisms can reduce the quality of incoming signals reducing the likelihood that they will be efficiently registered. So difficulties at this stage may contribute to reducing older people's learning proficiency but not account for them significantly. We do not, of course, remember the stimulus itself but our interpretation of it, what it means to us.

Short-term memory: This memory process is to be distinguished from memory for recent events. e.g. 'What did I ask you to do five minutes ago?'. According to current thinking that information will already be in some form of long-term store. Short-term memory (STM) has a limited capacity and items are dealt with in a matter of a few seconds. They are held in awareness, and this part of the memory system is thought to have a controlling function for all thinking and remembering activity (Baddeley, 1992).

One way to measure STM capacity is by the serial memory span task which also forms one of the WAIS sub-tests. A person is presented, either visually or verbally, with a sequence of digits or letters at the rate of one every 2 seconds. Immediately, she has to repeat the list in the same order in which it was presented. Her score is the longest string of items that can be correctly reproduced.

Most people between 20 and 60 years of age can manage to reproduce six to seven items without any trouble. The average may drop slightly in the 60s and 70s to five to six items depending on the type of material to be remembered. It seems that, provided that the material does not have to be changed in any way, such as repeating it backwards (backwards memory span), this ability does not decline markedly in early old age, although it may do so in late old age.

These results suggest that STM capacity is only slightly affected by age (Welford, 1985; Craik and Jennings, 1992). The memory span tasks, however, reflect a rather passive form of storage and when more demands are placed on STM processes, such as that required by the backward memory span task, age-related decrements appear. Older people are likely to have difficulty in simultaneously holding and manipulating information being held in awareness. In practice this problem may be apparent in tasks such as mental arithmetic or in keeping track of who said what in a group discussion (Rabbitt, 1981).

This tendency can be explained in terms of the working memory model of STM where STM is thought to be made up of several sub-processes. They comprise a central executive supplemented by various slave systems all with limited storage capacity. One of these is responsible for rehearsing verbal material and another for maintaining visuo-spatial material in awareness. The central executive itself probably exerts an overall controlling function as well as being able to store limited amounts of material. This model is summarized by Baddeley (1992), and Stuart-Hamilton (1994). The central executive's storage capacity may well decrease with age, if so the reduction in processing resources may affect many aspects of mental performance.

Encoding: the perceived material is encoded into a memory trace for long-term storage. To encode the material it must be stored briefly while it is manipulated simultaneously in some way such as rehearsing it, reorganizing or regrouping it.

The more elaborately items are encoded, i.e. the more information about them that is processed, and the more effective the strategies developed for organizing the material, then the more efficiently it will be retrieved at the fifth stage. For example encoding verbal material in terms of its meaning leads to it being retrieved more easily than if it were processed in terms of its sound. For this reason rote learning is an inefficient learning strategy. Old people do not seem to engage spontaneously in the most effective encoding strategies and when they are instructed how to do so the outcome is still not as good as that of younger people (Hulicka and Grossman, 1967).

Also, compared to younger people, it appears that old people are more easily distracted. Kay (1951) showed that if an old person makes an error in a learning task, he or she may persist in making the same mistake over and over again. Old people seem to have difficulty in eliminating previous errors.

Encoding operations require additional mental space. From one perspective it appears that the available space in terms of working memory capacity may decrease in old age but in turn this may be related to slower information processing speed.

Long-term storage: the long-term store probably has a huge, even unlimited, capacity. The memory traces maintained there are not in awareness. Old people probably have few problems at this stage as they do not appear to forget more readily than younger people.

Retrieval: old people have difficulties in retrieving material from long-term store. The more material they have to recall, the worse they are compared with young people. However, under certain conditions their performance does not differ very much from that shown by young people.

Remembering items learnt by rote is hard at any age but becomes even harder in old age. This is particularly true of people's names (Maylor, 1996). The difficulty with names is understandable. There is no reason, apart from my parents' whim why I was given the name I have, there is nothing about my face that dictates that I should be called Janet, other people just have to rote learn the connection between me and my name. In contrast most other information that we need to recall is embedded in a rich network of related material allowing alternative paths of access.

Old people often perform as well or better than young people when it comes to using external memory aids in prospective memory tasks, i.e. memory for planned action such as remembering to telephone the researcher at his or her office during the next week. Their secret is that they are readier than young people to make use of notices, diaries, etc., but when they are not allowed to use such props they perform at the same level as young people (Maylor, 1990). Overall, elderly people are at a disadvantage when they have to rely on internal cues. They benefit from another form of prompt – retrieval support. In a free recall memory test the subject has to remember as much of the material he or she has learnt as possible and report it in any order. In a recognition memory test, however, he or she has to identify this target material, by distinguishing it from new items that were not presented at the pre-test. Both young and old people are much better when they are tested by recognition than by free recall. But although the young are still better than the old, the difference between them is less than under free recall conditions. Thus old people benefit most from the retrieval support offered by the recognition condition.

Retrieval support means that the array of possible items to be recalled is reduced, so the subject does not have such an extensive search to find the required information. Old people can, like young people, benefit from cueing which also offers retrieval support. For example giving the first letter or syllable of the word to be recalled ('My name begins with "J" ') or hinting at the category of material to be recalled (for apple: 'You can eat it', 'Its a fruit'). Therapists can make good use of retrieval support in appropriate circumstances.

Retrieval support benefits old people even more than young ones. So part of their memory difficulty may arise from actual retrieval deficits such as inefficient searching of the memory store. But, as we have seen, even with retrieval support they still do not recall as much as younger people. It seems, therefore, that old people's difficulties with recall also arise from poor encoding at Stage three. If material is not elaborately encoded, especially in terms of meaning, then it is more difficult to locate and retrieve.

Working with older adults

Inexperienced therapists, like novice doctors, are often baffled by the multiple pathology presented by frail old people (Young, 1989; Simpson, 1993). Furthermore, an old person's apparent lack of enthusiasm for rehabilitation can result in therapists shrugging them off as 'not being motivated', but the problem is more likely to lie with therapists who lack the knowledge and skills to elicit their elderly patients' cooperation.

It often helps us to understand old people to think in terms of processing capacity or resources available for mental activity. As we have seen, these resources, like those for physical activity, are likely to decrease in later life. Starting with changes in the nervous system, a chain of events appears to lead to slowed information processing and on to restricted working memory capacity. In most day-to-day business, however, this restriction may be of little consequence, the elderly person can cope within his or her available capacity. However, if he or she becomes tired, feels unwell or is stressed in some other way, his or her coping resources may be overloaded to the extent that performance suffers. In a similar situation a younger person, who will have more reserves of resources may not suffer a noticeable deterioration in performance.

Therapists, therefore, should be alert to an older client's needs in these respects. For example it might make a difference whether or not a client has been able to have a nap on his or her bed after lunch or has just been left to doze in an armchair. Some elderly in-patients, who are often woken quite early, have been known to fall asleep on the exercise bed in the physiotherapy department because they have been so tired!

There are two main strategies to avoid overloading mental resources:

1. Allow the older person plenty of time to carry out a task.
2. Do not ask an older person to do more than one thing at a time.

Also taking account of elderly people's deficits in attention (possibly also attributable to slower information processing), it is advisable to avoid distractions.

A client's habitual style of conversation is often a guide to his or her capabilities. If he or she answers questions with sensible, lengthy and complex utterances rather than monosyllabic ones (but beware confabulation which can sound normal to the novice), it suggests that his or her working memory can cope with processing lengthy, complex utterances from the therapist.

If this does not appear to be the case the therapist is advised to speak to the client in short, simple phrases. For example, 'Mrs Jones' (pause to catch client's attention), 'please sit here' (indicate, pause), 'please sit on the side of your bed' (repeat as necessary). All unnecessary words are dropped, the key phrases stand out, they are not embedded in a matrix of extraneous niceties. The tone of the therapist's voice should be friendly and pleasant and the therapist should smile at Mrs Jones. We can convey politeness and empathy by our manner and touch even if our words may sometimes have to be pared down to essentials. Whereas it would usually be inadvisable to put your arm around the shoulders of a younger out-patient or in-patient and give that person a hug, old people may appreciate the warmth this gesture conveys. They often lack physical contact especially if they do not have any living friends or relatives. But we cannot assume that all old people would welcome such intimate contact!

To any elderly person, learning a new skill such as manoeuvring a wheelchair or walking with a frame may be stressful if the teaching is rushed. To avoid stress on mental resources, it is advisable to keep instructions short. Provide one chunk of information at a time and then allow time for each chunk to be encoded before adding the next one. For example, the instructions for relearning a familiar activity such as standing up from a chair can be overwhelming if quickly listed in one go: 'Please move your bottom to the front of the seat and put your feet well underneath you and push up from the arms of the chair with your hands'. In this situation the rapidly incoming information may interfere with the processing of items already being held in working memory. The client is effectively being asked to perform two tasks at the same time, take in the new information while still dealing with the previous chunk.

In a group discussion, the participants also have to do several things at once. They have to remember what was said, and who said it as well as work out what they may wish to contribute. Rabbitt (1981) found that older people often had difficulties even when they had perfectly good hearing. He advises younger people unostentatiously to up-date elderly participants about what is going on if they appear to have lost track of the proceedings. Rabbitt's work suggests it may be inadvisable to arrange activities for large numbers of old people grouped together, probably six or eight is most satisfactory.

Showing an interest in the person's previous job or hobbies often fosters self-esteem and building choices into the treatment session encourages feelings of personal autonomy (Weinberg, 1995). These feelings together with an agreed achievable treatment goal (Cott, 1995), increase the likelihood that the person will cooperate in what might appear to be a painful and strenuous task. As Rodin (1986) and Coleman (1986) also make clear, old people risk developing feelings of incompetence. Most of their achievements are behind them and they are faced with failure more often than are young people even in the simplest of daily activities. Obviously this risk increases if the person has a mobility problem. The rehabilitation therapist can bolster his or her elderly client's self-esteem, and hence more easily elicit his or her cooperation in several ways. In particular:

1. Show respect for the person's past achievements.
2. Recognize and acknowledge current achievements and successes.
3. Set achievable mobility goals.

Further guidance on working with elderly people is available: Peterson (1989) reviews research findings on learning in old age and draws implications for physiotherapy practice, Orange and Ryan (1995) advise on effective communication and in Chapter 6 of this book French discusses the implications of ageism.

Conclusion

However trivial the patient's success may appear to the physiotherapist or however small an achievable goal may seem, the old person may have had to expend considerable energy to reach it and may also have had to overcome pain, fatigue and fear. Our elderly patients should not fail at their rehabilitation tasks, if they do so, it may be the therapist's fault. Familiarity with cognitive changes that occur to all of us as we grow older and their concomitant implications for working with this client group facilitates success for both participants.

References

Baddeley A. D. (1992) Working memory. *Science* **255**: 556–559.

Birren J. E., Fisher L. M. (1995) Aging and the speed of behaviour: possible consequences for psychological functioning. *Annual Review of Psychology* **46**: 329–353.

Birren J. E., Morrison D. F. (1961) Analysis of the WAIS sub-tests in relation to age and education. *Journal of Gerontology*, **16**, 363–369.

Busse E. W. (1969) Theories of aging. In *Behaviour and Adaptation in Later Life*. (Busse E. W., Pfeiffer E., eds). Boston: Little Brown, pp. 11–32.

Cerella J. (1990) Aging and information-processing rate. In *Handbook of the Psychology of Aging* (3rd edn) Birren J. E., Schaie K. W., eds). London: Academic Press.

Coleman P. (1986) *Ageing and Reminiscence Processes: Social and Clinical Implications*. Chichester: John Wiley.

Cott C. A. (1995) Goal planning. In *Physiotherapy with Older People* (Pickles B. *et al.*, eds). London: W. B Saunders.

Craik F. I. M., Jennings J. M. (1992) Human memory. In *The Handbook of Aging and Cognition* (Craik F. I. M., Salthouse T. A., eds). San Diego: Lawrence Erlbaum.

Elias M. F., Robbins M. A., Schultz N. R., Pierce T. W. (1990) Is blood pressure an important variable in research on aging and neuropsychological test performance? *Journal of Gerontology*, **45**, 128–135.

Fozard J. L., Vercruyssen M., Reynolds S. L. *et al.* (1994) Age differences and changes and reaction time: The Baltimore Longitudinal Study of Aging. *Journal of Gerontology*, **49**, 179–189.

Hayslip B. Jr, Panek P. E. (1993) *Adult Development and Aging* (2nd edn). New York: Harper Row.

Holden U., Woods R. (1995) *Positive Approaches to Dementia Care*. Edinburgh: Churchill Livingstone.

Hulicka I. M., Grossman I. L. (1967) Age group comparisons in the use of mediators in paired associate learning. *Journal of Gerontology*, **22**, 44–51.

Hultsch D. F., Hammer M., Small B. J. (1993) Age differences in cognitive performance in later life: relationship to self-reported health and active life style. *Journal of Gerontology*, **48**, 1–11.

Hunt A. (1978) *The Elderly at Home*. London: HMSO.

Kay H. (1951) Learning of a serial task by different age groups. *Quarterly Journal of Experimental Psychology*, **3**, 166–183.

Kunanec S., Simpson J. M. (1995) Psychiatric problems. In *Physiotherapy with Older People* (Pickles B. *et al.*, eds). London: W. B. Saunders.

Maylor E. A. (1990) Age and prospective memory. *Quarterly Journal of Experimental Psychology*, **42A**, 471–493.

Maylor E. A. (1996) Older people's memory for the past and the future. *The Psychologist*, **9**, 456–459.

Orange J. B., Ryan E. B. (1995) Effective communication. In *Physiotherapy with Older People* (Pickles B. *et al.*, eds). London: W. B. Saunders.

Perlmutter M., Nyquist L. (1990) Relationships between self-reported physical and mental health and intelligence performance across adulthood. *Journal of Gerontology*, **45**, 145–155.

Peterson D. A. (1989) Older adult learning. In *Physical Therapy of the Geriatric Patient* (2nd edn) (Jackson O., ed.). New York: Churchill Livingstone.

Pomeroy V. (1995) Dementia. In *Physiotherapy in Mental Health: A Practical Approach* (Everett T., Dennis M., Ricketts I., eds). Oxford: Butterworth-Heinemann.

Rabbitt P. (1981) Talking to the old. *New Society*, 22 January, 140–141.

Rabbitt P. (1986) Memory impairment in the elderly. In *Psychiatric Disorders in the Elderly* (Bebbington P. E., Tacoby R., eds). London: Mental Health Foundation.

Rodin J. (1986) Aging and health: effects of the sense of control. *Science*, **233**, 1271–1276.

Salthouse T. A. (1985) Speed of behaviour and its implications for cognition. In *Handbook of the Psychology of Aging* (2nd edn.) (Birren J. E., Schaie K. W. eds). New York: Van Nostrand Reinhold.

Schaie K. W. (1990) Intellectual development in adulthood. In *Handbook of the Psychology of Aging* (3rd edn) (Birren J. E., Schaie K. W., eds). London: Academic Press.

Siegler I. C., Botwinick J. (1979) A long-term longitudinal study of intellectual ability of older adults: the matter of selective subject attrition. *Journal of Gerontology*, **34**, 242–245.

Simpson J. M. (1993) Quality physiotherapy for people of all ages (Editorial). *Physiotherapy*, **79**, 3–4.

Simpson J. M., Revell G., Dyer J. (1993) Rehabilitation of elderly people: What should physiotherapist students learn on clinical placements? *Physiotherapy*, **79**: 628–632.

Stuart-Hamilton I. (1994) *The Psychology of Ageing* (2nd edn). London: Jessica Kingsley.

Weinberg I. C. (1995) Applications of perceived control and learned helplessness. In *Physiotherapy with Older People* (Pickles B. *et al.*, eds). London: W. B. Saunders.

Welford A. T. (1985) Changes of performance with age: an overview. In *Aging and Human Performance* (Charness N., ed.). Chichester: John Wiley.

Young A. (1989) There is no such thing as geriatric medicine, and it's here to stay. *Lancet*, **ii**, 263–265.

15

Cognitive and perceptual deficits following brain damage

M. Jane Riddoch

The main objective of physiotherapy is the restoration of function in the patient to as near a premorbid level as possible. In this chapter, the focus will be on the effects of brain damage on normal perceptual and cognitive abilities and how deficits in these abilities may affect the standard treatment of people with neurological deficits by the physiotherapist.

The effects of brain damage on human behaviour are often profound and long lasting. Traditionally, assessment of impairment by the physiotherapist has focused on disorders of tone, sensation, balance and movement (Bobath, 1970; Davies, 1985) and relatively little emphasis has been given to more central disorders (for example, perception, planning, memory, language comprehension and production). This may be because assessment of cognitive and perceptual performance is not seen to fall within the remit of the physiotherapist but is thought to be more appropriate for the clinical psychologist, occupational or speech therapist. However, while physical deficits may often be the primary restriction of a patient returning to normal daily living, frequently it is the cognitive and behavioural defects that most impair the capacity to return to work and maintain social activities. Also, it has been shown that cognitive and perceptual problems may significantly affect rehabilitation (Andrews *et al.*, 1982; Denes *et al.*, 1982; Wade *et al.*, 1985; Blanc-Garin, 1995; Jeffery and Good, 1995; Riddoch *et al.*, 1995a), in that patients with impaired perception and cognition fare worst at rehabilitation. Hence it is important that the physiotherapist should have some idea about the varieties of perceptual and cognitive deficit that may occur as a result of brain damage. Such knowledge would, at the very least, enable the therapist to refer the patient to the appropriate specialist. More significantly, some knowledge of perceptual and cognitive problems may help the therapist to devise more appropriate treatments for individual patients (see Riddoch *et al.*, 1995b).

To give some idea of the effects of a perceptual deficit on normal everyday functioning, let us consider the case of a young soldier wounded by a machine gun bullet during the First World War (Holmes and Horrax, 1919). The sophisticated techniques we have available today to locate precisely areas of brain damage were not available at that time, however, Holmes and Horrax indicate that the bullet entered the brain through the posterior portion of the right angular gyrus and left via the upper part of the left angular gyrus. The soldier regained consciousness after several days and was observed to be alert and intelligent. He showed no trace of weakness, incoordination or disturbance of muscle tone and could move his limbs easily and naturally. Yet, although he showed no obvious abnormality of gait, he would typically walk with short, slow steps with his hands held out in front of him. Furthermore, despite being able to see, he would collide with obstacles in his path always to his great surprise and discomfort. On questioning, he explained that he had not realized that the objects were so near to him. He was not blind. He did have defective vision in the lower part of his visual field, but this could not account for his behaviour since visual acuity was normal in the upper portions of the visual fields. The young soldier's difficulties were the result of an impaired perception of depth and the distances between objects.

This case provides a very clear example of how important normal depth perception is to everyday functioning, with the patient's difficulties resulting from a very circumscribed lesion. It is of course possible to argue that a physiotherapist would never actually encounter a patient such as this in the normal course of clinical work since the soldier was documented as having had no sensory/motor disability. However, many of the brain damaged patients typically encountered by the physiotherapist are likely to have diffuse rather than localized damage as a result of a stroke, head injury, viral infection, etc. Such diffuse damage is quite likely to implicate the motor and/or sensory areas of the brain; it is also conceivable that areas of the brain necessary for normal cognitive and perceptual functioning are implicated *additionally*. So, for instance, therapy sessions which emphasize the restitution of normal motor performance may fail if allowance is not made for perceptual and cognitive deficits. A patient may have a motor impairment in addition to a depth perception deficit. Concentrating on the physical impairment will not help the patient in his or her attempts to negotiate the everyday world. Furthermore, if the physiotherapist fails to appreciate and understand perceptual and cognitive problems, the patient may be classified as 'difficult' or 'uncooperative'; such labelling is likely to make the everyday life of the patient even more problematic.

A further, and all too frequent problem, is that after brain damage, patients may be unable to explain their impaired perceptions either to themselves or to the therapist. Brain damage can precipitate people into a strange and confusing world, and even if language functions are not directly affected, patients may lack the words to describe their new state. It is therefore imperative that therapists working with brain-damaged people should have some idea of the nature of normal cognitive and perceptual abilities and how they may be affected as a result of damage to the brain. Such knowledge may not only improve approaches to rehabilitation, but may also allow the therapist to help the patient understand, to some degree, failures in the performance of seemingly simple tasks.

We have many complicated perceptual and cognitive abilities. We are able to recognize a friend from a crowd of other people with no apparent effort, we can communicate our feelings to others by either the spoken or written word, we can traverse a town with a maze of apparently similar streets and arrive at a predetermined destination etc. However, this apparent ease of everyday functioning leaves us at a loss to explain cases where patients fail to recognize the therapist or even members of their own families from one day to the next; why the patient can understand a complex sentence (such as 'what is the name of the instrument we use to tell of the passage of the hours?') but will fail to understand a simple sentence such as 'put the pen on the pencil' (e.g. putting the pencil on the pen instead); or why the patient gets lost on the short route from the ward to the physiotherapy department. How can these abilities be classified and interpreted?

The traditional neuropsychological approach has been to ascribe different functions to the different lobes of the brain (i.e. the occipital lobes are concerned with vision, the parietal lobes are concerned with spatial abilities, the temporal lobes are concerned with memory and some language functions, while the frontal lobes are concerned with executive functions, such as the selection of which task to perform and also some language functions). More recently, a slightly different approach has emerged – often labelled cognitive neuropsychology. Its aim is to identify the component parts and processes of complex perceptual and cognitive behaviour by analysing the performance of both brain-damaged and non-brain-damaged subjects. The accounts of cognitive functions derived by cognitive neuropsychologists were not initially specified in terms of underlying brain structures. However, recently developed techniques in brain imaging (e.g. Functional Magnetic Resonance Imaging and Positron Emission Tomography) are now being used by cognitive neuropsychologists in order to study the patterns of brain activity that underlie higher mental function.

While it is useful to have some appreciation of the major functions of the brain regions (see Figure 15.1), it is important to appreciate that many

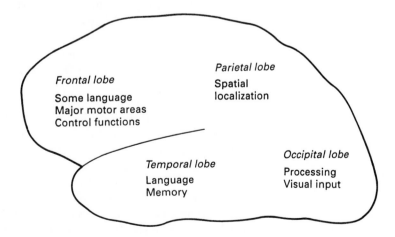

Figure 15.1 A schematic diagram of the lateral view of the brain demonstrating the positions of the lobes.

complex functions require the integrated working of a number of different brain areas. For instance, in front of you is a book, in order to name the book you need to be able to process the relevant visual input (occipital lobes), match the results of that processing to your memories of similar items (temporal lobes) and name the item (temporal and frontal lobes). If you were to pick up the book prior to naming it, you would need to locate its position in space relative to your own position (parietal lobes) and initiate the appropriate action routine for picking it up (parietal and frontal lobes). Study of the isolated functions of the individual lobes is not really appropriate when considering some of the complex abilities which we possess. To understand these complex abilities requires an in-depth account of the different processes involved in different tasks, and how these processes interact. This is the emphasis given by cognitive neuropsychologists. Unfortunately, it will not be possible to deal in depth with cognitive neuropsychological accounts of all perceptual and cognitive abilities, and interested readers should pursue some of the references to cognitive neuropsychological texts given at the end of the chapter. Instead, I will concentrate on our ability to deal with visual stimuli, covering processes involved in selecting, perceiving, recognizing and acting in relation to the visual environment.

Selecting

Our everyday environment contains many objects, each of which could serve as the target for a particular action. We would have a very confusing existence indeed if we were to respond to all the sensory input to which we are exposed. We need to select those sensory stimuli which are important and/or relevant and which require further processing. As a result of brain damage, the ability to select may be impaired – this type of selection problem is often associated with frontal lobe damage. Consider here the case of L.E., who suffered occlusion of the left posterior anterior cerebral artery at the age of 52 (see Shallice et al., 1989). Following the lesion, he behaved in a very bizarre manner. For instance, he was found one morning wearing someone else's shoes, going around the house, moving furniture, opening cupboards and turning light switches on and off. This form of behaviour is consistent with an inability to be selective to various forms of input. Seeing a pair of shoes, he was instantly 'stimulated' to put them on, seeing a switch, he was 'stimulated' to operate it regardless of the appropriateness of such actions to his current situation.

At the other extreme, selection may be too specific; so, some patients have enormous difficulty dealing with more than one thing at a time. This problem can be confined to dealing with visual stimuli, where it is termed 'simultanagnosia', a problem in processing simultaneously presented stimuli. Its effect on everyday life may be profound. Thus, I.R., who suffered bilateral occipital damage appeared to behave like a blind man despite the fact that his visual acuity was normal (Luria et al., 1963). When ascending a staircase (with his eyes fixed on the stair), he could not perceive a person approaching him and avoid a collision. If he was looking at a picture containing many items, he would always say that he could only see one object. When looking out of the window of a car, he was able to see one car, then a second, and then a third, but only one at a time.

The cases of L.E. and I.R. illustrate the importance of being able to select objects from our everyday environment to which we can respond in a coherent and planned way. Problems can occur either because patients are quite unselective (as a result of frontal lobe damage) or because selection is restricted to just one item (a condition which may result from occipital lobe damage). Both forms of deficit may profoundly affect normal everyday behaviour.

How may the therapist approach rehabilitation in these instances? For the over-selective patient, one approach may be to de-emphasize vision, implicating a training regimen which emphasizes the learning of verbal instructions. To ensure that a patient does not become diverted in a required task (e.g. entering the gym, selecting the appropriate plinth and getting undressed ready for treatment), the task could be divided into its component stages which the patient would be required to learn:

> e.g. As I enter the gym, I look for the green plinth;
> I sit on the green plinth;
> I take off my shoes, socks and teeshirt;
> I lie down.

If this method is successful with the one task (and it may take some time to achieve success), then other activities may be treated in the same way.

A different treatment strategy may prove more appropriate for the patient who is only able to select one item at a time. Improved scanning may help such patients. Therapy sessions could include exercises on scanning to the left and right of the environment initially in a predictable way ('move your eyes along the wall in front of you to the left corner, now move your eyes along the wall in front of you to the right corner'), followed by a more unpredicatable sequence of commands ('move your eyes to the left until they reach the green plinth, move a little further to the left until they reach the wall bars, move your eyes to the right until they reach the sink, move back to the left until they reach the left corner ...'). Emphasizing quickness and accuracy of the actual eye movements may prevent fixation on individual objects.

Processing

In some patients, the selection process may be intact, but there may be some form of impairment to the processing of the sensory input. Peripheral problems in the processing of sensory input are relatively easy to understand, as when a patient is blind due to damaged retinas or cataracts. Indeed there exists a wealth of sophisticated clinical tools available to assess the peripheral disorders in the various modalities (audiometry, optometry etc.), where examiners may be interested in whether a patient can *detect* a particular stimulus. Unfortunately, there are few satisfactory tests that examine processing of sensory signals in the brain. Take, for instance, the case of R.R. who had a ten year history of language disturbance (EEG showed abnormal activity in the left temporal region, a brain scan was normal). Despite having normal spontaneous speech, R.R.'s ability to comprehend spoken language was very impaired. His constant complaint was that he could hear the sound of the voice but could not understand what was being said (Denes and Semenza, 1975; Franklin, 1989). It is important to note here that auditory function was *quite normal* in this patient. He was somehow unable to attach meaning to the sounds that he was hearing. This disorder is known as word deafness. Detection of sensory input was normal (as assessed by audiometry), but the recognition of speech clearly requires more in the way of processing than simple detection. Further processing which links the perception of sounds to knowledge of what those sounds mean is necessary.

Analogous deficits may also occur in the other modalities. In the visual modality the process of linking sensory input to meaning may be impaired. For instance, H.J.A., as a result of a stroke affecting both occipital lobes, was unable to give the name (or indeed, demonstrate any other form of recognition) of many items in his visual world (Riddoch and Humphreys, 1987a). It was not that he could not *see* things, he was able to produce very accurate copies of the things he could not recognize; nor was it the case that he had an impaired memory. He was able to produce very good drawings from memory and his descriptions of items included many visual characteristics of that item, in addition to functional and associative knowledge.[1]

The case of H.J.A. is important in showing that the processing of visual input is complex and involves more than simple detection. His visual acuity was normal when he wore his glasses, and yet he was unable to recognize the items he saw. It was not that he could not remember what the names of the items were; indeed, he had no memory impairment since he had no difficulty describing or drawing items from the past. His deficit lay somewhere along a processing continuum which allows a match between an item registered by the eyes with knowledge about that item or similar items stored in memory. H.J.A.'s case has been very important in informing theoreticians about the nature of our visual processes in immediate perception, but what relevance has his case to the practising clinical therapist? H.J.A. was fortunate in that he had no physical problems as a result of his stroke; however, other stroke victims may not be so lucky and recognition difficulties may co-occur with physical problems. As noted earlier, while it may be easy to understand physical deficits (they are observable and one can account for failures to perform functional tasks in terms of motor impairment), it is not easy to communicate about higher cognitive deficits. How can you account for a recognition failure to your friends? Do you think they would understand if you were to say that you could no longer recognize things? H.J.A.,

---

[1] This may be illustrated by his definition of a lettuce. 'A lettuce is a quick growing, annual plant, cultivated for human consumption of its succulent, crisp, green leaves which grow during the younger stage of the plant, tightly formed together in a ball-shaped mass. Widely cultivated, lettuces are of many varieties and of absolutely no value as a food. They do however, enable one to eat delicious mayonnaise when using a knife and fork in polite places'.

although an intelligent articulate man, was unable to convey the nature of his difficulties to his doctors, who decided that he was suffering from 'postoperative confusion'. It was only after he returned home, after a month of hospitalization, and as a result of strong pressure from his wife, that more detailed investigations were initiated. If the therapist is able to detect a problem, he or she can support the patient and relatives at least with a simple explanation.

Problems, such as that suffered by H.J.A., can also have severe effects on normal everyday functioning. H.J.A. was unable to live by himself because for instance, he was unable to recognize the foods in the kitchen so he could not prepare himself a meal. He could not recognize his environment or other people.[2]

I have described two patients in this section, and we should be aware that, in both cases, the impairment is *modality* specific. H.J.A., for instance had no difficulty in understanding what people said to him and was usually able to recognize things if he was able to touch them. Such modality specificity has important implications for therapy. If a patient is severely impaired in one modality, and restitution of function in that modality appears unlikely, therapy should be particularly directed towards the intact modalities to facilitate the development of compensatory strategies.

Recognizing

In some cases, patients may have completely intact sensory processes, but they may still fail to recognize objects. The implication here is that the impairment has the effect of either preventing access to the stored knowledge that each individual builds up through a lifetime of different experiences (as is the case for R.R. and H.J.A., described above), or there may be some impairment within the patient's stored knowledge. Again, the situation with disorders of stored knowledge is likely to be complex. For instance, it is possible for patients to lose stored knowledge of what objects look like, but still to know what objects should be used for, or how they associate with other objects. For instance, D.W. reported that a giraffe looked like a horse and that it was coloured black, but also that it lived in Africa and ate leaves from trees (Riddoch and Humphreys, 1992). Constrastingly, patients can also lose access to functional knowledge about objects while having intact 'stored knowledge'. For instance, they may discriminate between familiar and unfamiliar objects, but not know whether a cup and saucer should be classed together and separately from (say) a knife (Riddoch and Humphreys, 1987b). This shows that we probably have a number of different types of stored knowledge about objects (visual, functional, and perhaps many other forms). Also, these different forms of knowledge can be selectively impaired. Disorders of functional knowledge are likely to be particularly disruptive to everyday living,

---

[2] He relates an anecdote of an occasion when he was helping his wife with the shopping. Thinking to make himself useful, he started to pack the shopping into a basket only to have a sharp voice ask what he thought he was doing. He was only able to say 'I thought you were my wife' to the stranger, having failed to recognize that she was *not* his wife and that he was packing the wrong shopping.

since patients will be impaired in using objects appropriately. Therapy in such cases needs to be addressed to the particular types of knowledge affected. In terms of the physiotherapist, it should be understood that it is possible that a patient fails to dress appropriately because he or she has lost the functional knowledge of, for example, what a shoe is for. It need not mean that the patient is simply being difficult!

Locating

So far I have discussed some of the processes involved in recognizing objects. However, that is only part of the story of how we successfully negotiate visual environments; the other part is concerned with our ability to direct action to (or from) objects.

Disorders of eye movements

Accurate location of an object in space is necessary if we are to make any form of action towards or with the object. For instance, we need to make accurate eye movements to a location in space in order to focus on an object and recognize it. We also need to locate accurately the position of an object relative to ourselves in order to make a movement towards it. Patients with parietal lesions may have defective oculomotor exploration. In the acute phase post stroke, the gaze may be permanently deviated towards the side of the lesion, and patients may be unable to display intentionally their gaze beyond the midline and explore the side of space opposite the lesion (Jeannerod, 1988). When involved in rehabilitation programmes with patients with stroke, it is worth assessing the ability of the patient to scan actively to the left and to the right of space. If difficulties are observed, active eye movement training exercises, described above, may need to be incorporated into the rehabilitation programme.

Disorders of spatial coding

Relating the spatial location of an object to our own spatial location is itself a complex feat, involving the interaction of a number of sensory processing modalities (e.g. vision, proprioception, audition), each of which may be separately impaired as a result of brain damage. Typically, following parietal lesions, some form of proprioceptive impairment may be observed during the course of neurological assessment. For instance, patients may make large errors when asked to point to an imaginary spot in space directly in front of them if their eyes are closed but not when their eyes are open, presumably because they are not using proprioceptive information (Heilman et al., 1983). Such a deficit may be successfully remedied by the use of a treatment regimen which encourages the patient to attend to the affected side. In a study by Dunning (1990) patients were encouraged to massage the affected limb with talcum powder. This had *visual* effects (it was easy to see areas which had not received any powder), *olfactory* effects (the powder had a pleasant smell), and *social* effects (sessions were conducted with groups of patients and social interactions were encouraged). The measured degree of proprioceptive deficit did not change; however, there was a marked change in the patient's awareness of the affected limb. When blindfolded, the patients found it much easier to find the affected hand than they had prior to the therapy sessions.

We may contrast a proprioceptive deficit with a similar visual deficit. Patients with optic ataxia (which occurs as a result of lesions to the parietal and occipital lobes) will demonstrate mispointing when they are actually looking at the target. If they are cued to a location by a sound, or if they are asked to point to a particular place on their own body, they have no difficulty. Such a deficit will again have profound effects on normal every day functioning. Damasio and Benton (1979) describe a woman with bilateral parieto-occipital lesions as a result of a drug over-dose. She had no visual or motor problems and was able to walk inde-pendently. However, she had difficulties in reaching for objects with her hands and behaved like a blind person in her attempts to approach objects. However, movements which did not require vision (such as buttoning and unbuttoning a cardigan, or bringing a cigarette to the mouth) were performed quite normally.

Dunning (1990) was able to demonstrate that a proprioceptive deficit could be compensated for successfully. It is unclear how a similar compensatory strategy could be taught in the visual modality, perhaps one can only teach such patients to compensate by using the intact modalities (i.e. proprioception and audition).

Disorders of spatial attention

Disorders of spatial attention or unilateral neglect are commonly encoun-tered by the physiotherapist. Such disorders are usually associated with lesions of the right parietal lobe (although neglect has been observed as a result of lesions to other brain areas including the frontal lobes, the occipital lobes, midbrain structures and the brainstem (see Riddoch and Humphreys, 1987c). The deficit is characterized by a failure to attend to the side of space contralateral to the lesion. The exact nature of the deficit is likely to depend on the locus of lesion. Thus patients with parietal lesions typically fail to complete drawings on the neglected side (a simple clinical test is to ask the patient to draw a clock, usually the outer circum-ference of the clock is drawn, but either the digits on the neglected side will be omitted or all the digits will be crammed on to the non-neglected side). Such patients will only eat food from one side of their plate, if they are able to walk they will bump into things on the neglected side.

A different picture may be observed in patients with frontal lesions. Here the neglect is not of a particular side of space but of one side of their body. Such patients need not have motor or sensory problems; they may catch a ball thrown to them with either hand but when asked to perform a simple task, such as to get off a bed, great difficulties ensue because the patient 'forgets' one of the lower limbs and instead of swinging it over the bed with the other limb, leaves it resting in its original position (Laplane and Degos, 1983; Coslett et al., 1993; Tegnér and Lerander, 1991).

There is much debate currently as to the exact nature of the neglect deficit, and in particular, parietal neglect (see Riddoch, 1992, for a review). Frontal neglect has not been so extensively researched. Parietal neglect may be the result of a failure in the ability to direct attention to the contralesional side either because attention cannot be oriented in that direction or because attention cannot be released from stimuli on the ipsilesional side (Humphreys and Riddoch, 1990); Whatever the case, for the practising clinician the implications for therapy are similar. It is important to make the environment on the contralesional side as stimulating as possible so that the patient is encouraged to attend to that side, and conversely, attempts should be made to reduce the stimulation on the ipsilesional side. Everybody involved with the patient, from relatives to medical personnel, should be encouraged to approach the patient from the contralateral side. In general, therapeutic approaches which emphasize stimulation of the affected limb should be employed.

For patients with frontal neglect the rehabilitative technique used by Dunning (1990) described above may prove useful, but this has yet to be investigated.

Acting

Once an object has been located in the environment, it may be necessary to perform some action in relation to it. For instance, when dining, different actions are required for the appropriate use of the varied utensils available. Different functions are performed by a knife and a fork, and these disparate functions require actions which may be quite dissimilar from each other. The cutting action of the knife and the piercing action of the fork may involve similar grips by the hands, but quite different motor movements of the arms. These actions are so familiar to us, and are performed so frequently, that we give no thought to their individual complexities. Brain damage may significantly impair the ability to perform these simple everyday tasks *even if* there is no sensory or motor impairment. Take the case of C.D. who suffered a stroke at the age of 54 following a period of hypertension (Riddoch *et al.*, 1989). He had minimal weakness of the arm on the right (affected) side, but found that he was frequently unable to use simple household objects. For instance, C.D. went into the bathroom one morning and found that he was unable to perform the familiar shaving action with his razor; he could pick it up, knew it was a razor, but was somehow unable to initiate the usual motor action. These difficulties could not be accounted for in terms of any motor weakness, since if he was asked to pantomime the use of the item, he had no difficulty. Also, C.D.'s impairment was restricted to the right hand; he had no difficulty in using objects with the left hand.

There is much to learn from C.D.'s problem. First, we should note that the ability to perform simple actions may be impaired even when the patient can recognize what the objects are, and strength, sensation and tone are virtually normal. This implies that in order to perform particular motor actions, the motor areas of the cortex must receive some form of stimulation. Thus, by actually *seeing* the object (e.g. a knife), the appropriate grasp is initiated and the limb is in readiness for the appropriate action. There must be other ways of stimulating the motor cortex. C.D., if asked to pantomime an action, was able to do so. In this circumstance, presumably the verbal request triggers the stored knowledge of a knife in memory which then allows activation of the actions appropriate to it. In C.D.'s case, this route was intact, but he did not seem to be able to use it *automatically*, that is when he experienced difficulties on actually seeing the object, there was no evidence of a spontaneous use of the intact 'verbal' route. Fortunately for C.D., his condition quickly resolved and there was no need for a formal rehabilitation programme. However, therapists may encounter similar patients and a possible therapeutic strategy may be to facilitate performance in the damaged modality by reinforcement from the intact modality. For instance, on presenting a knife to the patient, verbalization of performance should be encouraged. ('That is a knife. It is used for cutting. Cutting is a backwards and forwards motion …').

Other patients may show the reverse deficit; that is, they may not be able to pantomime the use of an object but will have no difficulty in actually using the object (Rothi and Heilman, 1985). This may be the result of impaired comprehension of the command or a failure to access stored knowledge on how objects may be used via the 'verbal' action route. If patients have difficulties in verbal comprehension, use of the verbal modality by the therapist should be reduced and simplified as much as possible and a greater emphasis should be placed on the use of the visual modality to elicit performance (i.e. demonstration of an action by the therapist).

While C.D. (see above) was able to perform simple gestures well with his left hand, when he was asked to perform actions which required the integrated use of both left and right hand functions (e..g pouring a cup of tea, tying a tie, etc.), errors were again made. Another interesting point is that while C.D. was frequently unable to demonstrate the use of an object with his right hand, his ability to do so with his left hand was unimpaired. Also, once he had successfully performed an action with the left hand, he was able to perform the same action with his right hand (Riddoch et al., 1989). These two aspects of C.D.'s performance illustrate the strong reciprocal connections between the motor areas of the two hemispheres (see Goldberg, 1985). The use of the intact parts of the brain to facilitate performance of the impaired regions is not a new idea and formed the basis of the influential approach to the treatment of hemiplegia advocated by Brunnstrom in the 1960s (Brunnstrom, 1970).

However, other therapists have disputed this approach and strongly argued that immitation and reinforcement of associated reactions on the affected side were counterproductive to normal functional recovery (Bobath, 1970; Davies, 1985). What unfortunately appears to have been lost in these competing ideas is the notion of the complementary roles of the two hemispheres. We should also be aware that normal functional activity requires the intact functioning of both hemispheres. While attempting to elicit movement on the affected side during therapy sessions, the required movement should be performed by the unimpaired limb. This will have the result of allowing the damaged cortical areas to receive input from the unaffected motor areas via the callosal links (Goldberg, 1985). Additionally, motivational input as a result of the patient's wish to perform the action (via the cingulate cortex) and verbal input as a result of processing the therapist's instructions (via the temporal lobes) may be implicated. Maximizing the amount of stimulation of the damaged areas may have a facilitatory effect on movement.

Conclusion

The above account shows that brain damage can have profound effects on human perception and cognition, and that perceptual and cognitive deficits may co-occur with physical deficits. In order for rehabilitation to be effective, consideration must be given to the role of perceptual and cognitive processing. Figure 15.1 illustrated some of the functions thought to be associated with the different lobes of the brain. Some of the major functions of the brain (selection, processing, recognizing, locating, acting and memory) were then considered and it is clear that many of these abilities can be impaired as a result of lesions to a number of different brain areas. A most positive way to consider brain anatomy is therefore in terms of *connections* in addition to specific brain areas. This approach is illustrated in Figure 15.2. For instance, from this diagram we can see that normal motor action may be impaired as a result of a lesion to the occipital lobes where visual stimuli are properly processed, but the feed-forward pathways are interrupted to the parietal lobes, resulting in a failure to locate the object's spatial position correctly, or to the frontal lobes where the main motor centres are located. Designing appropriate therapy depends on understanding the different ways in which actions to objects can be disrupted.

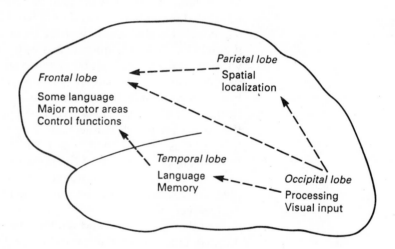

Figure 15.2   A schematic diagram of the lateral view of the brain demonstrating possible pathways of information through the brain.

Acknowledgements

This work was supported by a grant from the MRC. I would also like to thank Glyn Humphreys for his help with earlier drafts of this chapter.

References

Andrews K., Brocklehurst J. C., Richards B., Laycock P. J. (1982) Recovery of severely disabled stroke patients. *Paper presented at the 9th Scientific Meeting of the Society of Research in Rehabilitation*. Bristol.
Blanc-Garin J. (1994) Patterns of recovery from hemiplegia following stroke. *Neuropsychological Rehabilitation*, **4**, 359–385.
Bobath B. (1970) *Adult Hemiplegia: Evaluation and Treatment*. London: Heinemann.
Brunnstrom S. (1979) *Movement Therapy in Hemiplegia: A Neurophysiological Approach*. New York: Harper and Row.
Coslett H. B., Bowers D., Fitzpatrick E., Haws B., Heilman K. M. (1990) Directional hypokinesia and hemispatial inattention in neglect. *Brain*, **113**, 475–486.

Damasio A. R., Benton A. L. (1979) Impairment of hand movements under visual guidance. *Neurology*, **29**, 170–178.

Davies P. M. (1985) *Steps to Follow*. New York: Springer Verlag.

Denes G., Semenza C. (1975) Auditory modality-specific anomia: evidence from a case study of pure word deafness. *Cortex*, **11**, 401–411.

Denes C., Semenza C., Stoppa E., Lis A. (1982) Unilateral spatial neglect and recovery from hemiplegia. *Brain*, **105**, 543–552.

Dunning M. (1990) *Unpublished MSc Dissertation*. London: Polytechnic of East London.

Franklin S. (1989) Dissociations in auditory word comprehension: evidence from nine fluent aphasic patients. *Aphasiology*, **3**, 189–207.

Goldberg G. (1985) Supplementary motor area structure and function: reviews and hypotheses. *Behaviour and Brain Sciences*, **8**, 567–616.

Heilman K. M., Bowers D., Watson R. T. (1983) Performance on hemispatial pointing task by patients with neglect syndrome. *Neurology*, **33**, 661–664.

Holmes G., Horrax G. (1919) Disturbances of spatial orientation and visual attention. *Archives of Neurology and Psychiatry*, **1**, 385–407.

Humphreys G. W., Roddoch M. J. (1990) Interactions between object and space systems revealed through neuropsychology. In *Attention and Performance XIV* (Meyer D. E., Kornblum S., eds). Hillsdale, NJ: Lawrence Erlbaum.

Jeannerod M. (1988) *The Neural and Behavioural Organisation of Goal Directed Movement*. Oxford: Clarendon Press.

Jeffery D. R., Good D. C. (1995) Rehabilitation of the stroke patient. *Current Opinion in Neurology*, **8**, 62–68.

Laplane D., Degos J. D. (1983) Motor neglect. *Journal of Neurology, Neurosurgery and Psychiatry*, **46**, 152–158.

Luria A. R., Pravdina-Vinarsaya E. N., Yarbus A. L. (1963) Disorders of ocular movement in a case of simultanagnosia. *Brain*, **86**, 219–228.

Riddoch M. J. (1992) Towards an understanding of unilateral neglect. In *Cognitive Neuropsychology and Cognitive Rehabilitation* (Riddoch M. J., Humphreys G. W., eds). London: Lawrence Erlbaum.

Riddoch M. J., Humphreys G. W. (1987a) A case of integrative agnosia. *Brain*, **110**, 1431–1462.

Riddoch M. J., Humphreys G. W. (1987b) Visual object processing in optic aphasia: a case of semantic access agnosia. *Cognitive Neuropsychology*, **4**, 131–185.

Riddoch M. J., Humphreys G. W. (1987c) Perceptual and action systems in unilateral neglect. In *Neurophysiological and Neuropsychological Aspects of Visual Neglect* (Jeanerrod M., ed.). Amsterdam: Elsevier Science Publishers B.V.

Riddoch M. J., Humphreys G. W. (1991) The smiling giraffe. In *Mental Lives* (Campbell R., ed.). Oxford: Basil Blackwell.

Riddoch M. J., Humphreys G. W., Price C. J. (1989) Routes to action: evidence from apraxia. *Cognitive Neuropsychology*, **6**, 437–454.

Riddoch M. J., Humphreys G. W., Bateman A. (1995a) Stroke: Issues in recovery and rehabilitation. *Physiotherapy*, **81**, 689–694.

Riddoch M. J., Humphreys G. W., Bateman A. (1995b) Cognitive deficits following stroke. *Physiotherapy*, **81**, 465–473.

Rothi L. J. G., Heilman K. M. (1985) Ideomotor apraxia: gesture discrimination, comprehension and memory. In *Neuropsychological Studies of Apraxia and Related Disorders* (Roy E. A., ed.). Amsterdam: Elsevier Science Publishers B.V.

Shallice T., Burgess P. W., Schon F., Baxter D. M. (1989) The origins of utilisation behaviour. *Brain*, **112**, 1587–1598.

Tegnér R., Levander M. X. (1991) Through a looking glass: a new technique to demonstrate directional hypokinesia in neglect. *Brain*, **114**, 1943–1951.

Wade D. T., Wood V. A., Langton-Hewer R. (1985) Recovery after stroke: the first three months. *Journal of Neurology, Neurosurgery and Psychiatry*, **48**, 7–13.

Further reading

Campbell R. (ed.) (1992) *Mental Lives: Case Studies in Cognition*. Oxford: Blackwell Publishers.

Campbell R., Conway M. A. (eds) (1995) *Broken Memories: Case Studies in Memory Impairment*. Oxford: Blackwell Publishers.

Ellis A. W., Young A. W. (1988) *Human Cognitive Neuropsychology*. London: Lawrence Erlbaum Associates.

Humphreys G. W., Riddoch M. J. (1987) *To See But Not to See: A Case Study of Visual Agnosia*. London: Lawrence Erlbaum.

McCarthy R. A., Warrington E. K. (1990) *Cognitive Neuropsychology: A Clinical Introduction*. San Diego: Academic Press.

16

Dimensions of impairment and disability

Sally French

The ways in which people experience disability and impairment depend on many interacting factors including social status, personality, biography and environment. A flight of steps can, for example, create disability, and the effects of an impairment vary with the person's interests and employment. In this chapter the following four factors, which appear to be central to the experience of disability, will be discussed:

1. The point in life at which the impairment is acquired.
2. The visibility of the impairment.
3. The comprehensibility of the impairment and disability to others.
4. The presence or absence of illness.

Many of the psychological and social aspects of disability can be understood by analysing these and other factors. It is important to realize, however, that generalizations regarding impairment and disability merely provide ideas and possible explanations, never 'the truth' about any particular person.

The point in life at which the impairment is acquired

Impairment can arise at any time of life, it may be present at birth or be acquired later in childhood, in early adulthood, or in old age. The psychological and social effects of impairment, and the disability which may accompany it, are likely to differ according to the time of life at which it occurred.

If an impairment is present at birth or arises in early childhood, many areas of development are at risk of disruption or delay, even those not directly associated with the impairment. Consider, for example, children with cerebral palsy who are restricted in their ability to move around freely. This situation has the potential to affect their cognitive development as they are less able to learn through exploration. Perceptual development, such as the appreciation and understanding of spatial relationships, may also be affected adversely as its full development is partly determined by movement and actively manipulating the environment.

Emotional development, language development and social development, might also show delay in children with motor impairments; they may be dependent on adults for far longer than usual, and their restricted mobility may mean that fewer demands are placed upon them. Their needs may be anticipated so readily that language is delayed, and opportunities to play with other children may be limited or lacking (Lewis, 1987). Thus an impairment of the motor system threatens to disrupt many areas of development.

Whatever the impairment, a similar pattern holds. In the case of visual impairment a very important channel for learning is lost, this may be exacerbated by difficulty in moving safely and lack of incentive to move in the absence of visual stimuli. Lewis (1987) notes that blind children are delayed in many aspects of their motor development including reaching forward, rolling and pushing up to sitting, as well as standing and walking independently. This lack of movement, as well as fear on the part of others that the child may come to harm, may disrupt social interaction and retard social development. The visually impaired child may be given insufficient opportunities to take responsibility and to make mistakes, with a subsequent delay in emotional development.

The visually impaired child's language development may also be delayed. Burlington (1979) found that the vocabulary of blind children develops more slowly than that of sighted children. The visually impaired child may have less experience of the world than other children and less to talk about. Lewis (1987) notes that visually impaired children have a qualitatively different experience of the environment than other people, including their parents and immediate carers. This may inhibit the acquisition of language as it is often heavily based on what we see, particularly when we interact with young children.

The notion that blind people have superior touch and hearing is a misconception. Lewis (1987) states that, '... there is no evidence to support the claim that the sensory apparatus of the blind child is actually more acute; she just uses the senses she has more effectively'. Lewis goes on to explain that blind children do less well than sighted children on a wide range of tactile and auditory tasks, although the differences lessen as the children get older. Sighted children, when blindfolded, tend to cope better than blind children on these tasks. Lewis suggests that this is because sight helps us to integrate information from all of our senses and to understand our other experiences; thus lack of sight clearly has the potential to delay the cognitive development of blind children. Murphy and O'Driscoll (1989) make a strong case for the involvement of physiotherapists in the lives of young visually impaired children and their carers.

One advantage of congenital impairment is that the brains of young children are physiologically and anatomically malleable and will tend to develop in such a way as to maximize function. Thus a young child who injures the area of the brain responsible for language has the potential to regain these language skills. This process is less successful when the brain is more mature. Similarly, the visual centre of the brain of a baby born with defective eyes is likely to develop in such a way as to maximize vision. This would not be possible if the same eye condition were acquired later in life. This is why it is so important that children be encouraged to function within their area of impairment, provided it does not become a burden to them or their families or so time-consuming and stressful that enjoyment of life is lost. It also explains why a temporary period of loss, for example of sight or hearing, can be so detrimental, for it may occur at a particularly critical stage in the development of the brain.

Walker and Crawley (1983) state that the development of disabled children can be normal, absent, delayed, abnormal or compensatory. In the last case children may find an unusual way of achieving their goals, for example using their feet to manipulate objects rather than their hands, or using audible signals, which most people ignore, to compensate for lack of sight. Examples of 'abnormal' development, according to Walker and Crawley, are rocking backwards and forwards, which is sometimes seen in blind children, and self-injurious behaviour, sometimes witnessed in children with learning difficulties. This type of behaviour can sometimes be explained in terms of an interaction between the impairment and the environment; blind children may rock because they are under-stimulated, and the self-injurious behaviour of children with learning difficulties may be a response to frustration or boredom. Until recent times many disabled children were subjected to impoverished environments which in themselves can give rise to many adverse effects and can be far more disruptive to human development than impairment (Potts and Fido, 1991; Humphries and Gordon, 1992). The disabling physical and social structures within society, such as lack of access to buildings, continue to impoverish the lives of many disabled people (Swain *et al.*, 1993).

The areas of development which can be disrupted or delayed in children with motor and visual impairments are summarized in Figure 16.1 below.

| Child with motor impairment | Social development
Language development
Emotional development
Cognitive development
Motor development
Perceptual development |
| Child with visual impairment | Social development
Language development
Emotional development
Cognitive development
Motor development
Perceptual development |

Figure 16.1 Diagram to show the area of development which may be disrupted or delayed in a child with a motor or visual impairment.

This sequence of events is not inevitable but rather depends upon the limitations imposed by the impairment, parental and societal attitudes and behaviour, the individual characteristics of the child, available resources, and the social and physical environment in which the child and his or her family are placed. The situation will, of course, be complicated if the child has multiple impairments. It is important to realize that having more than one impairment is far more disabling than the sum of the individual impairments (French and Patterson, 1995).

As well as the threat of disruption to all areas of development which an impairment imposes, disabled children are likely to be socialized into a particular role during their formative years (French, 1994). This, in turn, may have an adverse effect on their confidence and self-esteem well into adulthood (French, 1996) (For further information on the disabled role the reader is referred to Chapter 24.)

An important aspect of the physiotherapist's role is to minimize or prevent developmental delay by informing carers of the potential problems and working with them to devise developmental programmes specific to each child. For example, the carers of a blind child may be helped to enter into his or her experiences of touch and sound and relate to the child in terms of these senses. They can be helped to provide the opportunities for the child to mix with other children and encourage early language development so that the world can be explained more effectively. The carers of a child with a physical impairment may be shown ways of positioning him or her to provide maximum stimulation from the environment as well as encouraging any motor abilities which may be present.

The physiotherapist will need to have a sound understanding of the impairment and disability in all its aspects as well as a good relationship with the child and the family. There is a need to be innovative, imaginative and, above all, prepared to listen and learn from the carers and the child. It is essential to consult the family when suggesting interventions and devising developmental programmes to ensure that they fit into family routines and do not become stressful or too much of a burden for any family member.

People who acquire an impairment in later childhood or adult life, have the advantage that their development has been 'normal' up until that point in time. For example, when people become deaf in adulthood, they will already have acquired language and the ability to read and write fluently. Similarly those who lose their sight in later life will have full knowledge of the visual world on which to draw; their mobility and orientation will, in fact, frequently surpass that of congenitally blind people although skills such as braille reading tend to be more difficult to acquire.

People who become disabled in old age, by far the majority, may find their situation particularly difficult owing to the fact that they frequently have multiple impairments. Thus the older person who starts to go deaf may also have a visual impairment, and the person who becomes paralysed following a stroke may already have arthritis or a heart complaint. The older person who becomes paraplegic may simply lack sufficient physical strength to manage as a younger person might. It is important, however, not to be ageist, many older people cope with impairment and disability as effectively as younger people. (For further information on ageism and cognitive changes in older people, the reader is referred to Chapters 6 and 14.)

Although childhood is the period in life of most rapid development, it should not be forgotten that people continue to develop throughout their lives. Those who acquire an impairment in adulthood, therefore, may find their social, emotional and cognitive opportunities and development restricted. They may also suffer prejudice, discrimination and hostile reactions. A person with ataxia following a head injury, for example, may fail to find employment or to integrate fully in society because of the attitudes and behaviour of others. This may lead to isolation and loneliness.

Negative attitudes can, however, sometimes have a positive effect. Lonsdale (1990) points out that the assumption that disabled women are asexual has advantages and disadvantages; on the one hand it may affect adversely their self-image, but on the other it frees them from sexist expectations. In Morris' book (1989) several of the women interviewed said that disability had liberated their relationships. Vasey (1992) can also see advantages, she states:

> 'We are not usually snapped up in the flower of youth for our domestic or child rearing skills, or for our decorative value, so we do not have to spend years disentangling ourselves from wearisome relationships as is the case with so many non-disabled women'.

Sometimes the change to life an impairment brings is regarded as equally satisfying as life before it occurred. A disabled woman in Morris' book (1989) explains:

> 'As a result of becoming paralysed, life was changed completely. Before my accident it seemed as if I was set to spend the rest of my life as a religious sister but I was not solemnly professed so was not accepted back into the order. Instead I am now very happily married with a home of our own'.

The person who acquires an impairment moves from the role of non-disabled person to disabled person, often very abruptly. It has been suggested that this can give rise to psychological reactions similar to those of the mourning process. Kübler-Ross (1969) presented a five stage model of psychological adjustment to death and dying. The stages she described were denial, anger, bargaining, depression and acceptance. Burnfield (1985) and many others believe this process to be similar to the psychological reactions required to adjust successfully to acquired impairment. These reactions are by no means inevitable, however, and the assumption that they are has been strongly challenged by Oliver (1983). Silver and Wortman (1980) reviewed the literature on stage models of adaptation after traumatic events and found little evidence to support it. The disabled person may, in fact, report that life has changed for the better, or that difficulties may relate more to social and physical barriers than to the impairment itself (Briggs, 1993). Disabled health professionals, including physiotherapists, also report advantages as well as disadvantages to being disabled (French, 1988a, 1990).

People's reactions to impairment depend on many interacting factors including their personal coping strategies, the accessibility of the environment, the kind of life they want to lead, the degree of social support available, and the attitudes and behaviour of others. Lenny (1993) believes that disabled people can sometimes find themselves in a 'Catch 22' situation as happiness and contentment following disablement is sometimes viewed as a form of denial.

Many people who acquire an impairment suddenly, however, do report that the experience is profoundly disruptive and disturbing. John Hull (1991) states that he grieved for 4½ years over his lost sight and Maggie, a disabled woman in Campling's book (1981), recalls, 'I felt I had little to offer anyone and rather than face rejection, I avoided people. Grieving over the lively gregarious woman I had once been'. Similarly Barbara writes, 'The sense of numbed shock, of powerlessness, anxiety and loss of direction, was my first reasoned response when the realisation that I was partially paralysed penetrated my brain ... Anger – a feeling that my body was now flawed, no longer as God meant it to be – and frustration succeeded'.

Maggie believes that the intensity of her reaction was probably the result of negative attitudes she had acquired about impairment and disability as a non-disabled person. She states, 'Whichever way I turned to think, the negative answer that I was deaf seemed to destroy any shred of hope. I can only think that I learned to expect so little from my future because I somehow soaked up these prevailing attitudes towards women with disabilities as a hearing woman ...'.

It is clear from other accounts of disabled women in Campling's book (1981), that those with congenital impairments can also suffer a similar psychological upheaval when they grasp the implications of their situation. Micheline recalls the day when she realized she would always be disabled:

'That momentous day I suddenly realized ... I was going to be the same as I had always been – very small, funnily shaped, unable to walk. It seemed at that moment that the sky cracked ... The next two years seemed like a dark roller-coaster ride, sometimes happy, often plunging into despair. My main preoccupation seemed to be desperately trying to deny the awareness of my difference which had started on that day'.

Accounts such as these demonstrate that the notion of people with congenital impairments 'not knowing what they are missing' is untrue, and probably serves the purpose of making non-disabled people feel less responsible, as well as denying that anything substantial needs to be done to improve the lives of disabled people. It is obvious that visually impaired people *do* know what they are missing as they wait for a bus on a cold, dark night while everyone else gets into their cars, and that physically disabled people know what they are missing when denied access to the theatre, the library or the public toilet. As Wilkinson (1992) puts it, 'The "loss" does not concern what was ... but what could have been'. It is often said that disabled people have qualities and attributes to compensate for these losses, such as the 'sixth sense' of blind people, the cheerfulness of those with learning difficulties, and the bravery of people who use wheelchairs. Such notions are, however, false: disabled people possess the same range of attributes as non-disabled people.

People who acquire impairments frequently experience serious problems with their relationships, Burnfield (1985) mentions that marriages often break down under the stress of multiple sclerosis, especially if they were under strain beforehand, and Parker (1993) notes that the onset of disability can bring about considerable strain within marriage. The disabled person may need to build a new self-image, cope with greater dependency on others for everyday needs, and change direction in occupation and leisure activities. Though many of these adaptations would be unnecessary if society was less disabling. Shakespeare (1975) states:

'A handicap acquired later in life involves a somewhat different type of realisation, in general much more rapid than the realisation of congenital handicap. In this case the self-concept has to be altered and with severe disability a totally new one has to be acquired. Alongside this process, others who knew him before he became handicapped need to get to know him again. People in the position of becoming handicapped in later life generally report that interaction is easier with new acquaintances than with those who were known previous to the handicap'.

To suggest such a profound change in the individual following the onset of impairment is probably somewhat exaggerated. Morris (1989) found that for many of the women with spinal cord injuries she spoke to, life went on much the same as it had before their accident or illness. However, those who acquire an impairment, particularly if its onset is rapid, are probably more likely than those with congenital impairments or those who develop impairments more slowly, to feel an acute sense of loss and a need to change many aspects of their lives. Because of their past experience as non-disabled people, those who acquire an impairment in adulthood may comprehend their disadvantaged status in society more clearly than those who have always been disabled.

People with progressive impairments must cope continually with altered and diminished function. Even those with static impairments are more affected by the normal ageing process than their non-disabled peers (Zarb, 1993). Paralysed people, for example, may develop early and severe arthritis in their over-used joints, and visually impaired and hearing impaired people may be adversely affected by small losses in their already limited sight and hearing.

When attempting to assess and respond effectively to the psychological reactions manifested by disabled people, it is important to attempt to distinguish psychological reactions to impairment and disability, from psychological reactions resulting from the physiological and pathological changes brought about by the disease or injury. People following a stroke or traumatic head injury, for example, may become aggressive, forgetful or depressed. Psychological changes can also occur in diseases such as multiple sclerosis and Huntington's chorea. Sometimes it is the medications people are taking which produce these effects, while the physical and social environment can also have a profound effect on the individual's psychological state. These complex interactions are explored in more detail by Finkelstein and French (1993).

The visibility of the impairment

Various researchers have found that people with a less obvious or hidden impairment have more psychological difficulties than those with a more visible impairment. This is so even though the less obvious impairment is often less severe in terms of function. Gulliford (1971) found that children with severe impairments are better adjusted psychologically than those with less severe impairments, and Cowen and Bobrove (1966) found that both deaf and blind people are better adjusted psychologically than partially hearing and partially sighted people. The deaf and blind people saw themselves as being less rejected and more accepted than the partially hearing and partially sighted people, and showed less discrepancy in terms of themselves as they would like to be and themselves as they really are. Dodds *et al.* (1992) found partially sighted adults to have more negative attitudes towards visual impairment and a lower sense of personal effectiveness than blind adults.

Davis (1984) found that the more clearly defined and visible the impairment, the greater the facility with which disabled individuals and non-disabled people adjust to each other. Albrecht (1982) believes that the major factor in producing social distance between disabled and non-disabled people is the degree of disruption to social interaction. Drewitt (1990) reports that interaction with others became much easier once her impairments could be seen.

Disabled people with hidden impairments are in a position to decide whether or not to reveal them. In every situation they must determine how the impairment will be received, whether or not it is relevant to mention it, how likely it is to be discovered, and what the consequences of that discovery will be. People with more obvious impairments are only free to make such decisions if their communications are not face to face, for example when filling in a form or speaking on the telephone – provided that the impairment does not involve speech and language.

Revealing an impairment or hiding it, has the potential for both positive and negative outcomes as illustrated in Figure 16.2 below.

	Positive outcomes	*Negative outcomes*
Reveal disability	Disabled person is accepted	Disabled person is rejected
Hide disability	Impairment is never discovered	Impairment is discovered

Figure 16.2   Outcomes of revealing or hiding disability

In reality, hiding an impairment is rarely a positive experience, even if it is never discovered, because the process of hiding it is often very stressful; people cannot ask for what they need and must constantly try to avoid situations where the impairment may be discovered, or be ready with excuses and explanations if it is. The hearing impaired person, for example, may pretend to be absent-minded, the person with slight ataxia, clumsy, and the person with learning difficulties, who finds it difficult to cope socially, introverted. A psychological cost is, therefore, paid for silence. The more social stigma people feel, the more likely they are to try and conceal their impairments. The alternative labels (absent-minded, clumsy, etc.) are also derogatory but, for the people concerned, less so than their real impairments.

It is interesting to note, that on occasions people may portray themselves as having other, less discrediting, impairments. In the novel *Judgement in Stone* by Ruth Rendell (1978), for example, Eunice Parchman, who cannot read, pretends to be visually impaired and is in a constant state of anxiety in case her excellent vision and her real limitations are discovered. Similarly those found guilty of crimes may plead 'diminished responsibility' or amnesia as an alternative label to 'criminal', indeed this has been a feature of some famous murder trials. Sometimes hiding an impairment becomes so habitual that people start to enact the characteristics of the alternative label. Visually impaired people who avoid parties and outings in case their impairment is discovered may, over the years, become rather isolated and lacking in social skills. They may gradually start to view themselves as people who prefer to be alone.

Other problems which arise for those with hidden or less obvious impairments or disabilities, are that help is not always offered when needed, and is frequently inappropriate when given. Those with visible impairments are not entirely free of such problems either, as people are generally poorly informed about impairment and disability whatever its degree (McConkey and McCormack, 1983). However, there must be more potential for people to respond appropriately to a person's impairment if they can see what it is. This can make disguising impairments, for example by using elaborate prostheses, a problem and a psychological burden for some disabled people (Sunderland, 1981).

Given that concealing an impairment is a stressful and difficult process, but is, nonetheless, regarded as the best option by many for whom it is possible, it follows that the problems of having an obvious impairment must be equally as bad, or perhaps worse. The difficulty which people with obvious impairments face is the tendency of others immediately to label them 'disabled' with all the misconceptions and stereotypes that the label implies. The impairment is considered to be the person's most important attribute, obscuring all others. This can have serious consequences when trying to find employment, gain acceptance on a college course or make friends. The reactions of others can also be both humiliating and demoralizing. Sue, a disabled woman featured in Campling's book (1981) explains:

> 'My weak grasp on my identity was no real match for the massed forces of society who firmly believed themselves as "normal" and myself just as firmly as "abnormal". I found myself inhabiting a stereotype. I became my illness. I was of interest only because of it. And as a person in a wheelchair I elicited embarrassment, avoidance, condescension, personal questions … Going out became a nightmare, I was public property. People either staring intently into my face, or looking away'.

It should also be appreciated that many people with obvious impairments also have hidden ones. Take people with paraplegia, for example, although the fact of their praplegia is obvious, the associated problems of impotence and incontinence, which may be present, are hidden from view. Julie, a disabled woman featured in Campling's book (1981) explains, 'In intimate relationships there is always that first moment when the mechanics of your bladder management are revealed. This is the major test. How will he react to a mature woman who wears plastic knickers, pads and requires help going to the loo?'. Burnfield (1985) speaks of the hidden impairments associated with multiple sclerosis, such as fatigue, blurred vision and sensory disturbances. These problems are frequently misunderstood and made more incomprehensible by their fluctuating nature.

The situation for people with sporadic impairments, for example those with epilepsy, is rather different; they appear non-disabled most of the time but when their impairment manifests itself it may be either obvious to others or relatively hidden. Despite the fact that 80% of people with epilepsy have the condition totally or well controlled by drugs (British Epilepsy Association), it remains a very stigmatized condition which can lead to an urgent need to conceal it. Hevey (1990) refutes the idea that people with epilepsy are only disabled during their actual seizures, believing that the terror and fear of epilepsy, brought about by other people's reactions, can render them 'epileptics' all the time.

The comprehensibility of the impairment and disability to others

The functional ability of disabled people is often markedly affected by the situation they are in. Hearing impaired people, for example, may only understand speech in an environment free from background noise, and with voices of a certain pitch. They may communicate well on the telephone but not in social situations, be able to hear the voices of men but not women, and find voices too loud even though they cannot understand what is being said. Their situation is perhaps less easy to understand than that of profoundly deaf people who cannot hear speech whatever the circumstance. Visually impaired people may function entirely differently according to the lighting; rushing around confidently in overcast conditions but needing to be guided on bright sunny days (French, 1988b). Similarly people with heart complaints may use wheelchairs on some occasions but not on others.

These ambiguities can make it very difficult for disabled people to explain their situation to others or even to understand it themselves. Dodds et al. (1992) explain:

'The partially sighted clients we spoke to mentioned that they had difficulty in trying to make other people understand their disability. This is understandable, as partial sight can be very confusing to the sufferer as well as the onlooker. For example, a client who can read a newspaper but who is unable to move through the environment without using a cane may feel, as well as appear to be, a fraud ... the totally blind client can more easily fulfil a well established set of non-visual expectations'.

Because the functional ability of disabled people varies so much according to environmental circumstances, their situation is difficult to comprehend. This is a particular problem for those with relatively hidden impairments, although there is much confusion surrounding more obvious impairments too. The blind person, or the person with a unsteady gait, for example, are likely to function more competently in a familiar setting, and the person using a wheelchair will be less disabled in surroundings suited to his or her needs. The social environment must also be considered: the deaf person may cope with communication better if the atmosphere is friendly and supportive, and the person with a tremor may find that anxiety or lack of time tends to make it worse. All of this has major implications when assessing disabled people.

Because of the ambiguous nature of impairment and disability, the behaviour of disabled people is often interpreted in terms of intellectual or personality deficits. For example the child with slight ataxia may be reprimanded for being careless, or teased for being clumsy, or the hearing impaired person, who fails to reply, may be considered hostile and unfriendly. Shearer (1981) quotes a man with multiple sclerosis who found people kind and generous when he was eventually compelled to use a wheelchair but before he reached that stage they usually thought he was drunk.

To complicate the situation still further, impairments placed within the same category or arising from the same condition or disease, rarely produce identical manifestations. These manifestations can, in fact, be extremely diverse. Thus one visually impaired person may be able to see colour and rely on it a great deal, while another may be colour blind, the first person may function best in bright light but the second when the light is dim (French, 1988b). People classed as 'epileptic' have different types of fits, and the manifestations of those with head injury, or people diagnosed as having multiple sclerosis, can be entirely different. Further ambiguities and confusion can arise because conditions and diseases, which are not particularly similar, are often confused, for example mental learning disability and mental illness, rheumatoid arthritis and osteoarthritis, 'nervous' disease and 'psychiatric' illness.

The manifestations of impairment are poorly understood and tend to be individualized. This is epitomized in the notion that disabled people, with less severe disabilities, have an inner identity crisis, not knowing whether to associate with disabled or non-disabled people. As Shakespeare (1975) states:

> 'A basic dilemma of the handicapped person is that of which group he belongs to, whether he should identify himself with "the handicapped" or to what extent he should consider himself part of normal society. He finds he is a member of society but different from most other members. Hence he is often unsure where he belongs … it has been suggested that the severely handicapped experience less stress here, as they are clearly handicapped and have fewer opportunities of choice. The psychological position of the less severely handicapped has been referred to as "marginality", as they are between total disability and normality'.

Although some disabled people may believe this to be true, the roots of the problem almost certainly lie in the responses of non-disabled people, who cannot understand or cope with the complexities and ambiguities of disability. Shaw (1990) notes that when she tries to explain her disability, it is seen as 'embarrassing moaning', but when she keeps quiet about it people protest that they cannot help her if she will not inform them. Hevey (1992) found that every time he attempted to 'come out' about his epilepsy he was silenced and found himself capitulating. He realized that 'the hidden power contract was to stay like "us" or be obliterated'.

The presence or absence of illness

Many disabled people are extremely fit and healthy, but for others their impairment is associated with illness. Illness can be defined as the subjective feeling of being unwell and may include symptoms of pain, breathlessness, tiredness and vertigo. Some conditions which may give rise to impairment, for example, rheumatoid arthritis, and glaucoma, are associated with considerable pain. Pain, particularly when prolonged, has the potential to cause anxiety and depression. This can give rise to a vicious circle as both states of mind tend to heighten the perception of pain.

Prolonged pain, even if not particularly severe, tends to take the joy out of life. Even activities which previously seemed exciting become dull and uninteresting. This lack of activity means that time hangs heavily and depression is intensified. Peck (1982) believes that feelings of having little control over the situation also contribute to depression. Davison and Neale (1990) point out that anxiety and depression frequently coexist.

Pain is intrusive and people who experience it may find it very difficult to concentrate on anything properly or cope with physical or social demands. They will probably mix with other people less and have little to talk about, or talk only about their pain. In time their company may become less rewarding to others who may withdraw or cope with the situation by denying the reality of the pain. This can lead to a cycle of resentment and guilt, as well as feelings of anger and irritability on the part of both the people experiencing pain and their families and friends.

Morris (1989), in her book about the experiences of women with spinal cord injuries, devotes an entire chapter to the subject of pain. She states:

'One in four of us experience pain which is so serious that it curtails our activities or confines us to bed for all or part of the time. Pain does not seem to follow any set pattern for any particular level of lesion, whether cervical, thoracic or lumbar, or whether complete or incomplete'.

Anita, who is featured in this book complains that:

'The common reaction from professionals and lay people is: "If you can't feel, how can you have pain?" This is very upsetting. Most professionals know about the phantom pain amputees suffer, so why can they not accept that we have a great deal of pain, even though there may be no sensory feeling?'

Disabled people who cope with pain as well as disability, are clearly in a very different position to people who, though severely disabled, are free of pain. Yet people often 'learn to live' with pain to the extent that others may disbelieve that they are in pain and regard them as frauds. The way someone is behaving is thus not always a very good guide to the amount of pain, or other symptoms, they are experiencing. (For a full discussion of the psychology and sociology of pain the reader is referred to Chapter 10.)

Another symptom of illness is extreme fatigue which is felt, for example, by many people with multiple sclerosis. Burnfield (1985) reports on a Canadian survey of people with multiple sclerosis, where it was found that fatigue was the most distressing symptom for 40% of the respondents. Fatigue is, of course, relatively hidden which leads to a lack of understanding. Burnfield (1985) reveals that his wife thought he was trying to avoid working in the garden when he complained of fatigue. Sexual relationships, social life and work may all be adversely affected. Fatigue may also arise because of the effort required to function with an impairment. Dodds (1993) explains that visual impairment, 'involves the person in a lot of effort. Great amounts of concentration are required to extract useful information and this is tiring'.

Breathlessness, associated with conditions such as asthma and bronchitis, may also give rise to psychological and social problems. Rubeck (1971) interviewed people with chronic bronchitis and found that many of them reported feelings of choking or suffocation. One person said, '… your shoulders try to meet in front of you, tighter and tighter … you think you're going to choke … you gasp and gasp to get your breath, and then you panic …'. Morgan *et al.* (1983) found that the anxiety level of people with bronchitis was more predictive of their ability to walk a given distance than the function of their lungs.

As well as understanding the situation of disabled people who have symptoms of illness, it is vitally important to recognize that many disabled people are as fit and as free from symptoms as anyone else. Not only are impairment and disability frequently unassociated with illness, but there is often no link with a disease process either. The belief that disability is inevitably linked to illness and disease has given rise to many misconceptions about disabled people with far reaching effects such as reluctance to employ them.

Conclusion

In the last analysis, disabled people are individuals who respond to their situation in unique ways. However, by considering the dimensions of impairment and disability, it is possible to gain a greater understanding of the difficulties and barriers disabled people face. Other factors, such as whether or not the impairment is progressive, how certain the prognosis is, the gender ethnicity and social class of the individual, and how acceptable the impairment is to others, can also provide valuable insights. Without this knowledge there will inevitably be a lack of understanding between physiotherapists and disabled people which will interfere with the success of treatment and rehabilitation. This chapter provides a few leads but the best way of learning about disability is to talk to disabled people themselves.

References

Albrecht G. (1982) Social Distance from the stigmatised: a test of two theories. *Social Science and Medicine*, **16**, 1319–1327.
Briggs L. (1993) Striving for independence. In *Disabling Barriers – Enabling Environments* (Swain J., Finkelstein V., French S., Oliver M., eds). London: Sage.

Burlington D. (1979) To be blind in a sighted world. *Psychoanalytic Study of the Child*, **34**, 5–30.

Burnfield A. (1985) *Multiple Sclerosis: A Personal Exploration*. London: Souvenir Press.

Campling J. (ed.) (1981) *Images of Ourselves: Women with Disabilities Talking*. London: Routledge and Kegan Paul.

Cowen E. L., Bobrove P. H. (1966) Marginality of disability and adjustment. *Perceptual and Motor Skills*, **23**(5), 869–870.

Davis S. (1984) Deviance disavowal: the management of strained interaction by the visibly handicapped. In *The Other Side* (Becker H. S., ed.). Illinois: Free Press.

Davison G. C., Neale J. M. (1990) *Abnormal Psychology* (5th edn). New York: John Wiley and Sons.

Dodds A. G. (1993) *Rehabilitating Blind and Visually Impaired People*. London: Chapman and Hall.

Dodds A. G., Ng L., Yates L. (1992) Residential rehabilitation 1: client characteristics. *The New Beacon*, **76**(901), 321–325.

Drewitt J. (1990) Disabilities no-one can see. *Disability Now*, November, 11.

Finkelstein V., French S. (1993) Towards a psychology of disability. In *Disabling Barriers – Enabling Environments* (Swain J., Finkelstein V., French S., Oliver M., eds). London: Sage.

French S. (1988a) Experiences of disabled health and caring professionals. *Sociology of Health and Illness*, **10**(21), 170–188.

French S. (1988b) Understanding partial sight. *Nursing Times*, **83**(3), 32–33.

French S. (1990) The advantages of visual impairment: some physiotherapists' views. *The New Beacon*, **74**(872), 1–6.

French S. (1994) The disabled role. In *On Equal Terms: Working with Disabled People* (French S., ed.). Oxford: Butterworth-Heinemann.

French S. (1996) Out of sight, out of mind: the experience and effects of a 'special' residential school. In *Feminism and Disability* (Morris J., ed.) London: The Women's Press.

French S., Finkelstein V. and Patterson S. (1995) Enabling interventions. Workbook 4 of the Open University Course *Disabling Society – Enabling Interventions*. Milton Keynes: The Open University.

Gulliford R. (1971) *Special Educational Needs*. London: Routledge and Kegan Paul.

Hevey D. (1990) Hidden disabilities: help or hindrance. *Disability Now*, October, 14–15.

Hevey D. (1992) *The Creatures Time Forgot: Photography and Disability Imagery*. London: Routledge.

Hull J. (1991) *Touching the Rock: An Experience of Blindness*. London: Arrow Books.

Humphries S., Gordon P. (1992) *Out of Sight: The Experience of Disability 1900–1950*. Plymouth: Northcote House.

Kübler-Ross E. (1969) *On Death and Dying*. London: Tavistock Publications.

Lenny J. (1993) Do disabled people need counselling. In *Disabling Barriers – Enabling Environments* (Swain J., Finkelstein V., French S., Oliver M., eds). London: Sage.

Lewis V. (1987) *Development and Handicap*. Oxford: Basil Blackwell.

Londale S. (1990) *Women and Disability*. London: Macmillan.

McConkey R., McCormack B. (1983) *Breaking Barriers: Educating People about Disability*. London: Souvenir Press.

Morgan A., Peck D., Buchaman D. (1983) Psychological factors in chronic bronchitis. *British Medical Journal*, **286**, 161–173.

Morris J. (1989) *Able Lives*. London: The Women's Press.

Murphy F. M., O'Driscoll M. (1989) Observation of the major development of visually impaired children. *Physiotherapy*. **75**(9), 505–508.

Oliver M. (1983) *Social Work and Disabled People*. London: Macmillan.

Parker G. (1993) *With this Body: Caring and Disability in Marriage*. Buckingham: Open University Press.

Peck C. (1982) *Controlling Chronic Pain*. London: Fontana.

Potts M., Fido R. (1991) *'A Fit Person to be Removed': Personal Accounts of Life in a Mental Deficiency Institution.* Plymouth: Northcote House.

Rendell R. (1978) *A Judgement in Stone.* London: Arrow Books.

Rubeck M. F. (1971) *Social and Emotional Effects of Chronic Bronchitis.* London: Health Horizon Limited.

Shakespeare R. (1975) *The Psychology of Handicap.* London: Methuen.

Shaw G. (1990) Hidden disabilities: help or hindrance. *Disability Now*, October, 14–15.

Shearer A. (1981) *Disability: Whose Handicap?* Oxford: Basil Blackwell.

Silver R. L., Wortman C. B. (1980) Coping with undesirable events. In *Human Helplessness* (Garber M., Seligman M. E. P., eds). New York: Academic Press.

Sutherland A. T. (1981) *Disabled We Stand.* London: Souvenir Press.

Swain J., Finkelstein V., French S., Oliver M. (eds) (1993) *Disabling Barriers – Enabling Environments.* London: Sage.

Vasey S. (1992) Disability culture: it's a way of life. In *Disability Equality in the Classroom: A Human Rights Issue* (Rieser R., Mason M., eds). London: Disability Equality in Education.

Walker J. A., Crawley S. B. (1983) Conceptual and methodological issues in studying the handicapped infant. In *Educating Handicapped Infants: Issues in Development and Intervention* (Gray Garwood S., Fewell R. R., eds). Rockville: Aspen Systems Corporation.

Wilkinson H. (1992) A step out of denial. *The New Beacon*, **76**(903), 418–419.

Zarb G. (1993) The dual experience of ageing with a disability. In *Disabling Barriers – Enabling Environments* (Swain J., Finkelstein V., French S., Oliver M., eds). London: Sage.

Section 3

Communication in Physiotherapy Practice

17

Interpersonal communication

John Swain

Communication is one of those terms which have an intuitive and obvious meaning but are hard, if not impossible to define precisely. It is part of our social existence as human beings, as much as the air we breathe is a part of our physical existence. The provision of physiotherapy, in these terms, is a form of communication and the whole process is one of communication between the client and the physiotherapist, between the physiotherapist and colleagues, including other physiotherapists, doctors and so on, and also between the physiotherapist and members of the client's family. Nevertheless the possibility of a clear concise definition of 'communication' seems to slip inexorably through the fingers like sand as soon as questions are raised.

How do we communicate? Perhaps most people's lists of the ways in which we communicate would start with speech, and language is, indeed, a much studied, significant and highly complex medium for communication (Greene and Coulson, 1995). It is important to recognize, too, that physiotherapists work with people whose first language is not English, including people who use a sign language. Looking beyond language the list becomes seemingly endless. Everything about people and everything they do can convey messages: the way they wear their hats; a wave of the hand; a raising of the eye-brows; the style of their hair; their accents; and the way they stand. A touch of the hand, for instance, can convey feelings which an hour of conversation might never reach. We have to complicate the list even further by adding written communication, drama, music, and the ever expanding technology of communication through faxes, e-mail, computers and so on. As the list lengthens, it seems pertinent to ask when we are *not* communicating, at least in any encounter between two or more people. Dickson *et al.* (1989) argue that 'in situations where two people are present and one is aware of the other, communication is taking place.' Communication is inevitable in encounters between people. Silence can 'say' more than words. Even falling asleep can send messages, particularly in the middle of a lecture session.

The next question that can be raised, 'What is communicated?', further exposes the elusive and ephemeral nature of communication. What is communicated depends on more than one participant: it happens *between* people. An act of communication can have many different meanings for both the sender and the receiver. A smile might be an act of communication, but depending on the context, the same act can convey anything from affection, to threat, to lack of understanding, to embarrassment, as well as mixed messages. The question of what is communicated has at least three components: the meaning as intended by the sender; the meaning as understood by the receiver; and the degree to which these meanings are shared. The notion of intentionality is important here. A look on someone's face, or touch or wave of the hand can convey a whole array of messages about feelings and attitudes of which the sender is unaware, or at least did not mean to convey. This is evident in what is sometimes called 'leakage' (Ellis and McClintock, 1994). This occurs when messages we are intentionally sending, usually verbally, are contradicted or changed by other signals, usually non-verbal. For instance, leakage would be occurring when a person tells you that he or she is feeling relaxed and happy, but his or her whole posture and tone of voice tells you otherwise.

There is another question before we look at specific definitions: 'Why communicate?'. In relation to the provision of physiotherapy the importance of communication is highlighted in studies which suggest that health care professionals can be deficient in their abilities to communicate and also studies which suggest that ineffective communication can significantly affect both the processes and outcomes of health care. In their review of relevant research, Davies and Fallowfield (1991) include the following in a list of deficiencies in professional communication skills, though it is important to note that this does not imply that all physiotherapists have inadequate abilities all the time.

1. Failure to greet the patient appropriately, to introduce themselves, and to explain their own actions.
2. Failure to elicit available information, especially major worries and expectations.
3. Acceptance of imprecise information and the failure to seek clarification.
4. Failure to encourage questions or to answer them appropriately.
5. Avoidance of information about the personal, family and social situation, including problems in these areas.

Studies also suggest that the consequences of such poor communication include: dissatisfaction for both clients and professionals; inaccuracies in assessments; clients not adhering to the treatment or advice given by professionals; and as Davies and Fallowfield (1991) state, 'poor communication must affect treatment outcomes both physically and psychologically'. Improved communication, on the other hand, is associated with: increased client knowledge and recall; increased client satisfaction; genuinely informed consent; increased client compliance; and quicker recovery from illness (Ley and Llewelyn, 1995).

Looking in more general terms, rather than specifically at the practice of physiotherapy, questions about why we communicate reach beyond the specific purposes of professional practice. They reach, for instance, into what we are as human beings. How we communicate and what we communicate are not just a set of learned behaviours or skills which are deployed more or less effectively. Personal identity is, at least in part, established and determined in communication with others.

Given the complexity of communication, it is hardly surprising that there are numerous definitions, almost as many as people who provide definitions. The following are a couple of examples.

> 'Communication is the process of sharing information using a set of common rules.' (Northouse and Northouse, 1992)

> 'Responses which the person makes intentionally in order to affect the behaviour of another person and with the expectation that the other person will receive and act on that message.' (Keirnan *et al.*, 1987)

One way to look at such definitions is that they are themselves a form of communication directed at specific audiences for specific purposes. The first of the above is taken from a book aimed at helping health care professionals develop effective strategies of communication, while the second is from a manual for professionals working with people with learning difficulties. The following definition of my own suits the purposes of this particular chapter:

> 'communication is a dynamic process of sharing meanings within the specific context of the practice of physiotherapy'.

The processes are constructed by the questions raised above: why we communicate; how we communicate; and what is communicated. The specific context may seem easier to define, but as all practising physiotherapists know, every session is different and for a variety of reasons. One way to look at the context is along three dimensions. The first is as interaction between people (rather than physiotherapist and client). Marková (1987) writes:

> 'Interpersonal communication is one of the most significant expressions of self- and other-awareness. Its quality and kind depends very largely on the participants' ability to assess each other's feelings, thoughts and intentions, and on their reactions to each other's messages'.

Communication is closely related to concepts of self, self-awareness and awareness of others. This has three elements:

1. First, the messages we intentionally attempt to convey are shaped by self-awareness of thoughts, feelings and sensations. For instance, to convey intentionally the message that you are feeling anxious about a certain situation relies, in the first instance, on you being aware of feelings of anxiety.
2. The act of communication can in itself increase self-awareness. Thus, for instance, I might not know how I feel about a certain situation until I have talked it over with a confidante.
3. Furthermore, our conceptions of ourselves, self-image and self-esteem, are at least in part determined by the responses of others.

A second dimension of the context of communication is the relationship between the two people involved. In general terms, communication has meaning in the context of relationships. This is easy to see: you need only compare one of those long difficult conversations in which you remain 'in the dark' with a 'look in the eyes' of an intimate partner which conveys a whole world of meaning. Looking more specifically at the relationship between physiotherapist and client, it is evident that their relationship is shaped and defined in certain ways inherent in the practice of physiotherapy. One approach to thinking about this is in terms of the roles of both the physiotherapist and the client. This concept of 'role' is used to describe the expectations that are attached to a position. Clients will have expectations about how physiotherapists act and how they themselves should act in a 'patient role', and these explanations will affect the flow of communication.

Physiotherapists have their own expectations, of course, which include notions of what it means to be a professional. Roles become part of personal identities and are integral to how we see ourselves and how we see others. They are also governed by rules, both formal and informal, which shape behaviour and communication (Strawbridge, 1993).

Finally, in this list of aspects of the context, broader issues must come into play. Communication is shaped by the whole social and historical context. It is culturally defined: a way of dressing or a hand gesture, for instance, can have quite different connotations in one culture than in another.

The purpose of this chapter, then, is to provide a foundation, which can only be introductory in such a complex area but will facilitate physiotherapists in their reflections on the dynamic processes of communication in the context of physiotherapy practice. The particular focus is on face-to-face, or interpersonal, interactions between physiotherapists and clients.

Processes: the how, what and why of communication

There are a number of important aspects to a process model of communication. Firstly, it is a rejection of models of communication conceived as the sending and receiving of information. Sending and receiving a message can be thought of as like the sending and receiving of a parcel. However, if I communicate a message to you I still have that message. To communicate is to share: to share thoughts, feelings, information and so on. Indeed, when two people communicate very effectively they are sometimes said to 'be of like mind': a sharing of minds.

A process model of communication is also dynamic in the sense that communication is seen as a *transaction* constructed between people. It is an interplay between people in which participants are both active agents, affecting the interplay, and re-active agents, affected by the interplay.

A process model of communication addresses the close interrelationship between how we communicate, what is communicated, why we communicated and the context of communication. Two crucial points emerge at this stage. First, there is no simple one-to-one correspondence between acts of communication and the meaning expressed. The context is all-important. Even signals which usually have a well-defined meaning, such as raising the hand to signal 'stop', depend on the context of the two-way flow. If accompanied by a smile, for instance, the raising of the hand could be meant as and understood to be a joke. Furthermore, there are differences between cultures in the actual behaviours used and their possible meanings. Unlike British children, for instance, American blacks, Puerto Ricans and Japanese children tend to avert their eyes when listening to another person. This can be understood by British adults to be a sign that the child is not listening or, even worse, is purposely showing that he or she is not listening. Similarly white British and Americans require a much larger personal space and they also touch less than people from some other cultures. Such generalizations are difficult, however, particularly in cosmopolitan societies, and there is variability within as well as between cultures. Thus, there is plenty of room for misunderstanding and the need for feedback and reflection to check understanding is essential.

It is in this light that we look next at what might seem the most straightforward of the processes: reasons for communicating.

With purpose

Why do we communicate? The question is so basic that it defies answers. As Dalton (1994) says:

> 'Spoken and written language are the media through which we learn to co-operate with one another and organise ourselves socially'.

Yet the question of why is crucial in that the purposes of communication determine both what is communicated and how it is communicated. Perhaps the most fundamental barrier to communication is the lack of a reason to communicate.

Purpose in communication can be looked at in terms of what a person consciously wishes to communicate to another. There are times when it seems useful to consider what we intend to communicate, for example when preparing a report. Indeed, intentional communication tends to be given priority in education and literature aimed at health care professionals. In physiotherapy practice such instrumental communication can be found, for instance, in assessment procedures for gaining information to formulate aims and goals for therapy to select means by which aims and goals are to be achieved; and to devise detailed programmes of treatment (Parry, 1985).

French (1994) recognizes four aims of nurse–patient communication which apply equally to physiotherapist–client communication:

1. Establishing a relationship founded on trust, empathy and respect.
2. Determining clients' needs as perceived by them, and helping them recognize their other needs as perceived by the health professional.
3. Providing factual information on which clients can structure their expectations.
4. Assisting clients to use their own resources and those offered to them.

As recognized in this list, the content dimension of communication is only half the story. The other dimension is the social interplay between people (Watzlawick *et al.*, 1967). Penman (1980) makes the distinction

between functions associated with the activity/concerns of the participants (activity-orientated) and functions associated with the relationship
between the participants (relation-orientated). Both sets of functions, or
dimensions of communication, are served at the same time in any process
of communication. He suggests three activity-orientated functions:

1. the task to be accomplished;
2. the problems/concerns of the participants;
3. the expansion of available alternative solutions.

He also identifies three relation-orientated functions:

1. defining;
2. maintaining;
3. or redefining the social relationship.

In physiotherapy practice, as in all forms of communication, whatever
the activity-orientated dimension of communication, such as assessment,
planning or evaluation, there is *always* a relation-orientated dimension.
Relationships between physiotherapist and client are defined or maintained through all the communication between them. To illustrate this,
consider the following statement: 'Please do these exercises at least twice
a day, though stop if it gets too painful'. (You will have assumed, I
presume, that the statement is made by the physiotherapist to the client).
In this example, using Penman's categories, the activity-orientated
function is 'the task to be accomplished', specifically the treatment
regime as planned by the physiotherapist. The relation-orientated
function will obviously depend on the existing relationship between the
physiotherapist and the client as to whether it is being defined, maintained or redefined. The crucial point is that the relationship dimension
provides the context for the meaning of the content dimension. The
content can be interpreted in many ways by the client. If, for instance
there is a trusting relationship, the client may interpret this as a useful
suggestion with which he or she should comply. If, on the other hand,
their relationship is distant and the client feels the physiotherapist has no
real knowledge of him or her as a person this might be seen as a rigid
directive more to do with the physiotherapist complying with the expectations of the professional role.

By all means

There are numerous channels of interpersonal communication. The most
obvious is verbal communication: as expressed in the meaning of words.
Important as this is, however, many people who investigate communication come to believe that the most important channels for conveying
meaning are non-verbal. One way of categorizing all the different types
of non-verbal behaviour is to separate into three groups (Trower *et al.*,
1978): vocal; changing behaviours; and stable behaviours.

The 'vocal' category is often referred to as 'paralanguage'. This covers
all those aspects of speech and the sounds we make which convey
meaning other than the words actually spoken. 'It's not what you say its

the way that you say it.' This includes: loudness, pitch, intonation, emotional quality, stress and accent. For instance, the question 'Does this hurt?' will have different implications depending which word is stressed. A stress on 'does' might suggest a disbelief that it hurts at all. A stress on 'this' suggests a comparison with another movement or pressure point. A stress on 'hurt' also could suggest a comparison, between causing pain rather than, say, discomfort.

There is little research evidence concerning non-verbal communication within the specific context of physiotherapy practice. It is not surprising, however, that Huntingdon (1987) found a direct link between the tone of a doctor's voice and the relationship with patients. Research suggests that a warm, friendly tone encourages patients to discuss their concerns and ask questions, and this is associated with a higher degree of trust in the doctor's diagnosis and greater commitment to carry out instructions. In general, paralanguage cues, such as rate and pitch, can affect the health professional's communication with clients. How things are said influences both the client's perceptions of the physiotherapist and his or her understanding of the physiotherapist's messages, information and feelings (Niven, 1994).

The second category of non-verbal behaviours, 'changing behaviours', tends to be the best known and talked about. Eyes, for instance, have been called 'the window to the soul', and eye contact is an extremely expressive means of non-verbal communication. All the emotions, including affection, anger, fear and joy, can be there in the eyes. Facial expression is also a powerful channel with, generally, a tremendous range of expressions for conveying messages, responses, attitudes and emotions.

One highly complex channel of communication, which is particularly pertinent to the practice of physiotherapy, is touch. An interesting taxonomy of touch suggests that there are a number of different types of touch which depend on the situation and on the relationship that people have: functional-professional touch; social-polite; friendship-warmth; love-intimacy; and sexual arousal (Heslin, 1974, cited in Northhouse and Northouse, 1992). Useful as these might be as categories, however, it is a model which over-simplifies the communication process. Meanings of touch depend on gender differences, cultural norms and the whole context of the two-way flow of communication accompanying touch. A touch with a smile can be quite different from a touch with an impassive facial expression. Though there is little relevant research, the evidence suggests that touch is an important aspect of the communication between health care professionals and clients. One relevant study, for instance, conducted by McCann and McKerna (1993), suggested that touching a patient whilst communicating emotional information usually indicates warmth and concern.

Another channel of communication which is particularly relevant to physiotherapy practice is proximity. This is the way in which people structure and use physical space between them. In a review of research Burgoon et al. (1994) explain:

'It is clear that people have strong spatial needs and strong reactions to violations of their personal space or territory. As a result, proxemic variations can serve as a very powerful communication vehicle. The ways in which people define and defend territories, the distances they adopt from others and the arrangements of space that they create can all act as messages'.

The third category of non-verbal behaviours includes those which generally remain the same throughout a period of interaction, including dress and hairstyle. We clearly make judgements about the nature and personality of individuals based on their appearance on first meetings (Kleinke, 1986). Clothing, accessories such as jewellery, and cosmetics have been found to be important in communication to others (Burgoon et al., 1994). Frank and Gilovich (1988) found, for instance, that sports teams wearing black kits were judged to be tougher and more aggressive than teams wearing other colours. In physiotherapy, then, uniforms and the accessories of professionals, such as goniometers, badges, stereoscopes and uniforms send messages. It is important to remember too that physiotherapists, from their side, will make judgements about clients on the basis of their physical appearances, clothes and so on. As Porritt (1990) suggests, in effective communication it is helpful to suspend judgements made on initial meetings and to remain open to other possibilities on future occasions.

With meaning and feeling

Having reached this stage in this exploration of communication, it will come as no surprise that there is a rich diversity of answers to the question 'what is communicated?'. We shall concentrate here on non-verbal communication. First, non-verbal behaviours accompany, elaborate on and manage speech. For instance, Ekman and Frieson (in Hall and Hall, 1988) distinguish between three types of hand gestures:

1. Those which can be directly translated into words or phrases, such as 'hello', 'stop' or some ruder examples which are well known.
2. Those which add directly to the meaning of speech, e.g. by adding emphasis or pointing out directions being given verbally.
3. Those which are self-orientated, such as stroking your hair, pulling your ear, or scratching.

Non-verbal communication manages the flow of communication. Eye-contact, for instance, can be involved in managing turn-taking, that is signalling when one person is going to stop speaking and the other person to start. Non-verbal behaviours also accompany speech by sending feedback signals of boredom, incredulity, joy and so on.

The same behaviours play a key role in expressing both interpersonal attitudes and emotions. In relation to the former, Trower et al. (1978), summarizing research at that time suggested that there are two dimensions of attitudes: superior/dominance and liking/disliking (or warmth/coldness). Attitudes of superiority/dominance can be expressed, for instance, through invasion of the other person's personal space or by staring. Liking/disliking can be expressed in eye-contact, touch, facial expression and so on. Emotional states, such as anger, depression, anxiety, joy and fear, can also find a communication outlet through non-verbal channels, whether or not the communication is purposeful. There is considerable evidence, for instance, that emotional states have a direct impact on the production of speech. Bodily changes, such as accelerated breathing rate and dryness in the mouth, result in changes in the voice. Evidence also suggests that the recognition of emotion from voice is as good or better than the recognition of emotion from facial expressions (Kappas *et al.*, 1991).

There are two crucial points to remember. First, there is no one-to-one correspondence between non-verbal behaviours and the meanings and feelings they convey. The context is all important. Second, it is also clear that there are numerous points in interactions in physiotherapy practice at which non-verbal behaviours, through intent or otherwise, can convey a hierarchical, de-personalised relationship. Clients' dependence, power-lessness and feelings of inferiority can be expressed and constructed by professionals through their dress, use of touch, proximity and so on.

In a two-way flow

As emphasized throughout this chapter, communication is an active and dynamic interplay between participants. It is constructed through listening and feedback as much as through expression. In general terms the importance of effective listening in helping is heavily emphasized within the literature with books devoted to the topic (Ellin, 1994). In relation to the work of health care professionals generally, again a heavy emphasis is put on listening skills. In an instructor's handbook, for instance, Dickson *et al.* (1989) quote the argument from Fritz *et al.* (1984): this skill is so important that the health practitioner who does not learn to listen effectively sets the course for a professional life filled with inefficiency, inaccuracy and shallow satisfaction'. Effective listening as discussed in this literature goes well beyond assimilating spoken information. Active listening is more than hearing the spoken word, as might be assumed. Deaf people listen.

Messages about how the person is feeling are often conveyed non-verbally. Yet it is more than this too. Good listening also includes listening to ourselves, our own understanding of and feelings about the messages the other person is sending. Furthermore, listening is part of interaction and a two-way flow of communication. Part of listening is the message sent by the listener to indicate that he or she is attending, or not, and understanding, or not, the messages being sent. Yet it is even more than this. There is a quality to the whole listening process which takes it beyond being a set of skills or processes in communication. When we are listened to by someone who is truly understanding, who takes the trouble to listen to us as we consider our problem and who acts on what we say, that experience can change our whole outlook on the world. There is little wonder, then, that people have found the actual word 'listening' inadequate as it sounds so mundane and such an easy process that we do not really have to think about it. The term 'active listening' is often used in an attempt to capture the full complexities and indicate that it is not a passive process. It is an intense personal involvement with another person and it is something we learn, rather than something we either can or cannot do, and learning requires self-reflection.

The context: barriers, dams and distortions

The complex, delicate and subtle processes of communication can be distorted and blocked in many ways:

1. The client's difficulties in expression, including a range of impairments including stuttering, lack of speech, lack of control over movements of the body, etc.
2. The client's difficulties in comprehension, including learning difficulties, hearing impairment, visual impairment, etc.
3. The physiotherapist's difficulties in expression, including use of jargon, patriarchal attitudes, etc.
4. The physiotherapist's difficulties in comprehension, including lack of time to listen, preconceptions, etc.

There can be barriers, for instance, in the expression of emotions. Physiotherapists encounter clients experiencing different kinds of trauma in their lives and complex and fraught problems. This includes clients who regularly experience physical illness and pain; who are terminally ill; who have recently become disabled; and clients who have experienced physical and mental abuse. These are contexts in which emotions can run high: fear, anger and hostility, shock and guilt, grief and anxiety. How each individual acts and reacts depends on numerous factors including cultural differences, differences in background and previous experiences. Two further general points can be added to this picture. First, the physiotherapist also has, and cannot help but have, emotional responses to encounters with clients, including the general stresses and satisfactions of the job as well as specific emotional responses towards clients, their experiences and feelings. Second, the communication of emotions and interpersonal attitudes is generally fraught with difficulties including threats to self-esteem, misunderstandings, denials and over-reactions.

Barriers to listening block or divert any two-way flow of communication. There are many lengthy lists of such barriers (see for instance Bolton, 1979; Porritt, 1990). The following seem to be most frequently cited.

Unhelpful context

Active listening requires a space to give undivided attention: a space of time, place and mind which is free, or relatively so, from all those distractions from within as well as from without. There is no attention to give if it is invested elsewhere. Lack of time is the most often quoted barrier, by professionals at least. The listener's attention is focused on another pressing appointment and his or her own need to limit the encounter. Other barriers to listening are often built on lack of time, such as selective listening, reassuring and advising. When time is felt to be pressing, for instance, it is quicker to offer a word or two of reassurance than to allow the other person to talk through his or her difficulties.

Listening to inner voices

The inner voice builds barriers when it is so loud it distorts, devalues and drowns the voice of the other person. It is a natural tendency to make judgements about other people and the messages they are sending. It is a natural tendency, too, to put your own point of view forward. You may have overheard, or indeed remember being part of, conversations in which each person is doing no more than speaking about his or her own concerns and interests. These barriers include selective listening, criticizing, labelling, praising evaluatively and diagnosing. Each is a violation of the voice of the other person which can channel the flow of conversation towards the judgements of the listener.

Criticizing is the inner judgemental voice of approval or disapproval. It can begin before a word is spoken. As mentioned above, judgements can begin from the way a person is dressed, from his/her make-up, hairstyle, gait, jewellery and so on. Deep-seated values, beliefs and prejudices can be a screen to listening to the individual. In some situations it is possible for the listener to put his or her judgements in abeyance and in some situations, too, they can be reflected and challenged by listening to the other person. Nevertheless, pre-conceptions and feelings can be so strong that criticism is an impenetrable barrier to listening.

Labelling and diagnosing are ways of categorizing people which can devalue them and what they are saying. Labelling can be seen as the making of presumptions, pre-judgements and prejudices about a supposed type or stereotype of person. There are, of course, many such labels: aggressive, chauvinist, disabled, deaf, and derogatory name-calling labels. It is not that labels are wrong in themselves. Indeed, they can be used to affirm positive identity ('Black is beautiful') and bring people together to challenge the discrimination and abuse they experience. In the context of these discussions, however, labelling can be a barrier to listening to another person as a unique individual.

Diagnosis does involve listening but a form of technical listening to pick up clues about conclusions being drawn. It might be concluded, for instance, that the other person is under stress or deceiving him or herself. Everything the other person says and does is sifted for signs to confirm the diagnosis. As you may have noted, labelling and diagnosing are part of the processes of physiotherapy. The dilemma for physiotherapists is that the techniques involved can thwart good listening.

Listening is not just internal to the listener: it is built into the whole two-way flow of communication. The inner voice can direct and subvert this flow. In selective listening only part of what the other person says and does is getting a response. One version of this is evaluative praise. This can be seen as a subtle manipulation of communication. To be positive towards the client can encourage self-confidence. When such praise is dictated by the inner voice, however, it is selected and given in accordance to the listener's judgements of what is important, right and required. It then becomes a dam in the flow of communication and the formation of mutual relationships.

Not following the other's path

In general, these are ways of responding which block, divert, distort and re-channel the track the other person is on. Interpreting builds directly on listening to inner voices, directing the flow of conversation in accordance with the listener's judgements and diagnosis about the other person. To tell the other person that he or she is being defensive, for instance, may actually make the other person be defensive, or change the subject to talking about the other person's supposed defensiveness.

Changing the subject is simply switching the conversation from the other person's to your own concerns. One source is avoidance of emotionally difficult concerns, such as death, sickness and personal conflicts.

Reassurance can also be a denial of strength of feelings. The rushed few words of support may be an attempt to show caring, but can be a means of closing down conversation. Clichés are a form of reassurance: 'time's a great healer' or 'you've got to take the rough with the smooth'. Such stock platitudes avoid rather than reflect the particular concerns of the other person.

Following your own path

In general terms, these barriers involve the 'listener' taking over and dominating the flow of conversation, deciding needs and solutions for the other person. These barriers have been labelled: advising, excessive questioning, ordering, defensiveness and telling your own story.

So why is advising sometimes a barrier to listening? It certainly has its place in physiotherapy practice as, for instance, in health education. It becomes a barrier, however, when stock advice pre-empts listening. It is easy to provide solutions without really knowing the problem.

Ordering is a form of advising backed with authority: 'you'll have to live with the consequences if you don't'. Such threats do not have to be explicit, but can be inherent in people's perceptions of physio-therapy.

Telling your own story can be a barrier in two ways. First, it can deny the individuality of experiences. For instance, the listener's experiences and feelings of grief following a death in the family will be quite different from those of the other person. Grief is an individual experience. Telling your own story can devalue the experiences and feelings of the other person. At an extreme, the listener does not have to listen because he or she supposedly knows what the other person has been through. Second, perhaps more obviously, it is the listener who is dominating and being listened to. Telling your own story simply denies the other person space to tell his or hers.

Defensiveness is a general barrier. Excessive questioning, advising, ordering and telling your own story can all be expressions of defensive-ness. They can be ways of putting up a screen of expertise which promotes the credentials of the professional. Such screens are strength-ened in our culture by expectations from both sides. Sometimes clients expect physiotherapists to be 'all knowing' and may lose confidence if screens are lowered. All the baggage of professional education, accountability, appraisal, client expectation and professional responsibility can help cement the wall between physiotherapist and client with defensiveness.

The context: opening channels

'Effective communication' has increasingly been recognized as a significant element of physiotherapy education. Students are even assessed on their ability to communicate with clients. From a dynamic model of communication, however, improving communication is not a simple matter of improving physiotherapists' skills of expressing and listening to information. Communication is 'meaning making' rather than 'information processing' and meanings are constructed between people. Communication is both based on and generates our perceptions, descriptions and understandings of the world or, more specifically, physiotherapy.

Anderson (1992), a family therapist, has developed a social construction of communication from understandings arising out of the practice of physiotherapy. He describes the work of a physiotherapist, stimulating patients to stretch out and 'open up' their bodies, to show the subtleties of interaction. Along with others (Swain, 1995), Anderson sees the process of opening channels as a process of reflection on the communication process. Opening up channels for people to express and explore their feelings, understandings and aspirations involves reflecting on questions of the why, what and how of communication.

Looking first towards reasons for communicating, the opening of channels is founded on openness about expectations. This requires professionals to be clear about their expectations of an open two-way flow of communication and mutuality in relationships, and conveying this to others. Dalton (1994) writes about the difficulties as a counsellor of people with communication problems:

> 'More difficult to approach … is the client's conviction that what is wrong is physical and only physical. They see the practitioner as there to "cure" the problem – to offer medicine, mechanical repair or exercises. Being asked about their feelings, their views of themselves and their place in their worlds is experienced as an intrusion and this must be respected'.

She goes on to say:

> 'If the counsellor/therapist (or physiotherapist) respects their wishes and works alongside them in their struggle for recovery, a degree of acceptance and understanding of their feelings that is at the heart of any counselling may be experienced'.

A similar statement could be made about the heart of communication in physiotherapy practice. People seem often to be happy about receiving physiotherapy as a straightforward physical form of treatment. Through the medium of physical treatment, however, they may express other concerns and feelings which present a fuller picture of the client as a whole person. Why do people feel they can open up and express their feelings, understandings and wishes? The answer usually lies, in part, in the effectiveness of the communication established between the physiotherapist and client.

Opening up what is communicated relies on listening to the meanings conveyed not only by what the client says but also all those non-verbal messages which express feelings, understandings and wishes. This is grounded in the professional's self-awareness of his or her own feelings, understandings, wishes and so on. Self-awareness is a topic discussed in Chapter 19.

Reflecting on modes of communication begins by questioning the dominance of spoken language. The recognition of touch and physical manipulation as alternative modes of communication is a good starting point for reflecting on the practice of physiotherapy. There are, as indicated above, many other possibilities which can only be mentioned here.

1. The use of sign language is the clearest example of a communication mode or channel other than speech. Sign languages, as developed by deaf people, are actual languages with their own syntax. Clients may be fluent in or use British Sign Language. The onus on physiotherapists is the difficult task, if they are not fluent themselves, to learn what is essentially a foreign language, or at least use the services of a translator. It is important, too, not to make simplistic assumptions. There is a linguistic diversity among deaf people and there are also pros and cons to using translators. The book by Corker (1994) provides an excellent introduction for anyone seeking greater self-awareness and skills in this area.
2. Slightly less obvious, but no less important, is the use of translators generally. Though a physiotherapist working, for instance, with a person with learning difficulties may have difficulties understanding him or her, it is often the case that others, including members of a young person's family, other professionals or an advocate, are 'tuned in' to him or her.
3. Writing is a mode of communication that is different from speech. Speech is of the moment, but writing can be more deliberate and intentional, and is more permanent, unless speech is recorded.
4. Dalton (1994) suggests that other media of communication are essential when working with clients who have what she calls 'impaired communication': 'drawing and painting, materials which can be handled, and music and movement'. All of these can open communication whether or not the client would be said to have impaired communication. In particular, materials or toys of various kinds can be very useful when working with children using play. Joining children in their play is an effective way of opening channels of communication.
5. Finally in this short list, we must include facial expressions and gesture. At their simplest such signals suggest negative or positive feelings towards people, events or experiences. With people who have profound and multiple impairments, for instance, expressions of discrimination and preference can be the basic level of communication within which the physiotherapist needs to be receptive.

Conclusion

With a dynamic, social construction model of communication everything interacts and is influenced by everything else. Any framework for analysing communication (such as verbal versus non-verbal) may further understanding but also distorts the complexities of the whole. The whole is greater than the sum of the parts. The ultimate challenge for physiotherapists wishing to understand and enhance communication in practice is to put the parts together to gain a holistic perspective (Porritt, 1990). The why, the what and the how of communication are interrelated in processes of interaction between physiotherapists and clients that require continuing reflection.

References

Anderson T. (1992) Reflections on reflecting with families. In *Therapy As Social Construction* (McNamee S., Gergen K. J., eds). London: Sage.

Bolton R. (1979) *People Skills: How to Assert, Listen and Resolve Conflict.* Englewood Cliffs, New Jersey: Prentice-Hall.

Burgoon M., Hunsaker F. G., Dawson E. J. (1994) *Human Communication* (3rd edn). London: Sage.

Corker M. (1994) *Counselling – The Deaf Challenge.* London: Jessica Kingley.

Dalton P. (1994) *Counselling People with Communication Problems.* London: Sage.

Davis H., Fallowfield L. (1991) Counselling and communication in health care: the current situation. In *Counselling and Communication in Health Care* (Davis H., Fallowfield L., eds). Chichester: Wiley.

Derlega V. J., Metts S., Petronio S., Margulis S. T. (1993) *Self-Disclosure.* London: Sage.

Dickson D. A., Hargie O., Morrow N. C. (1989) *Communication Skills Training for Health Professionals: An Instructor's Handbook.* London: Chapman and Hall.

Ellin J. (1994) *Listening Helpfully: How to Develop your Counselling Skills.* London: Souvenir Press.

Ellis R., McClintock A. (1994) *If You Take My Meaning: Theory into Practice in Human Communication* (2nd edn). London: Edward Arnold.

Frank M. S., Gilovich T. (1988) The dark side of self and social perception: Black uniforms and aggression in professional sports. *Journal of Personality and Social Psychology,* **54**, 74–85.

French P. (1994) *Social Skills for Nursing Practice* (2nd edn). London: Chapman and Hall.

Fritz P., Russell C., Wilcox E., Shirk F. (1984) *Interpersonal Communication in Nursing.* Norwalk, Connecticut: Appleton-Century-Crofts.

Greene J., Coulson M. (1995) *Language Understanding: Current Issues* (2nd edn). Buckingham: Open University Press.

Hall E., Hall C. (1988) *Human Relations in Education.* London: Routledge.

Huntingdon D. (1987) *Social Skills and General Medical Practice.* London: Allen and Unwin.

Kappas A., Hess U., Scherer K. (1991) Voice and emotion. In *Fundamental of Nonverbal Behavior* (Feldman R. S., Rime B., eds). Cambridge: Cambridge University Press.

Keirnan C., Reid B., Goldbart J. (1987) *Foundations of Communication and Language: Course Manual.* Manchester: Manchester University Press.

Klienke C. (1986) *Meeting and Understanding People.* New York: Freeman.

Ley P., Llewelyn S. (1995) Improving patients' understanding, recall, satisfaction and compliance. In *Health Psychology: Processes and Applications* (2nd edn) (Broome A., Llewelyn S., eds). London: Chapman and Hall.

McCann K., McKenna H. P. (1993) An examination of touch between nurses and elderly patients in a continuing care setting in Northern Ireland. *Journal of Advanced Nursing,* **18**, 38–46.

Marková I. (1987) *Human Awareness: Its Social Development.* London: Hutchinson.

Niven N. (1994) *Health Psychology: An Introduction for Nurses and Other Health Care Professionals* (2nd edn). Edinburgh: Churchill Livingstone.

Northouse P. G., Northouse L. L. (1992) *Health Communication: Strategies for Health Professionals* (2nd edn). Norwalk, Connecticut: Appleton and Lange.

Parry A. (1985) *Physiotherapy Assessment* (2nd edn). London: Chapman and Hall.

Penman R. (1980) *Communication Processes and Relationships.* London: Academic Press.

Porritt L. (1990) *Interaction Strategies: An Introduction for Health Professionals.* London: Churchill Livingstone.

Strawbridge S. (1993) Rules, Roles and Relationships. In *Health, Welfare and Practice* (Walmsley J., Reynolds J., Shakespeare P., Woolfe R., eds). London: Sage.

Swain J. (1995) *The Use of Counselling Skills: A Guide for Therapists.* Oxford: Butterworth-Heinemann.

Trowere P., Bryant B., Argyl M. (1978) *Social Skills and Mental Health.* London: Methuen.

Watzlawick P., Beavin J. H., Jackson D. D. (1967) *Pragmatics of Human Communication.* New York: Norton.

18 Clinical interviewing

Sally French

'An important responsibility of the physical therapist is to create an open, communicative atmosphere whereby information can be readily offered and received.' (Croft, 1980)

Interviewing the patient is an important aspect of the physiotherapy assessment and is an on-going process throughout treatment (Parry, 1988). It is often referred to as the 'subjective' part of the assessment, although the implication that the rest of it is 'objective' or that a dicotomy exists has been disputed (Grieve, 1988; French, 1993a; Stewart, 1995). Effective clinical interviewing is difficult but can be learned and improved by understanding and practising interviewing skills (Millar *et al.*, 1992; Newall, 1994). Froelich and Bishop (1977) believe that the purpose of a clinical interview is to gather information about the patient, to establish a relationship with the patient, to help the patient understand his or her illness and to support and direct the patient in his or her treatment.

Effective clinical interviewing is dependent on a variety of interpersonal skills which include proficiency in asking questions, the ability and motivation to listen and respond effectively and the capacity to understand and emit non-verbal cues (Millar *et al.* 1992; Newell, 1994; French, 1995). These skills are very similar to those used in counselling (Burnard, 1992; Swain, 1995). Hasler (1985) considers that the acquisition of interpersonal skills, in medical and paramedical education and practice, have been taken for granted and are thought to be largely a matter of common sense. He is opposed to this view and believes that consultations are only successful if communication, as well as the more technical components of the assessment, are correct. He points out that a poor consultation can have far reaching negative consequences in terms of patient satisfaction and compliance. Regarding interpersonal skills, Dickson and Maxwell (1987) believe that:

'It was generally assumed that such aspects of the professional role would be gradually and largely subconsciously acquired through increased clinical experience. However, this rather comfortable philosophy has gained little support from the available empirical evidence'.

Types of interview

There are many types of interview, ranging from those which are highly structured to the totally unstructured type. In structured interviews very specific questions are asked which can be coded easily, often by means of a standard chart or form. Conversely, with the unstructured type of interview there is little attempt to formulate the content which is written out in full. Most interviews conducted by physiotherapists fall somewhere between these two extremes and are said to be semi-structured.

What type of interview should physiotherapists use?

There are advantages and disadvantages to both structured and unstructured interviews. The degree of structure will depend on the beliefs and personality of the physiotherapist, the ideology of the institution where he or she works and the beliefs, personality and needs of the particular patient. A highly structured interview may run counter to an ideology of free expression or an holistic approach to patient care and may be inappropriate for certain groups of patients, for example young children, or people with complex problems. On the other hand some patients may regard an open-ended, holistic approach as an invasion of privacy. Norell (1987) points out that, according to their style, doctors are liable to be regarded either as uncaring or as intrusive.

The structured interview

The main advantages of the structured interview are that patients' responses can be categorized and coded relatively easily, irrelevant information can be avoided and timing can be kept under control. The coded information can be a useful source of statistics for managerial purposes and as data for quantitative research. There is a danger, however, of assuming that structured information is more factual and scientific than it really is. With this in mind, Goldfinger (1973) talks of the 'fallacy of misplaced concreteness' when discussing the problem orientated medical record. There is a tendency to believe that data which are presented graphically and expressed numerically are valid, but this is not necessarily the case (Huff, 1973; Slattery, 1986; French, 1988; Abberley, 1992).

Interesting and relevant information, falling outside the physiotherapist's frame of reference, may be lost with the structured interview. Much has been written about the differing definitions patients and health professionals have about illness and disability and the problems to which this can give rise (Abberley, 1993; Oliver, 1993; Silburn, 1993; French, 1994; French et al., 1995). In order for a consultation to be successful the clinician and the patient must have a shared understanding of the problem. If the interview is highly structured the physiotherapist's definition will dominate.

In attempting to code patients' responses precisely, they may be adjusted to fit a given category. Hyman et al. (1954) found that researchers tended to 'bend' subjects' responses to fit the categories provided. It is desirable that the coding systems used by physiotherapists are reliable; high reliability would exist if several physiotherapists or one physiotherapist, taking the same measurement on several different occasions, arrived at a similar result. There is, however, the danger that high reliability will be achieved at the expense of validity. Reliability is largely a technical matter whereas validity is concerned with the nature of reality; a test is valid if it is measuring what it purports to measure. It is possible for information to be highly reliable yet be incorrect or insignificant. In the quest to ensure high reliability the information gathered may become so simplified that its validity is reduced or lost.

There is a danger of this happening in physiotherapy interviews if a highly structured format is adopted.

In order to gain 'relevant' information the physiotherapist's questions are selective and focused. The emphasis is usually on the patient's signs and symptoms and their consequences, with little attempt to explore other aspects of illness behaviour. This issue leads to questions concerning the physiotherapist's role, but clearly if the major reason for becoming a patient is of a social or psychological nature, than a highly structured interview, following the medical model of illness and disability, will be insufficient. Pendleton *et al.* (1984) believe that consultations are unsuccessful unless the clinician manages to establish why the patient has come and Campkin and Jones (1987) warn that preoccupation with 'problems' and diagnoses may draw the clinician's attention away from the patient as an individual. A similar critique has been given by disabled people (Woolley, 1993; French, 1994).

Some patients may be alienated by a structured interview where their input is restrained and where the flow of conversation is interrupted by note-taking. Coates and King (1982) recommend that physiotherapists should not write while they are interviewing patients as it disturbs interaction. Some physiotherapists use a tape recorder when interviewing. Provided the patient is not intimidated by the machine, this will ensure that the flow of conversation is maintained without the risk of it being forgotten. It may also indicate to the patient that the physiotherapist is interested and taking seriously all he or she has to say. Bernstein and Bernstein (1980) point out that the question–answer format may imply that the professional has 'so specialized and mysterious a knowledge' that the patient will only respond to answering the specific questions posed.

There is a danger with the structured approach, particularly with students and inexperienced staff, that the exercise of filling in the assessment form correctly over-rides the importance of the patient/therapist relationship, with its considerable therapeutic effects (Newell, 1994; Burnard, 1995). The physiotherapist may become preoccupied with the mechanics of recording the interview data, or frustrated if the patient's responses are vague or confused. Unfortunately practice does not always make perfect; there is a tendency for people to develop rigid routines over time, whereby they adhere strictly to a given assessment format without considering its usefulness to the particular patient concerned. Parry (1988) warns physiotherapists against this tendency.

The unstructured interview

Most writers on the subject of clinical interviewing advocate a relatively unstructured approach. Bernstein and Bernstein (1980) believe that the therapist should avoid over-controlling the patient or he or she may feel intimidated and relevant information may be lost. They believe that the therapist should listen more than talk.

Samual (1987) believes that patients sometimes 'have to struggle quite hard to find a gap in the doctor's routine' and that they are often ready to talk at times when professionals are not ready to listen. Norell (1987) reminds us that:

'It is sometimes difficult to remember that the important thing for the patient is the opportunity to have his say, however falteringly. It is in creating an atmosphere in which the patient can feel secure enough to do this that the doctor makes a major contribution to a worthwhile consultation'.

Bernstein and Bernstein (1980) and Swain (1995) point out that helping is not necessarily dependent on talking or doing and Campkin (1987) warns that clinicians should not take refuge in 'respectable medical activities' in order to avoid listening to patients.

When the unstructured interview is used the advantages of the structured approach are lost; coding is difficult, timing can get out of hand and the patient may give a great deal of peripheral information. Despite these problems Samual (1987) believes that, 'The ability to accept muddle is invaluable'. The information from an unstructured clinical interview will not be easily quantified but it will certainly be rich and detailed and may provide useful data for qualitative research. Some patients, however, may object to enquiries which do not closely relate to their signs and symptoms and it has been argued by some sociologists and disabled activists, for example Illich (1984) and Davis (1993), that the tendency of health professionals to delve into social and psychological matters is expanding their empire and 'medicalizing' life. However, given that much illness stems from and incorporates psychosocial factors, ignoring them in favour of a purely biological model of illness would seem detrimental from the patient's point of view.

Most physiotherapists adopt a semi-structured approach when interviewing patients. This is favoured by Parry (1988) who states:

'... history-taking should not be a stereotyped routine even though answers to specific questions are needed. The physiotherapist must walk the thin line between conversation and formal consultation ...'

Practical considerations may limit the physiotherapist's choice of interview. The more 'open' it is the more time consuming it tends to be both to conduct and to write up and read the resulting notes, Millar et al. (1992) urge interviewers to be realistic over time. However, Norell (1987) believes the problems of time can be exaggerated and that 'achievements in consultation are not time-related but intensity-related', and Newell (1994) believes that professionals use lack of time as an excuse for poor interviewing. Weston and Brown (1995) believe that:

'The most common excuse given to avoid asking about patients' personal concerns is lack of time. But it is not efficient use of time to search for a disease that is not present or to ignore a major source of patients' distress, such as their fears or concerns'.

Brown et al. (1995) point to research which shows that interviews where patients are actively involved in asking questions take no longer than those where they are not.

The social psychology of the interview

Non-verbal communication

Whichever interview method is adopted the physiotherapist will come face-to-face with the patient (Millar *et al.*, 1992; Newell, 1994). The patient's non-verbal communication can be a useful additional source of information. By observing the patient's gait, posture and facial expression as he or she enters the treatment room, the physiotherapist can learn a great deal. Dimatteo and Taranta (1979) found that communication between doctor and patient was unsatisfactory unless the doctor could understand the patient's non-verbal cues and was able to emit them effectively him or herself. Thompson (1981) found that patients preferred medical students who were socially skilled in terms of their non-verbal behaviour and Wooley *et al.* (1978) note that interviewing skills, including non-verbal skills, correlate with patient satisfaction and compliance.

Dockrell (1988) investigated the use of verbal and non-verbal communication skills of final year physiotherapy students, by means of structured observation. The frequency of the following behaviours was observed and recorded; eye contract, tone of voice, listening ability, explaining, facial expression and responding with interest. The 29 students were observed twice while treating the same patient in the clinical setting. Questionnaires were also completed by the students to discover the importance they attached to each of these skills.

Facial expression, responding with interest and listening were demonstrated least often by the students. It was found that they had adequate knowledge of communication and rated all the skills as important but were not sufficiently proficient when using them and over-estimated the extent to which they did use them. It is likely that the behaviour of the students was affected to some extent by the fact of being observed, although the purpose behind the observation was not disclosed.

Non-verbal communication can distort verbal information as well as enhance it. Lack of facial expression or a monotonous voice, for instance, may disturb communication. Some aspects of non-verbal communication cannot be changed, the interviewer and the interviewee are affected by each other's age, race, sex and physical appearance. Accent is another relatively stable characteristic by which people are often evaluated (Honey, 1989). There is a tendency to make global inferences about people on the basis of very limited information, thus if the patient appears anxious he or she may be labelled as an anxious 'type', which may, in turn, be written into the medical records and consolidated into 'fact'. There is a tendency to minimize just how much people's behaviour is affected by the situation and environment they are in, especially if they perceive it as strange or intimidating as the physiotherapy department may be. Parry (1988) warns us not to take much notice of initial impressions. The more relaxed patients feel the more likely they are to show their usual behaviour.

Hargreaves (1987) points out that non-verbal signals, which are often emitted and received without full awareness, are more powerful than words if the two conflict, although the meaning of the message, in this situation, is often ambiguous and confusing. Fagerhaugh and Strauss (1977) found that physiotherapists and nurses tended to assess the severity of patients' low back pain by interpreting their behaviour rather than believing what was said. Saxey (1986) warns that we should not judge how much pain someone is in by his or her behaviour alone as many people learn to adapt to it and lead relatively normal lives even though their symptoms are quite severe. In addition non-verbal messages have different meanings according to culture (Newell, 1994).

The physiotherapist may influence what the patient says and how he or she behaves, by verbal communication, non-verbal communication and silence. If the physiotherapist only responds positively when the patient mentions improvement of symptoms, for example, the patient may become inhibited about admitting that his or her condition is static or worsening.

The physical arrangement of the furniture and the position and distance between the physiotherapist and patient are also important (Newell, 1994). If, for example, the physiotherapist sits some distance from the patient and interposes a desk between them, the atmosphere will tend to be rather formal especially if they are sitting directly facing each other. Patients are likely to feel rather vulnerable and anxious on their first visit so a less formal arrangement is preferable. This can be achieved by removing the table and sitting closer, though not too close, to the patient and at right angles rather than face to face.

Uniforms are another source of non-verbal communication; they give information regarding occupation and status and may also engender feelings of respect, fear or trust, or create a psychological distance between the health worker and the patient. Professional trappings, such as badges, stethoscopes and items of equipment can have similar effects. Such messages may or may not be helpful according to the setting and personality and beliefs of the patient. Uniforms have become less popular among those working with children where they may engender fear and in the areas of psychiatry and learning difficulties where the medical model of illness is being seriously challenged. Touch is a particularly ambiguous aspect of non-verbal communication which the wearing of uniforms and the professional setting helps to clarify. A great deal can be communicated through touch which can be very therapeutic (Newell, 1994; Poon, 1995; Swain, 1995). (For further information on non-verbal communication, the reader is referred to Chapter 17.)

The 'social desirability' effect

The 'social desirability' effect refers to the tendency people have to present themselves in a favourable light, a process which Goffman (1969) referred to as 'impression management'. The patient may feel that various aspects of his or her life will discredit him or her in the eyes of the physiotherapist, for example unemployment or personal habits such as smoking. Patients are unlikely to disclose discrediting information to the physiotherapist, at least until they know him or her better and only then if an empathic atmosphere which lacks anxiety and moral evaluation is provided. The social desirability effect has been shown to threaten the validity of research data and will operate similarly in the clinical interview.

Stimson and Webb (1975), in their research concerning the doctor/patient relationship, found that patients frequently felt disappointed in their performance after the consultation and that the consultation itself was characterized by feelings of nervousness and embarrassment. It is likely that some patients experience these feelings when communicating with physiotherapists. They may be anxious and self-conscious when discussing personal details and at not being able to answer the physiotherapist's questions through ignorance, forgetfulness or lack of understanding. Silences can also create tension and disrupt communication; the physiotherapist may break a silence too soon, not giving the patient sufficient time to think, or the patient may answer hurriedly and without due thought in order to avoid a silence. The research interview is sometimes viewed as being a good method for obtaining personal and delicate information, although some people prefer the more anonymous questionnaire (French, 1993b). Similarly many patients will respond favourably to the clinical interview if conducted well but others may prefer to give details of their problems in a written form or even to a computer.

The patient may believe that it is socially undesirable for his or her symptoms not to improve and may experience embarrassment and anxiety if they remain static or worsen despite painstaking treatment. Patients sometimes need encouragement to admit they are no better but can be further inhibited by the physiotherapist's verbal and non-verbal behaviour. For example rather than asking the patient how he feels the physiotherapist might say, 'You're looking better Mr Smith', making it all the more difficult for him to admit that no improvement has taken place. Lack of improvement can be difficult for health professions to accept and 'victim-blaming' may start operating whereby the symptoms are assumed to be 'all in the mind' or thought to persist because of lack of effort or adherence to advice (Posner, 1984). A strategy the patient may adopt, to avoid admitting a lack of improvement, is to concentrate upon a small, perhaps insignificant, area of progress while failing to mention or minimizing symptoms which are static or worsening. Physiotherapists may find themselves adopting this strategy too. Bernstein and Bernstein (1980) warn that patients tend to give socially desirable answers to the question 'why' and believe that 'why' questions should be avoided. Froelich and Bishop (1977) make the point that people's motives are often unknown even to themselves so they tend to give socially acceptable answers to the question, 'why?'.

The environment

When interviewing a patient, a quiet, private room free from interruption should ideally be used (Newell, 1994). Unfortunately such an area rarely exists in physiotherapy departments or wards where one patient is usually separated from the next by nothing more substantial than a curtain. This may well inhibit full and truthful discourse and rather undermines the notion of confidentiality. The physiotherapist should try to ensure that he or she is not interrupted by telephone calls, students, colleagues or other patients while conducting a clinical interview as interruptions give the impression that the physiotherapist has more important things to do.

Social class

It has been found in studies of the doctor/patient relationship that doctors tend to spend less time with working class patients than middle class patients, that they give them less information and assume they lack the ability to understand medical information (Fitzpatrick and Scambler, 1984). This may be one factor in what Tudor Hart (1971) referred to as the 'inverse care law', whereby those people who need medical care the most receive the least. Although there is no comparable research with physiotherapists it is possible that similar findings would emerge. Health professionals and middle class patients tend to share a common culture which helps them relate to each other more easily.

Defining the problem

The definition of the problem may vary considerably between the physiotherapist and the patient (Newell, 1994, French *et al.*, 1995). For example the physiotherapist may be delighted if there is an improvement in the patient's range of movement, but this may hardly interest the patient at all. The patient's definition of his or her problem must be taken seriously in the assessment, for it is difficult for rehabilitation to proceed unless some kind of consensus is reached (Brown *et al.*, 1995; French *et al.*, 1996). This takes time and it should not be assumed that the physiotherapist is inevitably 'right'; the patient may have lived with the impairment or illness for many years and is likely to have acquired a detailed understanding of his or her abilities and limitations (Swain *et al.*, 1993; Hales, 1996). Norell (1987) considers that 'problem solving' is an arrogant term and Croft (1980) believes that:

> 'The decision, although strived for through interaction by both participants in the process, should be primarily that of the patient. The therapist's inclination to solve the patient's problems, offer advice and approve or disapprove of ideas suggested by the patient must be controlled'.

Campkin and Jones (1987) believe that the professional's objectives, however worthy, should not be allowed to over-ride the patient's agenda during the consultation.

Questioning

Leading questions

Leading questions influence the direction of the patient's reply and, as a general rule, should be avoided. For example the question 'How did you get on with the exercises?' makes the assumption that the patient carried them out, which may or may not be so. Another example of a leading question is, 'Where is the pain?' before establishing whether the patient has any. A study was carried out by Loftus (1975) where one group of people were asked, 'Do you get headaches frequently and if so how many?' and another group were asked, 'Do you get headaches occasionally and if so how many?'. The first group reported an average of 2.2 headaches per week whereas the second group reported an average of 0.7 headaches per week. This study shows that by changing just one word patients' responses can be greatly altered. Hargie *et al.* (1980) note that leading questions are prohibited during cross-examination in court.

Leading questions can occasionally be used to advantage if the information sought involves behaviour which is socially disapproved of, leading to denial. A leading question may have the effect of indicating that such behaviour is normal and expected by the physiotherapist and that he or she will be unaffected by it and tolerant of it. For example, rather than asking the patient if he or she has taken time off work because of backache, the physiotherapist could ask how much time he or she has taken off. Leading questions of this type were used by Kinsey *et al.* (1948) in their study of sexual behaviour.

Multiple questions

Multiple questions, also referred to as double-barrelled questions, require two or more answers. An example of a multiple question is, 'Have you any pain or numbness in your arm?' Questions requiring two or more responses should be avoided as they are difficult to answer and confusing to both patient and therapist (Newell, 1994).

Loaded questions

Oppenheim (1968) describes a loaded word or phrase as 'one which is emotionally coloured and suggests an automatic feeling of approval or disapproval'. An example is, 'I hope you haven't forgotten to do your exercises today!'. The therapist expresses a judgement regarding what the patient should or ought to do. Questions and statements loaded with moral judgements and evaluations should generally be avoided because the patient is likely to respond to the emotional rather than the factual content (Porritt, 1990). It is not always easy to avoid such questions, however, because what is regarded as judgemental by one person may be viewed as neutral by another. Occasionally it may be appropriate for the physiotherapist to express disapproval in an attempt to alter the patient's behaviour.

Open and closed questions

Structured interviews are characterized by 'closed' questions and unstructured interviews by 'open' questions. Closed questions force the patient to reply in a specific way (Porritt, 1990). An example of a closed question is, 'Is your pain better or worse?'. This makes categorization of the response easy but the information gained is minimal. An alternative open question would be, 'Please will you describe your pain?'. The reply may be complex, rambling and difficult to categorize but nevertheless full and individualistic, perhaps reflecting the true nature of the pain experience. Roter and Hall (1987) found that patients give more information to doctors who use open-ended questions and that the amount of information patients give is related to how much information the doctor gives them. Closed questions are, however, useful for gathering factual information. They are easy to answer as they provide clarity and focus which may serve to relax the patient in the early stages of the clinical interview. It should also be appreciated that some patients are not sufficiently articulate to cope with open questions.

The ordering of questions

On most occasions it is best to begin the interview by asking for factual information of a neutral kind. When rapport with the patient has been established he or she is likely to feel more comfortable when giving personal details about work, home situation and life style. Sometimes the patient is very eager to explain certain aspects of his or her problem to the physiotherapist; in this situation the patient should not be restrained, for although this may throw the clinical interview out of sequence, making the physiotherapist's task more difficult, patients are unlikely to concentrate fully until they have had an opportunity to speak. It may also enable the physiotherapist to gain insight into how the patient views his or her illness or impairment. Samual (1987) believes that health professionals need 'to develop sensitivity to the subtle nuances of patients' feelings so as to keep in touch with the whole of their patient's condition' and that although this is initially time consuming it can save time in the long run as unnecessary investigations and treatments will be avoided. It is very important to encourage patients to ask as well as answer questions. Niven (1994) believes that the most important aspect of questioning is listening.

Asking sensible questions

It is not uncommon for the clinical interview to be characterized by rigid routines with some of the questions being entirely out of context. What is the purpose of asking a fit young person with a painful shoulder whether he or she lives alone? Even if the question is relevant it frequently ignores the complexities of social life. The question, 'Are you married?' when confronted with an elderly patient with a fractured femur, may seem reasonable, and yet we all know of husbands, wives, sons and daughters who live at home yet fail to help, and, conversely, of friends and neighbours who are tremendously helpful. We also know that people frequently live together without being married. The information required is probably, 'Do you have anyone to help you at home?' and, 'How much help are you receiving?'.

It is possible to use a psychosocial approach inappropriately when questioning patients. Weston and Brown (1995) explain:

> 'When a patient presented with concerns about her severe sore throat and about how long she was going to be off school, the resident interrupted her story, "Wait, I need to get to know more about your personal situation. Where did you grow up? What was your childhood like? Was there much conflict in your family?". These questions would be very useful in the appropriate context, but in this case they seemed unconnected with the patient's concerns about receiving effective treatment and getting back to school as soon as possible. The physician needed to be sensitive to any clues about how this patient's home and school situation were related to her illness, but not to impose a psychosocial agenda where it did not apply'.

When asking for non-medical information an explanation should be given of why it is needed. The question may be so worded that the explanation is implicit within it, for example, 'Are there any tasks at home which you find difficult to do now that you have sprained your wrist?', rather than, 'Are you managing to do your cleaning?'.

Many people find taking a social history difficult because it can feel like prying. Maguire and Rutter (1976), in their study of the interviewing skills of 50 senior medical students, found that 30% avoided asking personal questions, which led to a hurried and superficial approach. Weston and Brown (1995) believe that:

'Without practice, most young doctors feel uncomfortable inquiring about patients' personal lives. Often, the concern is that a patient will become emotional and perhaps cry or show anger; they worry that they will open up "a can of worms" they will not be able to handle'.

By asking sensible questions, which reflect the complexities of everyday life, and by explaining why such information is helpful, these awkward feelings are reduced and a meaningful social history can be obtained.

Probing and prompting

Probing questions ask for more detail or for clarification (Millar *et al.*, 1992). It is often very important in the clinical interview to ask such questions though it can be perceived as threatening if overdone. Maguire and Rutter (1976), in their study of the interviewing skills of 50 senior medical students, found that 62% failed to confront patients with inconsistencies or gaps in their stories.

Prompts are used to help or encourage the patient to reply. The physiotherapist may simply repeat the question or may rephrase it, perhaps in simpler language, if it is felt that the patient has not understood. The physiotherapist may convert open questions into a series of closed questions or help the patient to retrieve knowledge by reviewing information previously covered. For example, if the patient cannot remember the advice previously given the physiotherapist might say, 'Think of what we did in the gym last week'. A suitable period of silence may also serve as a prompt. These techniques are used extensively by teachers and enhance understanding and memory by making the learning process more active (French *et al.*, 1994).

Jargon

Every profession and occupation has its jargon and the physiotherapy profession is certainly no exception. It is a common mistake to use medical terms and jargon when questioning or communicating information to patients. The patient may not understand such terms which can lead to embarrassment and worry as well as wasting time. Examples in physiotherapy are, 'We'll try some suspension next time you come', or even 'Contract that muscle'. Care must be taken to avoid jargon, but at the same time it is important not to be patronizing. Bernstein and Bernstein (1980) believe that therapists should attempt to gauge the patient's verbal ability and adjust their verbalizations to that of the patient.

Patients have their own jargon when attempting to describe the signs and symptoms of illness. Examples are: 'I feel low' or 'It feels funny'. Parry (1988) warns physiotherapists not to take patients' pseudomedical jargon, such as 'slipped disc' and 'rheumatism', at face value but rather to try to clarify what they mean. Maguire and Rutter (1976) found that 92% of the senior medical students they studied failed to clarify patients' jargon and, in consequence, several were seriously misled about the nature of patients' problems.

Responding to patients

As well as asking patients questions the physiotherapist must also respond to their queries, suggestions and views. Bernstein and Bernstein

(1980) point out that health professionals are prone to respond by reassuring the patient. Although this can be appropriate behaviour it can also have the effect of denying that the problem exists and serves to shield the professional from discussing difficult issues, such as progressive illness and death, with which they feel ill-equipped to deal. Health professionals have, until recent times, been taught to distance themselves from patients' emotional concerns. Swain (1995) states:

> 'Reassurance can also be a denial of strength of feeling. The rushed few words of support may be an attempt to show caring, but can be a means of closing down communication. Cliches are a form of reassurance: "Time's a great healer", "You've got to take the rough with the smooth" or "Let bygones be bygones". Such stock platitudes avoid rather than reflect the particular concerns of the other person'.

Froelich and Bishop (1977) agree that there is no better way of closing a topic than offering reassurance and that it is much more reassuring to talk about a difficult problem than to be reassured. They believe that many questions are not requests for simple, factual information but rather reflect patients' anxiety and desire to understand fully their situation. For example the question, 'Do you think I thought to go back to see the doctor?' may indicate worry about lack of improvement.

Sometimes the patient's behaviour may be hostile (Newell, 1994). Bernstein and Bernstein (1980) suggest that hostility is normally an expression of fear and that the health professional should not respond with anger or a 'hostility–counterhostility' cycle may be set in motion. They believe that professional workers, 'cannot allow themselves the luxury of responding to disagreement or anger in kind'.

One aim of teaching interviewing skills is to help students adopt appropriate responses but Norell (1987) disputes its value or necessity believing that the desire to say always the right thing and respond in the 'correct' manner has become something of a preoccupation. He believes that a spontaneous response can be superior to the 'painfully laboured, contrived, self-conscious effort of the "trained" doctor' and that one measure of a good relationship is that it can survive disagreement. He states:

> '... the doctor who decides for instance not to conceal his disappointment or disapproval may be helping to develop a more productive relationship than if he were to assume the outward appearance of tolerance while fuming inwardly'.

It has also been argued that being excessively tolerant and 'nice' is a way of controlling patients now that an authoritarian stance on the part of the professional is considered inappropriate. Such a pose makes it very difficult for patients to express anger and dissatisfaction, to present opposing views or complain. In addition 'niceness' is often perceived as patronizing. Genuineness is an essential ingredient of all good human relationships.

Conclusion

It is clear from the above account that clinical interviewing is a very complex activity. It is little wonder that most people find it difficult. However, the skills of effective clinical interviewing can be learned and are now formally taught on many medical, nursing and physiotherapy courses. Although the effectiveness of the training is still a matter of dispute, most people who undertake it seem to find it helpful (Levins, 1984; Dickson and Maxwell, 1987). An understanding of the social psychology of the interview, along with vigilant practice of interviewing skills, such as questioning, is likely to bring about improvement in interviewing technique for even the most experienced physiotherapist.

References

Abberley P. (1992) Counting us out: a discussion of the OPCS disability surveys. *Disability and Society*, **7**(2), 139–156.

Abberley P. (1993) Disabled people and normality. In *Disabling Society – Enabling Environments* (Swain J., Finkelstein V., French S., Oliver M., eds). London: Sage.

Bernstein L., Bernstein R. S. (1980) *Interviewing: A Guide for Health Professionals* (3rd edn). New York: Appleton-Century-Crofts.

Brown J. B., McWilliam C. L., Weston W. W. (1995a) The sixth component: being realistic. In *Patient-centred Medicine: Transforming the Clinical Method* (Stewart M. *et al.*, eds). London: Sage.

Brown J. B., Weston W. W., Stewart M. (1995b) The third component: finding common ground. In *Patient-centred Medicine: Transforming the Clinical Method* (Stewart M. *et al.*, eds). London: Sage.

Burnard P. (1992) *Counselling: A Guide to Practice in Nursing*. Oxford: Butterworth-Heinemann.

Burnard P. (1995) *Learning Human Skills: An Experimental and Reflective Guide for Nurses* (3rd edn). Oxford: Butterworth-Heinemann.

Campkin M. (1987) Why don't you listen to me for a change? In *While I'm Here Doctor* (Elder A., Samual O., eds). London: Tavistock Publications.

Campkin M., Jones E. (1987) Conflict or collaboration? In *While I'm Here Doctor* (Elder A., Samual O., eds). London: Tavistock Publications.

Coates H., King A. (1982) *The Patient Assessment*. London: Churchill Livingstone.

Croft J. J. (1980) Interviewing in physical therapy. *Physical Therapy*, **60**(8), 1033–1036.

Davis K. (1993) The crafting of good clients. In *Disabling Barriers – Enabling Environments* (Swain J., Finkelstein V., French S., Oliver M., eds). London: Sage.

Dickson D. A., Maxwell M. (1987) A comparative study of physiotherapy students' attitudes to social skills training undertaken before and after clinical placement. *Physiotherapy*, **73**(2), 60–64.

Dimatteo R., Taranta A. (1979) Non-verbal communication and physician–patient rapport: an empirical study. *Professional Psychology*, **10**, 540–547.

Dockrell S. (1988) An investigation of the use of verbal and non-verbal communication skills by final year physiotherapy students. *Physiotherapy*, **74**(2), 52–55.

Fagerhaugh S. Y., Strauss A. (1977) *Politics of Pain Management: Staff/Patient Interaction*. Wokingham: Addison-Wesley.

Fitzpatrick R., Scambler G. (1984) Social class, ethnicity and illness. In *The Experience of Illness* (Fitzpatrick R., Hinton J., Newman S., Scambler G., Thompson J., eds). London: Tavistock Publications.

French P. (1995) *Social Skills for Nursing Practice* (2nd edn). London: Chapman and Hall.

French S. (1988) How significant is statistical significance? *Physiotherapy*, **74**(6), 266–268.

French S. (1993a) Setting a record straight. In *Disabling Barriers – Enabling Environment* (Swain J., Finkelstein V., French S., Oliver M., eds). London: Sage.

French S. (1993b) *Practical Research: A Guide for Therapists*. Oxford: Butterworth-Heinemann.

French S. (1994) (ed.) *On Equal Terms: Working with Disabled People*. Oxford: Butterworth-Heinemann.

French S., Neville S., Laing J. (1994) *Teaching and Learning: A Guide for Therapists*. Oxford: Butterworth-Heinemann.

French S., Finkelstein V., Patterson S. (1995) *Disabling Society – Enabling Interventions*. Milton Keynes: Open University Course.

Froelich R. E., Bishop F. M. (1977) *Clinical Interviewing Skills* (3rd edn). St Louis: C. V. Mosby.

Goffman I. (1969) *The Presentation of Self in Everyday Life*. Harmondsworth: Penguin Books.

Goldfinger S. E. (1973) The problem-orientated record: a critique from a believer. *New England Journal of Medicine*, **200**, 606–608.

Grieve G. P. (1988) Clinical examination and the SOAP mnemonic. *Physiotherapy*, **74**(2), 97.

Hales G. (1996) (ed.) *Beyond Disability: Towards an Enabling Environment*. London: Sage.

Hargie O., Saunders C., Dickson D. (1980) *Social Skills in Interpersonal Communication*. London: Croom Helm.

Hargreaves S. (1987) The relevance of non-verbal skills in physiotherapy. *Physiotherapy*, **73**(12), 685–688.

Hasler J. C. (1985) Communications and relationships in general practice. *Physiotherapy*, **71**(10), 435–436.

Honey J. (1989) *Does Accent Matter*. London: Faber and Faber.

Huff D. (1973) *How to Lie With Statistics*. Harmondsworth: Penguin Books.

Hyman H. H., Cobb W. J., Feldman J. J., Steinber C. H. (1954) *Interviewing in Social Research*. Chicago: University of Chicago Press.

Illich I. (1984) The epidemics of modern medicine. In *Health and Disease* (Black N., Boswell D., Gray A., Murphy S., Popay J., eds). Milton Keynes: Open University Press.

Kinsey A. C., Pomeroy W. B., Martin C. E. (1948) *Sexual Behaviour in the Human Male*. London: W. B. Saunders.

Levins M. F. (1984) Communication skills in physiotherapy students. *Physiotherapy Canada*, **36**(7), 32–35.

Loftus E. F. (1975) Leading questions and the eyewitness report. *Cognitive Psychology*, **7**, 560–672.

Maguire P., Rutter D. R. (1976) History-taking for medical students: deficiencies in performance. In *Basic Readings in Medical Sociology* (Tuckett D., Kaufert I.- M., eds). London: Tavistock Publications.

Millar R., Crute V., Hargie O. (1992) *Professional Interviewing*. London: Routledge.

Newell R. (1994) *Interviewing Skills for Nursing and other Health Care Professionals*. London: Routledge.

Niven N. (1994) *Health Psychology: An Introduction for Nurses and Other Health Care Professions*. Edinburgh: Churchill Livingstone.

Norell J. (1987) Uses and abuses of the consultation. In *While I'm Here Doctor* (Elder A., Samual O., eds). London: Tavistock Publications.

Oliver M. (1993) Conductive education: if it wasn't so sad it would be funny. *Disabling Barriers – Enabling Environments* (Swain J., Finkelstein V., French S., Oliver M., eds). London: Sage.

Oppenheim A. N. (1968) *Questionnaire Design and Attitude Measurement*. London: Heinemann.

Parry A. (1988) *Physiotherapy Assessment* (2nd edn). London: Chapman and Hall.

Pendleton D. A., Schofield T. P. C., Havelock P. B., Tate P. H. L. (1984) *The Consultation: An Approach to Learning and Teaching*. Oxford General Practice Series 6. Oxford: Oxford University Press.

Poon K. (1995) Touch and handling. In *Physiotherapy in Mental Health: A Practical Approach* (Everett T., Dennis M., Ricketts E., eds). Oxford: Butterworth-Heinemann.

Porritt L. (1990) *Interaction Strategies: An Introduction for Health Professionals*. Edinburgh: Churchill Livingstone.

Posner T. (1984) Magical elements in orthodox medicine: diabetes as a medical thought system. In *Health and Disease* (Black N., Boswell D., Gray A., Murphy S., Popay J., eds). Milton Keynes: Open University Press.

Roter D. L., Hall J. A. (1987) Physicians' interviewing styles and medical information obtained from patients. *Journal of General Internal Medicine*, **2**(5), 325–329.

Samual O. (1987) Search or serendipity? In *While I'm Here Doctor* (Elder A., Samual O., eds). London: Tavistock Publications.

Saxey S. (1986) Nurses' response to post-op pain. *Nursing Times*, **3**, 377–381.

Silburn L. (1993) A social model in a medical world: the development of the integrated living team as part of the strategy for younger physically disabled people in North Derbyshire. In *Disabling Barriers – Enabling Environments* (Swain J., Finkelstein V., French S., Oliver M., eds). London: Sage.

Slattery M. (1986) *Official Statistics*. London: Tavistock Publications.

Stewart M. (1995) Conclusion. In *Patient-centred Medicine: Transforming the Clinical Method* (Stewart M. *et al.*, eds). London: Sage.

Stimson G. V., Webb B. (1975) *Going to See the Doctor: The Consultation Process in General Practice*. London: Routledge and Kegan Paul.

Swain J. (1995) *The Use of Counselling Skills: A Guide for Therapists*. Oxford: Butterworth-Heinemann.

Swain J., Finkelstein V., French S. and Oliver M. (eds). (1993) *Disabling Barriers – Enabling Environments*. London: Sage.

Thompson J. A. (1981) Patient preferences and the bedside manner. *Journal of Psychosomatic Research*, **25**, 3–7.

Tudor Hart J. (1971) The inverse care law. *Lancet*, **i**, 405–412.

Weston W. W., and Brown J. B. (1995) Dealing with common difficulties in learning and teaching the patient-centred method. In *Patient-centred Medicine: Transforming the Clinical Method* (Stewart M. *et al.*, eds). London: Sage.

Wooley R. R., Kane R. L., Hughes C. C., Wright D. F. (1978) Doctor–patient communication on satisfaction and outcomes of care. *Social Science and Medicine*, **18**(269), 123–128.

Woolley M. (1993) Acquired hearing loss: acquired oppression. In *Disabling Barriers – Enabling Environments* (Swain J., Finkelstein V., French S., Oliver M., eds). London: Sage.

19   Counselling and the use of counselling skills

John Swain

Physiotherapy and counselling

It can be argued that a physiotherapist should no more provide counselling than a counsellor should provide physiotherapy. There are serious concerns here in that there is the possibility of the misuse of counselling skills to manipulate clients. Perhaps even more questionable would be 'dabbling in counselling', that is delving into clients' personal lives without their consent and against their wishes (Swain, 1995). Nevertheless, there are numerous texts such as Burnard (1994) which are specifically aimed at encouraging health care professionals to use counselling skills in their work and helping them do so. There is also evidence that training in counselling skills can enhance the practice of health care professionals (Ryden *et al.*, 1991).

So what relevance does counselling and the use of counselling skills have for physiotherapists? The purpose of this chapter is to answer this question and in doing so to begin to provide a basis for physiotherapists to reflect on themselves and their practice in this light.

The first question, then, is the meaning of the terms 'counselling' and 'use of counselling skills'. A widely accepted distinction is made between: (a) counselling in the formal sense of what counsellors do in their professional capacity; and (b) what is sometimes called 'use of counselling skills' in the more *ad hoc* sense of being part of the work of all carers and helpers, professional and informal, and including, of course, physiotherapists. As might be expected, however, there are contrasting definitions of counselling, in part because there are different approaches to the theory and practice of counselling (McLeod, 1993). Counselling, according to Burks and Steffire (1979), is a relationship which is, 'designed to help clients to understand and clarify their views of their lifespace, and to learn to reach their self-determined goals through meaningful, well-informed choices and through resolution of problems of an emotional or interpersonal nature'. The general orientation towards the empowerment of the other person as expressed in this definition is common to both the use of counselling skills and counselling *per se* (Bond, 1993). Both are grounded in respect for the other person's values, personal resources and capacity for self-determination. Physiotherapists can and do counsel clients in this 'informal' sense, and the word informal should not be taken to be derogatory or to diminish in any way the importance of this aspect of the physiotherapist's role. The distinction between the use of counselling skills and counselling as such is, then, not as straightforward as it might appear. Bond (1995) argues that a major distinction between formal counselling and the use of counselling skills is whether the contracting is explicit between the client and the professional. Thus for physiotherapists the use of counselling skills, as far as they and their clients are concerned, is not a matter of changing roles. The use of counselling skills is not a role in itself but a means whereby physiotherapists can enhance the performance of their role and develop their practice.

This chapter focuses first on the use of counselling skills as they are directly relevant to the practice of physiotherapy. The similarities and differences between some of the main theories of counselling are then briefly summarized, as these formal perspectives provide a background knowledge for physiotherapists to understand the work of counsellors and to consider situations in which referrals may be necessary.

The use of counselling skills

To focus on the use of counselling skills in physiotherapy practice is to focus on the relationship between the therapist and the client as people and their understanding of themselves and each other as people, rather than as 'therapist' and 'client'. There are four major elements to this.

1. The therapist is first and foremost a person. This may seem so self-evident it is not worth saying. Nevertheless, the dominant ideology in the literature, training and working context is addressed towards therapists as therapists, with all the expertise, responsibilities and expectations which define the role.
2. The same is true of the client. The physiotherapist, when thinking of the use of counselling skills, is not working with an illness, injury or impairment, or even with a patient or client, but rather with a person with all his or her values, feelings, aspirations, life style and human rights.
3. Physiotherapy is seen as a process of opening two-way communication and establishing empowering relationships between people. It is working *with* rather than *on* people through negotiation and cooperation.
4. The focus of therapy is the person rather than 'the problem': it is person-centred rather than problem-centred.

There are three widely discussed and accepted foundations for the use of counselling skills each of which will be discussed below in turn: self-awareness; professional–client relationships; and professional–client communication. These elements can be found in most books directed at professionals generally (Pratt, 1994), health care professionals (Burnard, 1994), and therapists (Swain, 1995).

Self-awareness

Pratt (1994) writes about a physiotherapist who he invited to talk to student physiotherapists about her work with incurably ill and severely disabled people. She began with the statement 'I start with myself', and then talked about therapy as a process in which she tried to be aware of herself and to promote and use that awareness in her work with clients.

Self-awareness, as Burnard (1994) states, is an essential component of the process of using counselling skills. He suggests a number of reasons why it is so important including the following. First, self-awareness enables professionals to be more secure within and about themselves and thus less likely to be swamped by clients' concerns or burden clients with problems of their own. Second, self-awareness enables the professional to make conscious use of personal resources in providing help for the client, as in the example given by Pratt above. Many texts provide exercises for health care professionals searching for self-awareness (Burnard, 1992).

Journeys into self-awareness take many forms, sometimes triggered by traumas. They are rarely comfortable 'sightseeing tours' and can often be expensive in psychological cost and energy. Research has shown, for instance, that severe or chronic illness can lead to greater self-awareness (Marková, 1987). Self-awareness is, in large part, constructed in communication with others. As Fontana (1990) says:

> 'Other people's behaviour doesn't happen in a vacuum. When they relate to us, they are relating to *us*, to the people we are. Their behaviour towards us is a response in no small measure, to our behaviour towards them. If I want to know why people are intimidated or confused or irritated by me, I need to accept that this says something about me as well as something about them'.

A process which can promote self-awareness is self-disclosure (Derlega *et al.*, 1993). It draws on both the 'I' that is acting and experiencing through disclosing, and the 'me' that is reflected on in disclosing. Self-disclosure is sometimes thought of as a technique used by counsellors, but it is also a process which is, to a degree, a part of all communication and relationships. It is the act of making yourself known, of being real, of revealing yourself to others. If communication is a process of sharing meaning, self-disclosure is a sharing of ourselves, and a route to self-knowledge. Tschudin (1991) emphasizes the idea of 'self-sharing'.

> 'Self-sharing can be tremendously liberating. Suddenly you feel equals, two human beings with each other, but the aim of self-sharing is not that *you* feel better, but that your client can move forward and perhaps feel less isolated'.

Niven and Robinson (1994) suggest that there are three levels of sharing: sharing opinions; sharing experiences; and sharing feelings.

Though valuable for both clients and physiotherapists, self-disclosure can be inappropriate and detract from or distort the relationship in various ways. Niven (1994) suggests four such effects: burdening the patient with one's own problems; seeming weak and unstable; domination of the patient, and 'doing it for yourself' – that is disclosing personal information for your own benefit as a means, for example, of seeking approval or affection.

Towards effective relationships

The central importance of relationships in the use of counselling skills, and counselling *per se*, is emphasized time and again in the literature. The necessary qualities of relationships are often referred to as 'core conditions' of counselling, particularly in person-centred approaches developed from the work of Carl Rogers (see below). Three such qualities have received considerable attention in the literature relating to practice and research (Mearns and Thorne, 1988). Apart from the first they are referred to by a variety of possible terms: empathy; genuineness/realness/congruence; and acceptance/respect/unconditional positive regard/trust/warmth.

Empathy

Empathy is a shared understanding and sensitivity between two people. 'Putting yourself in the shoes of another' and 'seeing through the eyes of another' are ways of describing empathy. It involves both feeling and understanding how the other person feels in particular situations. Rogers (1975) defines the process as involving:

> 'entering the private world of the other and becoming thoroughly at home in it ...' It includes communicating your sensings of his world as you look with fresh and unfrightened eyes at elements of which the individual is fearful. It means frequently checking with him as to the accuracy of your sensings, and being guided by the responses you receive ...'.

It is useful to distinguish empathy from the related term sympathy, particularly when this is based on one person thinking he or she had the same or similar experience as another. Empathy involves understanding the experience through the other person's eyes, rather than understanding an ostensibly similar experience through your own eyes. There is what has been called an 'as if' quality to empathy, that is feeling and understanding with the other person without ever losing the recognition that the feelings and understandings are uniquely his or hers and that you are a separate person in your own right with your own feelings and understandings. It is a growing together of minds while recognizing that you remain separate.

In their review of the relevant literature, Northouse and Northouse (1992) state:

> 'When a professional is able to empathise with another, he or she adopts a new frame of reference for the other. This new frame of reference in turn increases the probability that the professional will be able to interpret the other person's communication more accurately because the professional will be sensitized to the uniqueness and nuances of the other's point of view. Empathy assists professionals to see the problems of clients and other professionals more clearly'.

Genuineness/realness/ congruence

Genuineness involves the possibility of 'being yourself' in a relationship and in communication. Genuineness in communication involves the sharing of true feelings and attitudes, or mutual self-disclosure. In this sense, genuineness implies flexibility of expectations so that neither person is 'playing a role'. When the expectations of both participants are rigidly defined, communication is not genuine. Egan (1990) provides a list of suggestions for being genuine in helping clients, including the following.

(a) *Do not overemphasize the helping role.* This means not hiding behind the role or facade of being a physiotherapist and avoiding stereotyped behaviours of the role.

(b) *Be spontaneous.* This is being free to communicate 'here and now' feelings, but it does not mean expressing in an uncontrolled way negative thoughts and feelings which may be tactless, disrespectful and even hurtful to the client.

Acceptance/respect/ unconditional positive regard/trust/warmth

The third of these core conditions involves acceptance and trust in a relationship. It involves communicating that the other person is a worthwhile, unique and capable person. Acceptance in communication also involves accepting that the other person has a point of view which, whether you agree with it or not, is valid to that person and worth listening to. Rogers himself states:

> 'What I am describing is a feeling which is not paternalistic, nor sentimental, nor superficially social and agreeable. It respects the other person as a separate individual and does not possess him. It is a kind of liking which has strength, and which is not demanding. We have termed it positive regard'. (Rogers and Stevens, 1967)

Judgement is suspended and the therapist is in every way for and with the client and communicates this to the client. Trust is a widely used concept in applying this quality of relationships to the work of health care professionals. Northouse and Northouse (1992) suggest that there are two positive outcomes to trust in a professional–client relationship. First, trust engenders a sense of security and helps individuals feel that they are not alone in coping with their problems. It also creates a supportive climate in which individuals can be more open and genuine about their attitudes, feelings and values. Bennett (1993) provides a typical list of strategies for encouraging trust:

(a) Being sensitive to the person's needs and feelings.
(b) Demonstrating genuineness and sincerity.
(c) Being realistic, but optimistic, about people's abilities to get to grips with the problems they face.
(d) Maintaining confidentiality.
(e) Making a contract and keeping any agreements made.

Turning to the day-to-day realities of physiotherapy practice these qualities of relationships can seem unobtainable in the face of the expectations, roles and perceived responsibilities from both the client and the physiotherapist. It can be argued, too, that they are founded on values and assumptions which are white, western, middle class and even middle-aged. Corey and Corey (1993) provide examples of assumptions which may interfere with helping in multi-cultural situations, including the following:

1. *Assumptions about trusting relationships.* As a physiotherapist you may form relationships quickly and expect yourself and your clients to talk easily about issues which touch on personal lives.

This may be difficult for some clients from cultural backgrounds in which meaningful relationships are expected to be slow to form and where trust is to be earned rather than assumed.

2. *Self-actualization.* The belief in the importance of the individual is not shared equally across all cultures. Value systems can differ quite fundamentally in terms of whether self-worth is an individual or collective matter.

3. *Assumptions about directness.* Corey and Corey (1993) state:

   'Although the Western orientation prizes directness, some cultures see it as a sign of rudeness and as something to be avoided. If you are not aware of this cultural difference, you could make the mistake of interpreting a lack of directness as a sign of being unassertive, rather than as a sign of respect'.

4. *Assumptions about assertiveness.* The ideal of determining your own life and telling others what you think and feel is not shared across all cultures.

   The central issue in turning the ideals of qualities of relationship into practice in physiotherapy practice seems to emanate from the inequalities inherent in the physiotherapist–client relationship. As Northouse and Northouse (1992) state:

   'Control is important to clients primarily because they are experiencing the loss of it. For professionals, control is important because it is through the negotiation of control that they are able to effectively work with clients and with other health professionals'.

The barriers to equality are constructed in numerous beliefs and assumptions and approaches in the practice of physiotherapy. In such contexts equality in the physiotherapist–client relationship is difficult to achieve but can be worked towards. The elements or ingredients of such a relationship have been discussed by, among others, Davis (1993). In his 'partnership model' he includes: common aims; complementary expertise; mutual respect; negotiation; and flexibility. He suggests that what is required is 'an explicit understanding of the nature of the relationship for which we strive'. 'Working alliance' is also a widely used and developed term in the literature (Brechin and Swain, 1988). Woody *et al.* (1989), for instance, discuss three aspects of an alliance between professionals and clients: agreement over mutual goals; mutual understanding of the tasks of each person; and the bonds of caring and trusting.

Towards effective communication

Alongside developing self-awareness and empowering relationships, the development of effective communication lies at the heart of the use of counselling skills. Indeed, practical books aimed at helping health care professionals improve their communication skills cover much the same ground as books concerning the use of counselling skills (Porritt, 1990, being a much used example). There are different breakdowns of the skills involved, but listening is consistently seen as the most fundamental and is the focus here. It is thought to be of such central importance in some of the literature that it is given a preordinate position (Ellin, 1994).

Listening is a challenging and soul-searching process in which the listener not only meets the other person but also meets him or herself. There is no simple set of rules by which you can become a more effective listener. Listening is constructed in each encounter between people. A good listener not only shares the experiences and feelings of others, he or she confronts his or her own beliefs and emotions, and reflects back her understanding. Furthermore, the other person experiences 'good listening' and reflects this back to the listener. As Nelson-Jones (1982) says: 'The basis for listening to others is to be able to listen accurately to oneself'. This is a meeting of hearts and minds, not in agreement, but in sharing through a two-way flow of communication. There are many different frameworks or models of 'listening skills', but they are generally variants on the same theme. The breakdown below was initially taken from the work of Bolton (1979).

Listening, when there is face-to-face contact, is founded on being with the other person both physically and mentally. This is often called 'attending', though as usual the word seems inadequate for conveying the intensity of involvement. Directing your self, ears, eyes and heart in undivided attention to the other person begins even before the actual encounter. It starts by clearing the mind of distractions and worries and putting judgements into abeyance. This has been called a 'cleansing breath'.

> 'a deep breath helps clear yourself of muddled and distracting thoughts and helps "centre" yourself on the interaction that is about to begin'. (Kottler and Kottler, 1993)

The goal of listening is not just being with the other person, psychologically, though this is the essential foundation, but also to journey with the other person through his or her experiences and feelings. Following the other person's concerns involves helping him or her talk about whatever he or she wants to talk about, rather than what the listener wants to talk about or hear. This includes:

1. Staying out of the other person's way as he or she discovers and explores his or her own views, feelings and needs, by not proffering advice or being judgemental.
2. Picking up meaning and understanding of the other person's world and experiences from his or her viewpoint, so you can discover how he or she views the situation in his or her terms rather than yours.
3. Encouraging and facilitating the other person in his or her exploration.

As emphasized earlier, listening must be considered as part of the two-way flow of communication. Good listening involves not only understanding the other person's experiences and feelings, but also demonstrating to the other person that he or she is being understood and accepted. Reflecting can communicate understanding to the other person and, from the listener's side, checks understanding. Understanding can be seen as a guessing process. Language is imprecise and non-verbal communication is even more ephemeral. Furthermore, people often talk about safe topics rather than broaching real concerns. Indeed, we sometimes do not know what we think or feel until we have talked it over with someone who is really listening. The mirror that a good listener provides aids self-awareness and self-understanding. Reflection also helps the listener concentrate on what is actually being expressed: not what she is expecting, would like to hear, or the noise of her own thoughts and feelings. It is, then, a major part of building listening.

Contrasting theories of counselling

There is a whole array of theories and approaches in counselling, which may surprise someone relatively new to the field of counselling and can be threatening to the physiotherapist wishing to find a basis for developing his or her practice. There is no such thing as 'the theory of counselling' which physiotherapists can use to inform and develop themselves in their work. As Burnard (1989) states:

> 'no one school of psychology or theoretical approach to counselling offers *the* way of viewing the person. The approaches offer different ways of looking at the person and those ways of looking are not necessarily mutually exclusive'.

The following brief overview summarizes and contrasts some of the main theories. The theories are compared in terms of the overall direction they take in understanding the nature of human beings and the nature of helpful relationships, and also in conceiving problems and the aims of helping clients. Overall, the aim is to provide a framework for considering the nature of counselling and a sounding board of ideas to address your own beliefs, views and feelings in using counselling skills as a physiotherapist.

Three main approaches to counselling

Formal theories and approaches to counselling cannot be neatly compartmentalized. Indeed it could be said that there are as many theories as there are theorists. Furthermore, and to complicate matters further, many counsellors use more than one approach in their work (Culley, 1990; Egan, 1990). An eclectic approach to counselling is one in which the counsellor chooses the most appropriate ideas from a range of different theories, while an integrative approach brings together elements from different theories to create a new theory.

A summary of the basic characteristics of any approach to counselling will not be able to do justice to the range of opinions of people who espouse the approach. Nevertheless, it is generally recognized that there are three main orientations or broad approaches to counselling (Hough, 1994).

1. *Behavioural.* The historical basis of this orientation in counselling is learning theory. The specific approaches under this general umbrella are geared towards prediction and control in people's lives. In earlier 'behaviour modification' approaches what people do or say is the focus for prediction and control, while more recently developed approaches, such as cognitive counselling and rational-emotive therapy, take wider perspectives.

2. *Psychodynamic.* Of these three orientations, the psychodynamic is perhaps the most difficult to convey in a few words. It has been developed in many different directions by different theorists, but its origins lie in Freudian theory. A central concern is growth and development towards psychological and mental normality and health.

3. *Humanistic.* Humanistic psychology and counselling theory is a product of many individual efforts and an assimilation of many ideas. A specific perspective within this general orientation is the work of Carl Rogers. The central focus is the development of self as a unique and worthwhile individual.

It has taken people a lifetime's work and writing to develop the theories and practices of counselling that are briefly mentioned here. Two general texts which provide excellent overviews are Nelson-Jones (1995) and McLeod (1993). References are provided below for people wishing to read about specific approaches in more detail.

Rather than simply extending these briefest of summaries, the following is an exploration of some points of comparison and contrast between these three orientations to counselling. The similarities and differences between theories of counselling can be understood in various ways. Some points of contrast can seem so subtle as to be of negligible significance, while others pertain to such fundamental issues as the nature of human beings. The following discussion is organized around four points of comparison: the nature of human beings; concepts of 'problems', the aims of help; and the nature of help offered (see Table 19.1).

Human beings and their problems

Theories of counselling differ in the assumptions they make about our nature as human beings and in ways of understanding the problems people bring into the counselling situation. The essential starting point of a behavioural approach is what is believed to be the scientific study of people. This involves the application of techniques and principles of natural science in the ostensible objective study of human beings. People, and the whole social world we live in, can be understood in the same way as the physical world can be understood. Behaviourism seeks to explain and predict what happens in the social world by exploring what are thought to be regularities and causal relationships between 'facts'. There are two types of fact: events or 'stimuli' external to the person, including what other people do or say; and behaviours or 'responses' of the person, that is what the person does or says, but not what goes on inside his or her head. Both are by definition within this general orientation observable, measurable and can be manipulated. These facts are taken to be independent of meaning and interpretation. Behaviourism searches, as we all do, for rules which connect stimuli and responses, rules about how people learn: patterns between what people experience and how their behaviour changes. The essential rule is that behaviours that are followed by desirable events or stimuli, encouragement from others and so on, are more likely to be repeated or learned.

As perhaps is already apparent, this perspective incorporates a decidedly deterministic view of human nature and a behaviourist approach

Table 19.1 Comparison of approaches to counselling

Formal perspective	The nature of human beings	Concepts of 'problems'	The aims of help	The nature of help offered
Behavioural	Understood in terms of observable and measurable behaviour which is controlled in a predictable way by the environment	Inappropriate behaviours learned in responding to the environment and/or lack of appropriate behaviours	Learning appropriate behaviour and/or unlearning inappropriate behaviours	Helper changing environment to change the other person's behaviour or helping the other make the changes themselves
Psycho-dynamic	Shaped and determined by biological needs and drives and by early childhood experiences	Repressed unconscious thoughts and feelings leading to neurosis and mental disorder	Personality reconstruction and reorientation, making unconscious conscious	Helper analyses and interprets the behaviour of the other person
Humanistic	Each person is an individual of dignity and worth and strives to actualize, maintain and enhance the 'self'	Incongruence between self concept and experience and conditions of feelings of worth violated	Empowerment: self-direction and full functioning of other person	Relationship provides a context in which the other person can feel accepted as a person of worth whose aspirations and feelings are respected

can sound alienating. We are not chemicals: we are human beings. Yet this is a process of prediction and control which is part and parcel of being human. If we could not predict and control we would be lost. If I go into a supermarket, pick up a loaf of bread and take it to the cash till, the sales person will pass it across the electric eye and I will be asked for some money. If I pay I can walk out of the shop with my bread. Prediction and control are just part of daily living or, to extend the example, daily bread.

Like behaviourism, psychodynamic theory is essentially deterministic. A psychodynamic view of human nature is that everything we do is caused by factors within us, such as deep-seated desires, or in our environment. Slips of the tongue, for instance, are sometimes referred to as 'Freudian slips' with the connotation that they are not accidental but signify unconscious desires. The sources of our thoughts, feelings and actions lie in hidden or unconscious desires and conflicts, often derived from very early formative childhood experiences.

There are a number of common themes within psychodynamic theory (Cooper, 1984) which help to characterize the main sort of ideas.

1. Nothing of what we do or think is accidental. Something has always caused us to act and think as we do, though we might not know the causes ourselves.
2. Everything we think and do is purposeful or goal-directed. We are always working towards satisfying basic needs and motives whether we are conscious of it or not.
3. Mostly we are not conscious of these things. Our unconscious minds mould and affect the way we perceive ourselves and others. These are thoughts of a primitive nature, shaped by impulses and feelings within the individual of which he or she is unaware.
4. Early childhood experience is overwhelmingly important and pre-eminent over later experience.

Turning to the humanistic orientation, it is a multi-faceted perspective on human experience which focuses on each person's uniqueness. The following are probably the main characteristics of the work of most of those who maintain a humanistic perspective.

1. Attention is centred on the experiencing person and the emphasis is on meaningfulness and significance of experiences to the person.
2. The focus is given on such distinctive human qualities as making choices, creativity, valuation and self-actualization.
3. The ultimate concern is the dignity and worth of people and an interest in the development of the potential inherent in every person. Central to this perspective is the person, as he or she discovers his or her own being and relates to other people.
4. The person has one basic tendency and striving: to actualize, maintain and enhance the 'self'.

For Rogers the essential, fundamental difference between his work and that of Skinner or Freud lies in their conception of human nature. Rogers believes first and foremost that as human beings we are free, and our freedom can transcend all those forces, from within and without, which would determine ourselves and our lives. As in Sartre's existentialism 'existence comes before essence' and each person is 'responsible for the self one chooses to be' (Rogers, 1983). This rejection of the deterministic assumptions within behaviourism and psychodynamic psychology, and the declaration that 'people are free' is right at the heart of this perspective. Furthermore, freedom as self-actualization is not an underlying or implicit assumption, it is a fundamental, dynamic orientation essential to human survival and fulfilment. This perspective is not directed to such external, observable and measurable facts as 'stimuli' and 'behaviour'. Behaviour has meaning for the person in that it is intentional and the person is:

'... capable of evaluating the outer and inner situation, understanding herself in its context, making constructive choices as to the next steps in life, and acting on those choices'. (Rogers, 1978)

Aims and practices

In behavioural approaches, providing help focuses on changing the environment, including the behaviour of the helper, to change the behaviour of the other person. From this orientation, behaviour is learned and can also be unlearned. Help starts with identifying the problems in terms of the behaviours of the client which are deemed to be inappropriate or dysfunctional. Changing such behaviours, or 'behaviour modification', becomes the goal of counselling. This requires recognizing the stimuli which set, or lead to, and reinforce the undesired behaviours. Then, step-by-step, goals can be worked towards by engineering the environment, that is controlling what happens before and after the behaviours that are to be changed. Kanfer and Goldstein (1980) and Trower *et al.* (1988) provide useful further reading.

Help offered from a psychodynamic perspective would tend to:

1. highlight the relationship between past and present life events;
2. acknowledge that unconscious forces are at work that affect the client's behaviour;
3. encourage the expression of pent-up emotion (Burnard, 1994).

In the most general terms, help facilitates the development of self-awareness, the unconscious becoming conscious. Jacobs (1988) and Rowan (1983) provide good starting points for further reading.

Humanistic counselling seeks to facilitate and empower the person 'in the direction of increasing self-government, self-regulation and autonomy, and away from heteronymous control, or control by external forces' (Rogers, 1961). This perspective is directed towards the meaning of 'stimuli' for the person, the immediacy of experience, and the feelings and values that pervade all experience. The person creates tentative personal truths through action and interaction with the social world. Help, then, is primarily a process of facilitating people in defining their own problems and identifying their own solutions. For further reading try Rogers (1980) and Mearns and Thorne (1988).

Conclusion

Though physiotherapists are not counsellors in a formal sense, the use of counselling skills is integral to effective physiotherapy practice. Nevertheless, ideas from the theories and practices of counselling cannot be simply grafted on to physiotherapists' existing understandings and repertoire of specialist skills. The use of counselling skills involves physiotherapists in developing their self-awareness, and their relationships and processes of communication with clients. It can also involve addressing challenging questions which reach into the whole nature and process of therapy, the conception of 'problems', and assumptions underpinning aims and practices in working towards 'solutions'. Counselling and the use of counselling skills has relevance for physiotherapists when practice is seen as working *with people*, rather than on patients.

References

Bennet P. (1993) *Counselling for Heart Disease*. Leicester: British Psychological Society Books.
Bolton R. (1979) *People Skills: How to Assert, Listen and Resolve Conflict*. Englewood Cliffs, New Jersey: Prentice-Hall.

Bond T. (1993) Counselling, counselling skills and professional roles. In *Counselling and Psychology for Health Professionals* (Byrne R., Nicolson P. eds). London: Chapman and Hall.

Bond T. (1995) The nature and outcomes of counselling. In *Counselling in Primary Health Care* (Keithley J., Marsh G., eds). Oxford: Oxford University Press.

Brechin A., Swain J. (1988) Professional/client relationships: creating a 'working alliance' with people with learning difficulties. *Disability, Handicap and Society*, 3(3), 213–226.

Burks H. M., Steffire B. (1979) *Theories of Counselling* (3rd edn). New York: McGraw-Hill.

Burnard P. (1989) *Counselling Skills for Health Professionals*. London: Chapman and Hall.

Burnard P. (1992) *Know Yourself! Self-Awareness Activities for Nurses*. London: Scutari Press.

Burnard P. (1994) *Counselling Skills for Health Professionals* (2nd edn). London: Chapman and Hall.

Cooper C. (1984) Psychodynamic therapy: the Kleinian approach. In *Individual Therapy in Britain* (Dryden W., ed.). London: Harper and Row.

Corey M. S., Corey G. (1993) *Becoming a Helper* (2nd edn). Pacific Grove, CA: Brooks/Cole.

Culley S. (1990) *Integrative Skills in Action*. London: Sage.

Davis H. (1993) *Counselling Parents of Children with Chronic Illness or Disability*. Leicester: British Psychological Society Books.

Derlega V. J., Metts S., Petronio S., Margulis S. T. (1993) *Self-Disclosure*. London: Sage.

Egan G. (1990) *The Skilled Helper: Model, Skills and Methods for Effective Helping* (4th edn). Monterey: Brooks/Cole.

Ellin J. (1994) *Listening Helpfully: How to Develop Your Counselling Skills*. London: Souvenir Press.

Fontana D. (1990) *Social Skills at Work*, Leicester/London: BPS Books (The British Psychological Society) and Routledge.

Hough M. (1994) *A Practical Approach to Counselling*. London: Pitman Publishing.

Jacobs M. (1988) *Psychodynamic Counselling in Action*. London: Sage.

Kanfer F. H., Goldstein A. P. (eds) (1980) *Helping People to Change: A Textbook of Methods* (2nd edn). New York: Pergamon.

Kottler J. A., Kottler E. (1993) *Teacher as Counsellor: Developing the Helping Skills You Need*. Newbury Park: Corwin Press.

McLeod J. (1993) *An Introduction to Counselling*. Buckingham: Open University Press.

Marková I. (1987) *Human Awareness: Its Social Development*. London: Hutchinson.

Mearns D., Thorne B. (1988) *Person-Centred Counselling in Action*. London: Sage.

Nelson-Jones R. (1982) *The Theory and Practice of Counselling Psychology*. London: Holt, Rinehart and Winston.

Nelson-Jones R. (1995) *The Theory and Practice of Counselling Psychology* (2nd edn). London: Cassell.

Niven N. (1994) *Health Psychology: An Introduction for Nurses and Other Health Care Professionals* (2nd edn). Edinburgh: Churchill Livingstone.

Niven N., Robinson J. (1994) *The Psychology of Nursing Care*. The British Psychological Society, Leicester, in association with MacMillan Press, Basingstoke.

Northouse P. G. Northouse L. L. (1992) *Health Communication: Strategies for Health Professionals* (2nd edn). Norwalk, Connecticut: Appleton and Lange.

Porritt L. (1990) *Interaction Strategies: An Introduction for Health Professionals*. London: Churchill Livingstone.

Pratt J. (1994) *Counselling Skills for Professional Helpers*. London: Central Book Publishing.

Rogers C. R. (1961) *On Becoming a Person*. Boston: Houghton Mifflin.

Rogers C. R. (1975) Empathic: an unappreciated way of being. *The Counselling Psychologist*, 5(2), 2–10.

Rogers C. R. (1978) *Carl Rogers on Person Power: Inner Strength and its Revolutionary Impact*. London: Constable.

Rogers C. R. (1980) *A Way of Being*. Boston: Houghton Mifflin.

Rogers C. R. (1983) *Freedom to Learn for the 80s*. Columbus: Charles E. Merrill.

Rogers C. R., Stevens B. (1967) *Person to Person: The Problem of Being Human*. Layfayette, CA: Real People Press.

Rowan J. (1983) *The Reality Game: A Guide to Humanistic Counselling and Therapy*. London: Routledge and Kegan Paul.

Ryden M. B., McCarthy P. R., Lewis M. L., Sherman C. (1991) A behavioural comparison of the helping style of nursing students, psychotherapists, crisis interveners, and untrained individuals. *Archives of Psychiatric Nursing*, **5**, 185–188.

Swain J. (1995) *The Use of Counselling Skills: A Guide for Therapists*. Oxford: Butterworth-Heinemann.

Trower P., Casey A., Dryden W. (1988) *Cognitive-Behavioural Counselling in Action*. London: Sage.

Tschudin V. (1991) *Counselling Skills for Nurses* (3rd edn). London: Baillière Tindall.

Woody R. H., Hanson J. C., Rossberg R. H. (1989) *Counselling Psychology: Strategies and Services*. Pacific Grove, CA: Brooks/Cole.

20

The powerful placebo

Sally French

Spiro (1986) defines the placebo as, 'a substance or a procedure that is administered with suggestions that it will modify a symptom or sensation, but which, unknown to the recipient, has no specific pharmacological impact on the reaction in question'.

Until recent times the success of medicine depended very largely on the placebo. Spiro (1986) believes that since medicine has become more scientific the placebo effect has been undervalued and even something of an embarrassment to clinicians, who he thinks '... regard any deviation from the strictly scientific objective approach almost as religious thinkers regard sin'.

Engel (1977) agrees that scientific medicine has gained the status of a dogma and Lown (1985) believes that 'a pretentious "scientism" mars the physicians' perception of the power of the placebo'. The 'scientific fallacy' has, according to Spiro (1986), led to considerable resistance to the placebo on the part of clinicians. He urges them to consider how much their perceptions have been restricted by science and contends that, 'truth in medicine has moved from what the patient says to what the physician finds' and consequently, 'the more medical science does for disease, the less physicians do for patients'. Despite this resistance to placebos, Benson and McCallie (1979) remind us that they are safe and effective and, unlike most therapies, have stood the test of time. It is important to note, however, that there is little evidence at the present time that placebos affect the actual disease process. We cannot assume that just because symptoms are relieved that the underlying pathology has altered. Placebos can, however, influence physiological functions such as blood pressure and pulse rate (Griffiths, 1980; Richardson, 1995).

It is important to distinguish the non-therapeutic use of placebos, for example in clinical trials, from their therapeutic use. This chapter will concern the latter, though it is interesting to note how the therapeutic effect of the placebo is generally under-rated in clinical trials, despite its magnitude.

Placebos used in therapy can be pure or impure. A pure placebo is one with no known active ingredient whereas an impure placebo is a substance which contains active elements but, nonetheless, is thought to work through its symbolic power; an example of the latter is of antibiotics when given for viral infections. There is, however, a problem about regarding any substance as inert, for if the patient feels better after receiving it then clearly something must have happened. Spiro (1986) contends that, 'the physiological effect of gratitude has not been studied but that does not mean that it does not exist'. He thinks that impure placebos are used to deny, even to ourselves, that we are using placebos.

All treatments, given by physiotherapists or others, can be assumed to contain some placebo element. Weinman (1981) claims that even with pain associated with serious disease, more than one-third of patients report relief following treatment with a placebo, and Richardson (1995) claims that approximately 35% of people report pain relief from placebos. Melzack and Wall (1988) point out that the type of pain is important, for example they claim that 52% of headache sufferers are helped by placebos. Beecher (1959) found that severe postoperative pain could be relieved in 35% of patients by the administration of a placebo whereas morphine relieved pain in about 75% of cases. Parrott (1991) contends that the incidence of motion sickness can be reduced by 70% by the administration of placebos.

When placebos are used in clinical trials their effects tend to mirror those of the active drugs being tested. This has been found with regard to how long the placebo effect lasts (Seligman et al., 1953), the strength of the placebo effect (Evans, 1984), the time it takes for the placebo to work and its side effects (Ross and Olson, 1982). This is probably because the descriptions given to the research subjects are similar whether they are receiving the placebo or the active drug. Richardson (1995) also points out that active drugs become less effective if patients are told that they are receiving placebos.

Even the colour and brand names of drugs have been found to affect the placebo response (Shapiro, 1970; Braithwaite and Cooper, 1981). Melzack and Wall (1988) note that two placebo capsules are more effective than one, that large capsules are more effective than small ones and that placebos are more effective when given by injection than when given by mouth. Niven and Robinson (1994) note that placebos become less effective with repeated administration. Spiro (1986) points out that diagnostic procedures, surgery and even the words we speak to patients can all act as powerful placebos; furthermore, the placebo effect cuts across educational and social boundaries and can affect almost any area of the body (Benson and Epstein, 1975).

Dimond et al. (1960) report on an experiment carried out in the 1950s where half of a group of patients suffering from angina pectoris were treated by ligation of the internal mammary artery, which was a common procedure at that time. The remaining patients were given the same incision but, unknown to them, the operation was not carried out. Angina was improved in all the patients and in 86% the improvement was maintained, there was an increase in exercise tolerance and a decrease in the need for drug therapy. No significant difference existed between the two groups.

This type of experiment would now be considered unethical but it shows how difficult it is to assess the effect of treatments even as apparently objective as surgery. It is, however, possible that some improvement was due to factors other than the placebo, such as rest and changes in life style.

The placebo response varies greatly from one individual to the next

and in the same individual from time to time and according to circumstances (Richardson, 1995). Most people are susceptible to some degree.
As belief in the treatment or the person administering it is central to the
placebo response (Hanson and Gerber, 1990; Helman, 1994) the effectiveness of specific placebos will be culturally and temporally limited. Thus,
in our culture at the present time, taking placebos in the guise of drugs is
likely to be effective (Hanson and Gerber, 1990). Rachman and Philips
(1978) claim that placebos are more effective in people who are anxious,
sociable, conventional and dependable and are least effective in those
who are isolated and mistrustful. Melzack and Wall (1988) however,
believe that the only consistent difference is that placebo reactors tend to
have higher levels of trait anxiety. Hyland and Donaldson (1989) contend
that, 'It is incorrect to assume that placebo pain relief is more effective for
'neurotic' patients or those who have some psychological problem'. Ross
and Olson (1982) and Richardson (1995) believe that there is little
evidence that individual differences are strongly related to the placebo
response and that the research that exists tends to conflict.

Brill (1964) demonstrated that the placebo effect is not necessarily short
lived and Park and Covi (1965) found that the patient's belief in the
medicinal value of the treatment is not crucial. Park and Covi (1965) told
their patients that they were receiving 'sugar pills' but implied strongly
that the pills would help; they found that the placebo effect still operated.
People are not totally unaware of the nature of the placebo effect yet still
seem to find it helpful. They may, for example, take sleeping tablets even
though they have little belief in their medicinal value, or they may find
contact with a health professional invaluable even though their condition
is not improving. Health professionals probably under-estimate the
degree to which patients understand the placebo effect and may be
deceiving them less than they think. Spiro (1986) explains:

> 'The physician may not feel that he is doing very much for his patients, but
> somehow the active keeping in touch seems to keep things under control.
> Patients must realize this too even if unconsciously for a number of people
> have told me that they want another appointment "anyway" in three or
> four months. I assume that kind of medical contact provides a placebic
> therapy even if it is not intended in that way'.

It is likely that the placebo effect is enhanced or even produced by the
degree of understanding, empathy and enthusiasm of the clinician
prescribing or dispensing it, as well as his or her own belief in it
(Richardson, 1995). Helman (1994) states:

> 'Rapport, mutual confidence and understanding between prescriber and
> patient also contribute to the placebo effect. For this effect to be maximised
> there must be a congruence between the doctor's approach to therapy and
> the patient's attitudes towards illness and his expectations from treatment'.

Balint (1964) believes that the clinician can be a more powerful therapeutic agent than the treatment he or she administers. Morgan (1982)
states that it is the social relationship between doctor and patient that
engenders this powerful therapeutic effect and Richardson (1995)

believes that clinicians of high status are better able to engender the placebo effect than those of a lower status. Benson and McCallie (1979) report a 70–90% success rate in trials conducted by enthusiasts which reduced to 30–40%, the average placebo response, when conducted by sceptics. Novel treatments tend to be more effective than established ones, probably because of the enhanced enthusiasm of clinicians, thus new treatments have the power to render old ones less effective. Benson and McCallie (1979) quote Trousseau's remark, 'you should treat as many patients as possible with the new drugs while they still have the power to heal'. Despite the therapeutic power that clinicians possess, Shapiro (1969) believes that they prefer to view their success as due to less personal factors. Spiro (1986) states: 'The idea that the physician brings little benefit to his patients and his patient's disease except as he brings him pills and procedures has been growing since modern medicine began to become scientific and focus on disease rather than on the patient'.

If the patient thinks the treatment is more exotic than it really is he or she is also more likely to derive benefit from it.

The setting in which the treatment is given also has an effect (Parrott, 1991; Helman, 1994; Richardson, 1995). Uniforms, stethoscopes, the smell of disinfection and impressive-looking equipment may all act as powerful symbols of healing which can foster belief, according to the culture and expectations of the patient. Investigations of treatment carried out in the laboratory can show very different results from those conducted in the clinical setting. Spiro (1986) believes that, 'The patient who journeys to a world famous clinic or physician is as ready to be helped as a pilgrim who travels to a shrine'. Frank (1975) emphasizes how operating theatres foster belief in the efficacy of surgery. He explains that, 'These rooms contain spectacular machines that bleep and gurgle and flash lights, or emit immensely powerful but invisible rays, thereby impressively evoking the healing powers of science'. Brody (1980) refers to the setting as the 'healing context' and Helman (1994) states:

> 'Placebos, whether medications or procedures, are generally culture bound, that is they are administered within a specific social and cultural setting which validates both the placebo and the person administering it'.

Many of the machines used by physiotherapists look impressive and mysterious and one wonders how important this is in producing their therapeutic effects. Low (1994) believes that the placebo effect is likely to be present when treating patients with interferential current. He states:

> 'Since the placebo effect occurs in all treatments it would be surprising if it did not contribute to pain relief within interferential treatment, especially since the machines are technically impressive and produce an unfamiliar, although not unpleasant, feeling'.

Helman (1994) refers to the 'total drug effect' as being dependent on the following four factors:

1. The attributes of the drug itself.
2. The attributes of the person dispensing the drug.
3. The attributes of the person receiving the drug.
4. The setting in which the drug is administered.

These four factors apply equally to the success of many other types of treatment. Richardson (1995) believes that so much is involved in the placebo effect that it is an inadequate term which may restrict our thinking.

How placebos are used

Spiro (1986) contends that placebos can be used in various ways by clinicians, some of which are helpful but others destructive.

Placebo as a gift

The placebo can be considered as a gift when it is given to soothe the anxieties of a patient. Spiro (1986) believes that, though paternalistic, this aim can be considered generous.

Placebo as a challenge

In this situation the placebo is given to prove that the patient is wrong. Spiro (1986) states that, 'physicians often use placebos as a challenge to prove that the pain can be relieved by a placebo and therefore that it has no important origin'. Such a belief, however, is to under-estimate the power of placebos to relieve symptoms. Both Hyland and Donaldson (1989) and Sofaer (1992) point out that relief of pain from a placebo in no way invalidates the person's experience of pain.

Placebo as a ransom

Placebos may be given to get rid of demanding, difficult patients. Spiro (1986) believes that giving a placebo to such a patient provides the person with a negative label which indicates that he or she is beyond anyone's concern and help. Goodwin *et al.* (1979) believe that clinicians may also need to prove to themselves that anyone who causes them frustration and anger cannot be genuinely ill.

The intent of the clinician prescribing or administering a placebo is therefore an important ethical issue.

Many symptoms are not serious and are likely to resolve spontaneously. Placebos can be used to satisfy anxious patients while this process takes place. As Voltaire said, 'The art of medicine consists of amusing the patient while Nature cures the disease' (Andrews, 1987). Placebos also have the virtue that while the patient is taking them time is passing which gives the clinician the opportunity to think. Placebos, and any other form of treatment, can sometimes be given false credit as the symptoms remit or the condition spontaneously resolves.

Objections to the placebo

Various objections have been raised regarding the use of placebos in treatment. Most ethical objections hinge on the issue of truth telling. Bok (1978) thinks that deception regarding placebos merely falls into the category of 'white lies' and Spiro (1986) agrees that lying in association with placebos is relatively harmless. He states:

'There are lies and lies. Even the firmest ethicists will agree that some deceptions are trivial … they keep the social machinery oiled and do little harm … In looking at medical practice common sense should help us separate the trivial from the important. Reassuring a patient in acute pain who must undergo an emergency operation that everything will be all right hardly falls into the same category as telling a patient with a gastric cancer that he has a little ulcer'.

The clinician who tells the patient, when administering a placebo, that the treatment will work is not lying, for there is a good chance that it will. However, Bok (1978) believes that the context in which the words are spoken does deceive. Brody (1980) does not consider that the use of placebos is deceptive but Simmons (1978) takes a harder line believing that placebos should only be used if patients understand exactly what is going on. Parrot (1991) states that, 'it is unethical to administer a pharmacologically inactive substance while suggesting it is medicine' but Leslie (1982) is of the opinion that the deception involved in the use of placebos in treatment should be accepted, believing that, 'Deception is as integral to the placebo as copper is to bronze'.

The issue is complicated by the fact that the placebo effect is not confined to the drugs, equipment or techniques which are used in treatment but is integral to the relationship between the clinician and the patient and the setting in which the treatment is given. It is also the case that giving a placebo in which the patient believes increases the likelihood that he or she will comply with other treatments and that these treatments will be more effective (Melzack and Wall, 1988). Yet we do not feel obliged to disclose or discuss these aspects of the placebo effect with patients. It must also be appreciated that the placebo effect enters into all our treatments however objective and scientific they may seem. We cannot say how much it influences treatment outcome because we do not know enough either about how our treatments work or about the mechanisms of the placebo effect. Disagreements between ethicists and clinicians, regarding the use of placebos, is probably partly due to the fact that ethicists deal in generalities, usually at a distance, whereas clinicians are faced with individuals who want their immediate help. Jones (1989) believes that, 'If caring and truth are in conflict, then our duty becomes problematic and we face a dilemma'.

There are many ethical dilemmas which physiotherapists face in relation to placebos, they may be asked to give chest therapy to a patient who will not benefit from it, decide to continue treating a disabled person even though improvement has ceased, or to use a modality which is thought to have little therapeutic effect. There are further ethical dilemmas when considering the use of placebos in clinical trials. Should the patient be told that he or she is taking part in an experiment and may be given a placebo rather than an active treatment? If consent is gained is it really valid given that the person is ill, vulnerable and dependent on the people who have requested it? Physiotherapists may be asked to help conduct a clinical trial, or may wish to initiate their own research involving placebos. Thus the ethics of the placebo cannot be avoided.

Other dangers which have been raised are the physical effects of impure placebos, the possibility that the patient's beliefs in the efficacy of drugs will be increased, increased dependence of the patient on the clinican and the fear that the use of placebos may hide serious disease. Placebos may also be given as a way of managing a large number of patients in a short time, rather than providing counselling for example. It has been shown that placebos can have harmful side-effects, termed nocicebo effects (Parrott, 1991) though these may be confused with actual symptoms (Ross and Olson, 1982). These side-effects can be objective as well as subjective (Richardson, 1995). Griffiths (1980) reports that some people who take placebo tablets suffer sleeplessness, blurred vision and nausea. Some even report having hallucinations and other experiences associated with drug taking.

Other dangers are that if patients do not improve they may conclude that their condition is more serious than it really is and that if they find out that a placebo has been used their trust in the clinician will be destroyed. Another possibility, pointed out by Sim (1989), is that if the patient realizes that the clinician has not been totally truthful he or she may be less than truthful in return. Placebos have also been criticized on the grounds of cost, although their timely use may make other more expensive investigations and treatments unnecessary. Placebos should not be regarded as harmless or administered lightly. (For further discussion of ethical issues in physiotherapy practice the reader is referred to Chapter 22).

Understanding the placebo effect

Our understanding of the placebo effect is still very limited. It seems likely that a combination of factors operate to produce it. The main theories are given below. It is likely that several mechanisms are operating together, thus the theories are not mutually exclusive.

The release of endorphins

Endorphins are morphine-like substances which are produced by the brainstem and pituitary gland in response to pain and are thought to be stimulated by placebos. They are considered to be the body's natural opiates (Terenius, 1978; Mathews and Steptoe, 1988; Niven and Robinson,1994). Melzack and Wall (1988), however, regard the endorphin explanation as simplistic. They state:

'Clearly the placebo is produced by suggestion, personality and predispositions and other psychological factors. It is not due to any simple mechanism such as an out-pouring of the body's natural opiates'.

Kirsch (1985) believes that endorphins should be viewed as the effect of placebos rather than the cause of the effect.

Patients' expectations and beliefs

The patient's expectations and beliefs seem to be important in the placebo response. Even if the clinician tells the patient he or she is receiving a placebo it may still work well, perhaps because the patient assumes that the clinician would not give a useless treatment. People have various expectations of treatment from their past experience. For example they know that drugs generally take a while to work and that their effect wears off in time. Thus expectations, beliefs and knowledge from previous treatments may all be important in producing the placebo effect. Hanson and Gerber (1990) make the point that the beliefs of the patient's family and friends can also affect the placebo response.

One of the main functions of pain is to alert the brain that something is wrong. Niven and Robinson (1994) suggest that if a person takes a placebo and believes it will work the brain will send messages to inhibit the transmission of pain signals with a subsequent reduction or extinction of pain.

Reduction of anxiety and depression

The perception of pain is known to be associated with anxiety and depression (Melzack and Wall, 1988; Sofaer, 1992). It is likely that some patients who receive placebo treatment will feel less anxious and depressed with a subsequent reduction in their pain and other symptoms (see Chapter 11). In addition, the patient who feels that something is being done may concentrate on small areas of improvement while minimizing static symptoms or those which are worsening. Ambiguous symptoms may also be interpreted positively.

Compliance

Without any coercion on the part of the clinician, patients undergoing treatment are likely to feel some pressure to improve, it can be rather embarrassing not to do so when the clinician is making so much effort. Thus it could be that patients who receive a placebo as part of their treatment, or who receive a placebo in a clinical trial, report an improvement, not because of a genuine reduction of symptoms, but in order to comply or to please the clinician or researcher. No doubt this sometimes occurs, but an argument against this explanation is that objective changes can often be demonstrated, for example reduced blood pressure and heart rate.

Conditioning

It is possible that the placebo effect is a conditioned response – that is a response which has been learned. Most people have heard of the famous experiments by Pavlov (1960) where he paired food with the sound of a bell and in a relatively short space of time conditioned dogs to salivate at the sound of the bell alone. Similar conditioning occurs in humans, for example, if a person eats a particular food and is then ill it is sometimes the case that the person will feel ill again when eating or thinking about that food, even though the original illness was not caused by it. Similarly people with asthma who are sensitive to pollen may experience some discomfort when sitting near artificial flowers.

There have been many animal experiments which demonstrate that if they are made to feel ill, for example by the administration of a certain drug, they demonstrate the same signs and symptoms of illness if a placebo is administered in the same way (Reiss, 1958). Thus an unpleasant experience resulting from a previous treatment can give rise to the nocicebo effect so presumably a positive experience from a previous treatment can give rise to the placebo effect. Richardson (1995) points out that people may have learned that hospitals are associated with symptom relief and thus the hospital setting itself may bring about a conditioned response. It is often the case, however, that the placebo effect is produced even though the person has had no previous experience of a similar treatment or procedure.

Cognitive dissonance

Totman (1987) explains the placebo effect in terms of Festinger's theory of cognitive dissonance (Festinger, 1957). According to this theory, if people have a difficult choice to make they will inevitably be in a state of mental turmoil both before and immediately after the decision has been made, as they wonder which alternative to choose and whether their choice has been a wise one. Festinger (1957) termed this mental state 'cognitive dissonance'. In order to return to a more settled state of mind people try to find justifications for their decisions and will maximize the positive aspects of what they have chosen and the negative aspects of what they have rejected. Thus if someone has to choose between two jobs, both of which are appealing, he or she will actively search for justifications to support the decision and will emphasize the advantages of the chosen job and the disadvantages of the rejected one. If the choice is easy or if the person is forced into a decision, cognitive dissonance will not be experienced.

Totman (1987) believes that if a patient has a difficult decision to make regarding treatment, whether or not to subject him or herself to surgery for example, the person will wonder if it is all worthwhile and be in a state of cognitive dissonance. Similarly cognitive dissonance may be felt if a patient is having to make an awkward journey to the physiotherapy department several times a week, if the treatment is somewhat uncomfortable, or if the person is expected to spend considerable time carrying out exercises at home rather than doing something more enjoyable. In order to resolve this uncomfortable state of mind the patient will need to find justifications for his or her actions. This may be achieved, partly at a subconscious level, by experiencing an improvement in the symptoms for this will confirm that the decision to have the treatment was indeed the correct one. Totman (1987) reports that, 'The favourable consequences of a (dummy) treatment were substantially increased if patients had to make a difficult decision concerning whether or not to receive it'. He suggests that the experiment by Park and Covi (1965), mentioned above, where patients still responded to a placebo even though they were told that it was a 'sugar pill', may have been because they had to justify doing such a 'silly' thing as to take it. Unfortunately this experiment has not been replicated.

Thus it would seem that actively involving patients in their treatment, giving them the responsibility to decide whether to cooperate and even making life a little bit difficult for them, may be influential in harnessing the placebo effect, for by committing themselves to the treatment they have made a psychological investment. Janet (1925), talking of Lourdes, believes 'that the long arduous journey and the tedious waiting improves the prospects of a miracle cure'.

There is thus much speculation on how the placebo effect works, though Spiro (1986) questions the importance of knowing the mechanisms behind it. He states:

'Understanding the mechanisms will not help very much in understanding how, for whom, and if the placebo works. Do we not already know the remarkable feature, the triumph of the placebo, that one person can help another simply by trying'.

Conclusion

The placebo effect must surely be of interest to all physiotherapists. As noted above its influence is by no means marginal, it is inherent in every procedure physiotherapists use, and can be enhanced or reduced by their relationship with patients, their level of enthusiasm and the settings in which they work.

The use of the placebo in treatment and research does raise important ethical issues of which the physiotherapist should be aware. There is little agreement regarding the morality of using placebos in treatment or research and the physiotherapist must ultimately make up his or her own mind after careful consideration of the arguments. It may also be necessary, regarding research, for physiotherapists to have their ideas approved by the Health District's Ethics Committee.

A questioning attitude towards treatment, which is now encouraged in physiotherapy education, as well as an understanding of the placebo effect itself, may lead to a reduction in its power because the beliefs of the physiotherapist as well as those of the patient are influential in producing the effect. Furthermore, administering a placebo without the patient's full awareness contains an element of dishonesty which may run counter to present day beliefs that the patient/clinician relationship should be based on partnership and trust. It is, however, unlikely that the new patient/clinician relationship will destroy the placebo effect. As noted above, a good relationship with the patient can act as a powerful placebo in itself. Thus what we may lose by demystifying the treatment, we may gain by an improvement in communication.

Physiotherapists must decide whether to maximize the use of the placebo, avoid it, or ignore it. Even if it is ignored the effect will never be eliminated but its neglect may lead to less effective care. Orthodox practitioners are somewhat embarrassed by the placebo effect because it does not fit well with the image of medicine as a scientific enterprise. 'Alternative' practitioners are less concerned by this and it is interesting to note how popular their practices have become over the last decade. Katz (1984), who is sceptical of science, asks, 'Should placebos be left to faith healers and should physicians instead swear allegiance to new gods of science?'.

The profession of physiotherapy requires skills relating to both science and art and the placebo effect illustrates the tension between the two. Spiro (1986) believes that these two aspects of the clinician's role are not mutually exclusive and that we should not be afraid to turn to the 'magical' side of our work if we feel it will help our patients. Whether the placebo effect should be regarded as magical, however, is a matter of opinion, for no doubt its precise mechanisms will one day be explained. Whatever those mechanisms are, the placebo has proved itself to be an extremely powerful tool in the treatment of patients with a very wide range of conditions, leading Kaunitz (1985) to believe that, 'It is his (the clinician's) responsibility to influence to the best of his ability the patient's psychological mechanisms and external environment, so that nature's forces can bring to the fore the individual's underlying strength'.

Acknowledgement

This chapter is based on the article 'Magic Pills' (French S. (1990) *Nursing Times*, 25 April) and is reproduced here by kind permission of *Nursing Times*.

References

Andrews R. (1987) Quotation by Voltaire (1694–1778). *The Routledge Dictionary of Quotations*. London: Routledge and Kegan Paul.

Balint M. (1964) *The Doctor, His Patient and the Illness*. London: Pitman.

Beecher H. K. (1959) *Measurement of Subjective Responses*. Oxford: Oxford University Press.

Benson H., Epstein M. D. (1975) The placebo effect: a neglected asset in the care of patients. *Journal of the American Medical Association*, **232**, 1225–1227.

Benson H., McCallie D. P. (1979) Angina pectoris and the placebo effect. *New England Journal of Medicine*, **300**, 1424–1429.

Bok S. (1978) *Lying. Moral Choice in Public and Moral Life*. New York: Pantheon.

Braithwaite A., Cooper P. (1981) Analgesic effect of branding in treatment of headaches. *British Medical Journal*, **282**, 1576–1578.

Brill N. (1964) Cited in Rachman S. L., Philips C. (1978) *Psychology and Medicine*. Harmondsworth: Penguin Books.

Brody H. (1980) *Placebos and the Philosophy of Medicine*. London: University of Chicago Press.

Dimond E. G., Kittle C. F., Crockett J. E. (1960) Comparison of internal mammary artery ligation and sham operation for angina pectoris. *American Journal of Cardiology*, **5**, 483–486.

Engel G. L. (1977) The need for a new medical model: a challenge for biomedicine. *Science*, **196**, 129–136.

Evans F. J. (1974) The placebo response in pain reduction. *Advances in Neurology*, **4**, 289–296.

Festinger L. A. (1957) *A Theory of Cognitive Dissonance*. New York: Harper and Row.

Frank J. D. (1975) The faith that heals. *John Hopkins Medical Journal*, **13**(7), 127–131.

Goodwin J. S., Goodwin J. M., Vogel A. V. (1979) Knowledge and use of placebos by house officers and nurses. *Annals of Internal Medicine*, **91**, 106–110.

Griffiths D. (1980) *Psychology and Medicine*. London: Macmillan Press.

Hanson R. W., Gerber K. E. (1990) *Coping with Chronic Pain: A Guide to Patient Management*. London: The Guildford Press.

Helman C. (1994) *Culture, Health and Illness* (3rd edn). Oxford: Butterworth-Heinemann.

Hyland M. E., Donaldson M. L. (1989) *Psychological Care in Nursing Practice*. London: Scutari Press.

Janet P. M. (1925) Psychological healing: a historical and clinical study. Cited in Totman R. (1987) *Social Causes of Illness* (2nd edn). London: Souvenir Press.

Jones C. (1989) Little white lies. *Nursing Times*, **85**(44), 38–39.

Katz J. (1984) *The Silent World of the Doctor and Patient*. New York: Free Press.

Kaunitz P. (1985) The favourable prognosis. *Connecticut Medical Journal*, **49**, 453.

Kirsch I. (1985) Response expectancy as a determinant of experience and behaviour. *American Psychologist*, **40**, 1189–1202.

Leslie A. (1982) Letter. *Annals of Internal Medicine*, **9**(7), 781.

Low J. (1994) Electrotherapeutic modalities. In *Pain Management by Physiotherapy* (2nd edn) (Wells P. E. Frampton V., Bowsher D., eds). Oxford: Butterworth-Heinemann.

Lown B. (1985) Personal communication. Cited in Spiro. H. M. (1986) *Doctors, Patients and Placebos*. London: Yale University Press.

Mathews A., Steptoe A. (1988) *Essential Psychology for Medical Practice*. London: Churchill Livingstone.

Melzack R., Wall P. D. (1988) *The Challenge of Pain*. Harmondsworth: Penguin Books.

Morgan M. (1982) The doctor–patient relationship. In *Sociology as Applied to Medicine* (Patrick D. H., Scambler G., eds). London: Baillière Tindall.

Niven N., Robinson J. (1994) *The Psychology of Nursing Care*. London: Macmillan.

Park L. C., Covi L. (1965) Non-blind placebo trial: an experiment of neurotic patients' responses to placebo when its inert content is disclosed. *Archives of General Psychiatry*, **12**, 336–345.

Parrott A. (1991) Psychoactive drugs: efficacy and effects. In *The Psychology of Health: An Introduction* (Pitts M., Phillips K., eds). London: Routledge.

Pavlov I. P. (1960) *Conditioned Reflexes*. New York: Dover Press.

Rachman S. L., Philips C. (1978) *Psychology and Medicine*. Harmondsworth: Penguin Books.

Reiss W. J. (1958) Conditioning of a hyperinsulin type of behaviour in the white rat. *Science*, **51**, 301–313.

Richardson P. (1995) Placebos: their effectiveness and modes of action. In *Health Psychology: Processes and Applications* (Broome A., Llewelyn S., eds). London: Chapman and Hall.

Ross M., Olson J. M. (1982) Placebo effects in medical research and practice. In *Social Psychology and Behavioural Medicine* (Eiser J. R., ed.). Chichester: John Wiley and Sons.

Seligman A. W., Ferguson F. C., Garb S., Gluck J. L., Halpern S. L., Goodgold M. (1953) Evaluation of treatment in hypertension: effects of cinchona alkaloids. *American Journal of Medical Science*, **26**, 363–364.

Shapiro A. K. (1960) Attitudes towards the use of placebos in treatment. Cited in Spiro H. M. (1986) *Doctors, Patients and Placebos*. London: Yale University Press.

Shapiro K. (1970) Study on the effects of tablet colour in the treatment of anxiety states. *British Medical Journal*, **2**, 446–449.

Sim J. (1989) Truthfulness in the therapeutic relationship. *Physiotherapy Practice*, **5**(1), 121–122.

Simmons B. (1978) Problems in deceptive medical procedures: an ethical and legal analysis of the administration of the placebo. *Journal of Medical Ethics*, **4**, 172–181.

Sofaer B. (1992) *Pain: A Handbook for Nurses*. London: Chapman and Hall.

Spiro H. M. (1986) *Doctors, Patients and Placebos*. London: Yale University Press.

Terenius L. (1978) Significance of endorphins in endogenous antinociception. In *Advances in Biochemical Pharmacology*. Vol 18 (Coster E., Trabucchi M., eds). New York: Raven.

Totman R. (1987) *Social Causes of Illness* (2nd edn). London: Souvenir Press.

Weinman J. (1981) *An Outline for Psychology as Applied to Medicine*. Bristol: John Wright and Sons.

21

Teaching and learning in the clinical setting

Sally French and Susan Neville

'The supervisory role can be seen as a final stage in the development of the professional role – that of learning to teach the art that one has acquired oneself.' (Ford and Jones, 1987)

This chapter will consider the role of physiotherapists as educators in the clinical setting, with particular reference to those involved in the education of students. Sotosky (1984) contends that to educate others is part of the professional role and that the work of the physiotherapist can be defined as having three major functions: clinician; researcher; and educator. Higgs (1992), focusing on the role of clinical educators, states:

'In essence the primary roles of clinical educators are to provide competent clinical role models, to facilitate and manage students' learning and to empower students to learn and to take control of and responsibility for their learning'.

Coates (1986) believes that experienced, practising physiotherapists are better placed and better qualified than academic tutors to teach clinical skills to physiotherapy students. It is also likely that the attitudes and knowledge students acquire in the clinical situation are more profound and lasting than those acquired in the college setting. This places considerable responsibility on clinical educators.

The title of 'clinical supervisor' implies that physiotherapists are merely watching and directing the students' work. This diminishes their role, for in reality they are engaged in the complex and multi-dimensional task of teaching and helping students to learn. Thus the title 'clinical educator' is more appropriate (Cross, 1994) and will be used throughout this chapter. Over the past three decades, the role of the clinician in supporting the student during clinical practice placements has developed from that of clinical instructor in the 1960s to that of clinical educator in the 1990s (Cross, 1994). This reflects a change from the apprenticeship type of relationship, with its emphasis on instruction, to a more equal relationship with an emphasis on learning. The clinical educator is not merely assisting students to acquire facts and master procedures, but also to relate theory to practice and to develop appropriate attitudes and behaviour. The clinical educator must be able to motivate students and to modify the clinical environment to suit their needs. Students should ideally be stimulated but not over-anxious, be given adequate responsibility but not left to flounder, and be exposed to the realities of illness, disability and death without being overwhelmed by them. Individual differences between students and the stage they have reached in their education must also be considered.

Learning theories

There are many contrasting learning theories arising from different schools of psychology. Contemporary teaching practice is eclectic and the ideas presented in this chapter are drawn from various schools of thought. However, an outline of some of the main learning theories will be given.

Behaviourist theories of learning

The behaviourists view learning as resulting from stimulus–response connections. Beneficial responses to various stimuli tend to be repeated and to become established, whereas harmful or unsuccessful responses tend to diminish or disappear. Thus learning can occur through trial and error and is established through practice. It is also possible to influence the learning process by providing people with rewards and deterrents which 'shape' their behaviour in a given direction. Human beings are very sensitive to subtle signals of approval and disapproval from others and in this way we affect each other's behaviour and learning patterns. The behaviourists do not view the mental processes of the individual as important in the understanding of the learning process but rather concentrate on behaviour.

Cognitive theories of learning

Cognitive learning theorists view the learner as an active processor of information. They are interested in mental processes rather than behaviour, and place great emphasis on prior knowledge and assumptions. Over time our existing knowledge and experience of a given subject area become organized into a mental framework, often referred to as a 'schema' or 'set'. We tend to interpret new events, assimilate new information and approach new learning tasks in accordance with these schemas. Thus when students start their clinical education they already possess cognitive schemas, some of which may be rather sketchy but others very rich, in which to fit new knowledge. The more complex the existing schema, the easier it is to understand, assimilate, interpret and remember new information. For example, it will be less effort for a physiotherapy student to understand the pathological changes of pneumonia if he or she has knowledge of the respiratory system.

The clinical educator should be aware of the extent and complexity of the student's existing schema which will vary from one individual to another even at the same stage of their education. It is easy to over-estimate or under-estimate students' knowledge. Some students feel inhibited about asking questions, whereas others may be reluctant to reveal considerable knowledge and expertise for fear of being thought boastful or of causing embarrassment. The clinical educator should aim to help the student enrich his or her knowledge by linking new with existing material, challenging prevailing ideas and forming bridges between theoretical and practical knowledge. The more linkages made the easier it is for the student to remember the material. Thomas-Edding (1987) believes that clinical educators sometimes expect students to organize and assimilate information as efficiently as themselves: once knowledge-able on a subject it is very difficult to imagine or remember ignorance or confusion.

Prior knowledge, or an existing attitudinal 'set' may inhibit rather than enhance learning. People are motivated to maintain psychological homeostatis or balance and tend to resist knowledge if its incorporation gives rise to imbalance and the need to reorganize information and atti-tudes. If a piece of information or a treatment philosophy conflicts with an existing system of beliefs, the new knowledge may be rejected or distorted. Thus people do not merely assimiliate material which is presented to them but actively manipulate it. A dogmatic approach on the part of the clinical educator probably makes rejection of his or her ideas more likely.

The Gestalt theories of learning

Gestalt theorists believe that, 'the whole is greater than the sum of the parts'. Just as a whole symphony is greater than the sum of the notes, so the Gestalt theorists believe that mental processes, including learning, can only be comprehended in terms of their entirety. The concept of 'insight' is used by the Gestalt psychologists to describe the phenomenon whereby people experience a sudden flash of inspiration. They believe that this occurs as the result of a rapid reorganization of the learner's experiences. Controversy exists regarding whether tasks should be learned by breaking them down into parts or leaving them whole. Gestalt psychologists favour the later approach, though Pask (1976) believes the success of either approach varies according to the individual's learning style.

Learning by observation and participation

It is possible to learn a task by watching others perform it, and this may be very helpful to the student initially, but it is rarely sufficient in the learning of a new skill. There is considerable evidence to suggest that people learn best if they are actively involved. Thus it is important that students are given sufficient opportunities to carry out tasks themselves with adequate help. More passive methods of teaching do, however, have their place (Brown and Atkins, 1988; French et al., 1994). Repetition, to the point of over-learning, is necessary to become really proficient and also helps to substantiate the learning. Variety is, however, important to stimulate interest and avoid boredom. Ford and Jones (1987) point out that skilled workers often have a tremendous urge to intervene when students are attempting to learn a new task and that this increases the student's dependency.

In order to learn to 'be a physiotherapist' the student needs space to be alone with his or her patients and clients and develop rapport with them. Students vary in this respect and the clinical educator should aim to give the correct degree of help and support while allowing the student to gain confidence. This can be difficult if it is felt that the patient or client will suffer in any way. Many researchers have spoken of the conflict which clinical educators face when considering the needs of students as well as the needs of patients and clients (Scully and Shepard, 1983; Cross, 1995;

Maxwell, 1995). The number of patients and clients under their care may not be reduced to compensate for the extra work of teaching and they may have demanding administrative tasks to attend to as well. The Chartered Society of Physiotherapy (1994), in their *Guidelines for Good Practice for the Education of Clinical Educators*, provide a list of skills and abilities which clinical educators should acquire. These include teaching skills, knowledge of learning contracts, and the ability to help develop reflective practitioners and autonomous learners. However, these skills are not mandatory because the Society recognizes the difficulties physiotherapists experience in terms of workloads and the funding of clinical education.

Transfer of learning

Positive transfer of learning from one task to another is said to occur when the earlier learning task facilitates the later learning task. Negative transfer is said to occur when the earlier learning task hinders the later learning task. In general when two tasks are superficially similar though requiring different responses, transfer is likely to be negative (Child, 1986).

If someone learns to perform a task inaccurately it can be more difficult to correct his or her response than it is for a novice to learn the skill. A person who has learned to type with two fingers, for example, will probably find it more difficult to learn the correct method than someone with no experience of typing. Rogers (1989) believes that training exercises can adversely affect performance of the real task unless the two are very similar. It is obviously important for clinical educators to ensure that students learn tasks correctly the first time. Burnett *et al.* (1986) believe that transferring knowledge is more successful if students are taught through a problem-solving approach rather than a didactic approach.

Adult learning theory

Andragogy, the art and science of helping adults learn, has emerged as distinct from pedagogy, the art and science of teaching children. Andragogy is based on certain assumptions about adult learning and the climate in which learning is optimized (Knowles, 1983; Boud and Griffin, 1987). Adults are inclined towards behaviour which is self-directed and like to take responsibility for their own learning and apply it immediately, particularly when solving problems. They are, themselves, a rich learning resource and they function best in an environment which is collaborative and mutually respectful. Motivation to learn is derived more from an internal desire to achieve self-fulfilment than through external pressure from teachers (Knowles, 1984; Mezirow, 1985). Identification of learning goals and ways of achieving them, should, therefore, involve both the learner and the teacher, as should assessment of the extent to which the learning has been successful. This approach to teaching and learning is particularly appropriate in the clinical setting in the light of today's climate of continuing change and increasing complexity (Reed Ash, 1985; Higgs, 1992). (For a full discussion of learning theories, readers are referred to Brown and Atkins (1988) and Curzon (1990).)

Individual differences   Individual differences between students affect how well they learn and their preferred learning styles. No one factor in isolation is particularly predictive of success in higher education.

Intelligence and prior academic performance   There is a low positive correlation between IQ scores and academic success at degree level with a similarly low correlation between 'A' level GCE grades and degree success (Beard and Hartley, 1984). Rheault and Shafernich-Coulson (1988) found no correlation between the academic and clinical grades of physical therapy students, though their findings conflict with those of Pickles (1977). It is important that the clinical educator should not prejudge the student on the grounds of his or her academic achievement as this may not relate to clinical ability. Jobling (1987) points out that success in higher education is as much a function of personality as of intellect.

Extroversion and stability   There is a tendency for introverted students to achieve higher grades at degree level than their more extroverted peers (Entwistle, 1975). This is probably because introverts tend to have better study habits and are more tolerant of solitary activities such as essay writing and research. They also differ regarding the teaching methods they prefer. Extroverts are sociable and tend to like group discussion and working with others, whereas introverts often prefer lectures and working alone. Thus the traditional teaching practices of higher education may favour the more introverted students. Introverts do not contribute readily when in a group but if asked to deliver a paper or run a seminar the quality of their work is usually very high. There is no evidence that people who do not contribute to group discussions learn less. Stability is another personality characteristic which seems to be predictive of success in higher education.

It is interesting to note that the occupational stereotype of the physiotherapist, when measured by Eysenck's Personality Inventory (Eysenck, 1967), is one of a slightly neurotic extrovert (Child, 1974; Jobling, 1986). With the growing concern for academic excellence and research activity in the physiotherapy profession, perhaps candidates of more diverse temperament should be selected and encouraged to apply.

Cognitive styles   Messick (1978) states that, 'Each individual has preferred ways of organizing all that he sees and remembers and thinks about'. These preferences are termed 'cognitive styles'.

Honey and Mumford (1982) devised a questionnaire which identified four learning styles; those of activist, reflector, theorist and pragmatist. The activist likes activity and new experiences, thrives on challenge and enjoys crises. The reflector, on the other hand, likes to ponder, is thorough and cautious and prefers to stay in the background. The theorist is rational, has a logical step-by-step approach to learning and is concerned with basic concepts. The pragmatist is eager to initiate action and likes to try out new ideas.

Most people have one or two preferred cognitive styles. No styles can be said to be superior to any other, but rather each is suited to learning different tasks or aspects of a task. Thus individuals may seek to avoid certain areas of learning or activity according to their preferred cognitive styles. The theorist, for example, may be loathe to apply his or her knowledge and the pragmatist may not fully understand the basis of his or her actions. Although at first glance the pragmatist may appear to suit the role of physiotherapist best, all four styles are relevant to physiotherapy practice.

The clinical educator will have his or her own preferred style or styles of learning and may find it difficult to help or respond positively or adequately to students with different styles. This is a problem for all teachers. Honey (1988) concludes that people with all four styles within their repertoire are best equipped to teach but, unfortunately, only a minority of people are so versatile.

Clinical educators should to some extent adapt to the differing learning styles of students but should also encourage them to learn and perform in ways they find more difficult in an attempt to increase their overall effectiveness. At the same time clinical educators should analyse their own preferred learning styles and try to widen their repertoire so as to teach more effectively. This is no easy task for cognitive styles are firmly rooted within our personalities (Messick, 1978). However, adopting a facilitative teaching style, and encouraging students to direct their own learning, is likely to allow for individual differences among students (McMillan and Dwyer, 1990).

Many other cognitive styles have been described. Hudson (1966) made the distinction between the 'converger' and the 'diverger'. The converger enjoys thinking about technical, impersonal matters, likes argument to be clearly defined and logical and to know whether he or she is right or wrong. The converger is not interested in probing into topics of a personal, emotional nature, nor in controversy. The diverger is the reverse, he or she enjoys controversy and uncertainty but is not interested in technical matters. Hudson found that convergers tend to specialize in physical sciences whereas divergers favour the arts, law and business where decisions are made on the basis of probabilities. Beard and Hartley (1984) contend that divergers are difficult for teachers to cope with as they tend to think outside the structures provided for them.

Pask (1976) described the cognitive style of the 'holist' and the 'serialist'. Serialists like to take a step-by-step approach when solving a problem, whereas holists like to look at the problem in its entirety. Another style is 'field dependence' versus 'field independence'. According to Messick (1978) the field independent person is able to isolate factors from their global context, is analytical and has an impersonal orientation. The field dependent individual, on the other hand, tends to view situations globally, lacks competence in analytic functioning, has a social orientation and is socially skilled.

Only the minority of people tend to extremes, most showing a slight tendency to adopt some learning styles rather than others. All learning styles have advantages and disadvantages and are beneficial to physiotherapy practice in their different ways, their effectiveness varying according to the task. The individual's preferred learning styles, though deeply rooted in personality structure, are not fixed and can be modified and extended.

The student's state of mind

The student's state of mind will have a large effect on his or her ability to learn and the clinical educator will often be in a position to influence this. An important consideration is the student's level of anxiety. Brown and Atkins (1988) believe that 'significant learning only takes place in non-threatening environments'.

Trait anxiety, the individual's general tendency to be anxious, and state anxiety, the individual's level of anxiety in particular situations, though positively correlated are distinct. Thus the environment can be modified to alter the anxiety level of the student. The Yerkes-Dodson Law (1908) states that if arousal is either very high or very low, performance and learning of complex tasks is adversely affected. If arousal is too great the student is unable to concentrate and apply him or herself to the task and if it is too low the student will tend to be apathetic and under-stimulated. The level of a person's anxiety is not very easy to assess as various measurements – physiological, behavioural and self-report – tend to correlate poorly.

The task of the clinical educator is not to eliminate the student's anxiety but to prevent it from becoming debilitating. Various studies have shown that physiotherapy students feel anxious about the clinical aspect of their education. Cupit (1988) asked physiotherapy students to say in a word how they felt about starting clinical work. Words such as 'petrified', 'scared', 'worried' and 'uncertain' were very common. She also found that many students doubted their knowledge and were worried about harming patients or clients. Ramsden and Davitz (1972) found that physiotherapy students were both apprehensive and excited about the prospect of embarking on clinical work. They were worried about their level of knowledge and their ability to relate well to patients and clients as well as staff. Walish *et al.* (1986) interviewed 20 physiotherapy students and found they were most concerned about interpersonal relationships; worries about treatment techniques and administrative procedures were also expressed.

Being in a familiar place with familiar people reduces anxiety. Thus the clinical educator can help the student control his or her level of stress by giving clear instructions and information and taking care to orientate him or her within the hospital and department or community unit (Stengelhofen, 1993). The information given should be paced so that the student is able to assimilate and retain it. Probably the most important factor is for the clinical educator to create an atmosphere where students feel able to ask questions even if they feel they ought to know the answers or have been told before. This type of relationship is very helpful to clinical educators too as they will receive feedback which will enable them to understand the students' difficulties and limitations as well as improve their own performance. On rare occasions students may lack sufficient anxiety to stimulate action and learning; in such a situation it may be necessary to increase their level of anxiety a little.

The relationship with the student may also create various anxieties for clinical educators. They may be anxious about assessing students, afraid that their limitations will be exposed or that their ideas and practice will be challenged. Such feelings usually diminish as clinical educators become more experienced but can lead to an authoritarian, over-controlling attitude and style in order to protect themselves. A more equal relationship between the clinical educator and the student requires learning needs to be identified in collaboration and the learning outcomes to be jointly assessed. This can work well and may reduce anxiety for clinical tutors and students provided they are both ready to subscribe to the approach.

Any emotional problems the student may have are also likely to interfere with learning. There is a tendency to view the student years as a happy and carefree time but it can be a difficult period when many adaptations have to be made as the individual reaches full adulthood. Many students are now 'mature' and may have families to consider as well as other commitments. Maslow (1943) believes that the desire to achieve intellectually and reach one's full potential can only be realized when more basic needs are satisfied. He expressed this idea in terms of a hierarchy of needs where those needs at the bottom of the hierarchy, i.e. physiological, safety and social needs, must be satisfied before high level needs, such as the need for intellectual achievement and self-fulfilment, can be addressed. Although this model can be criticized – some people achieve a great deal despite tremendous odds – it is nevertheless useful.

The clinical educator should be aware that events in the student's life may bring about fluctuations in his or her ability to learn and should be prepared to counsel the student if the need arises. Some problems may relate to the work itself, for example difficulty in accepting terminal illness, or feelings of powerlessness when treating patients and clients with progressive diseases. It is very difficult for people to learn if they are overwhelmed by such feelings. Booy (1986) believes that clinical educators should possess counselling skills.

Motivation

The will to learn depends on internal motivators, for example, interest, enjoyment or wanting to achieve, and external motivators, for example praise, money or passing examinations. Internal and external motivators do, of course, interact, for example being praised may increase interest and being paid for a task may increase its enjoyment. Thus although internal motivators tend to be more powerful, they may be enhanced or diminished by external factors. External motivation has little effect if internal motivation is seriously lacking but happily this is not a common circumstance with physiotherapy students.

The clinical educator is very well placed to enhance internal and external motivation although it is important that students should take some responsibility for their own motivation and learning (Higgs, 1992). Cross (1996) explains the use of learning contracts within physiotherapy clinical education which she describes as '… a written agreement between a learner/student and a teacher/facilitator which details what is to be learned, the strategies and resources which may be used to assist in learning, and the evidence or criteria which may be used to demonstrate that learning has occurred'. Learning contracts serve to individualize learning, to foster independence, to engender a sense of ownership and to develop successful self-directed learning (Cross, 1996).

Positive reinforcement

Motivation is increased by giving praise and encouragement to desired behaviours. In British society we have a tendency to congratulate others and ourselves rather too infrequently. Bendall (1975) surveyed student nurses and found that most of the reinforcement they received came from the patients. Positive reinforcement enhances the individual's self-concept which can have a large effect on achievement (Baron and Byrne, 1991). If praise is given it must be genuine or the student will receive false feedback and will lose confidence in the clinical educator and respect for him or her.

Negative reinforcement

Negative reinforcement refers to criticism, disapproval or failure to reward a response. Criticizing specific acts can be effective in enhancing learning but a general attitude of criticism and punitiveness is likely to affect adversely the student's motivational state. It is unusual for a student's performance to be wholly bad and criticism can be tempered with praise and suggestions for improvement. Criticism should be related to specific problems which can be changed, rather than directed at the learner's personality as a whole. Booy (1986) believes that it is very important to be objective and specific especially now that the student can appeal against an assessment decision and that clinical assessment grades are taken into account when classifying students' degrees. It should also be appreciated that the way the student performs may be greatly influenced by the clinical educator's presence.

By giving reinforcement, either positive or negative, the clinician will be providing valuable feedback to his or her students enabling them to adjust to requirements and improve their performance. Although improvement can occur without knowledge of results it is greatly enhanced if feedback is given. Feedback is most useful if given immediately and regularly, it can then be easily related to the behaviour it concerns and gives the student time to improve. Students should always be given the opportunity to discuss or disagree with what is being said. Unresolved misunderstandings and suppressed resentments only serve to demotivate both educator and student and sour the relationship.

Success

Success is highly motivating and will facilitate learning, thus the clinical educator should attempt to ensure high levels of success in his or her students. The pace of learning should ideally be adjusted to suit the individual student so that success is assured. As well as succeeding most students like to feel they are being stretched intellectually or there is a danger of boredom.

Interest and enjoyment

Interest and enjoyment were cited above as internal motivators. The clinical educator should try to ensure high levels of interest and enjoyment in his or her students. This can be achieved in many ways: by providing a varied case load, teaching new techniques, involving the students in in-service education, and organizing visits to other departments. Most students lose interest if their work is too routine. The general atmosphere of the department – how approachable the staff are, how welcome students feel – is vitally important regarding their level of enjoyment.

Competition and cooperation

Competing and cooperating with others can be highly motivating and can enhance learning. Cooperation is more relevant to the clinical situation than competition. It is important that the clinical educator creates a situation in which the student feels he or she belongs and is contributing meaningfully to the work of the department. Although it is important to consider the effect of motivation on learning and achievement, it is interesting to note that the correlation between student motivation, as measured by students themselves, and achievement, is quite low (Entwistle et al., 1971). People who work the hardest are not necessarily the most motivated nor satisfied (Vroom and Deci, 1970). Thus the behaviour of students is not a perfect indicator of their attitudes or feelings. This is not too surprising when we consider the many constraints on the way we behave.

If the student appears to be uninterested, unmotivated or achieving poorly there is a tendency to spend less time with him or her and to be more critical, with the possibility or worsening the student's state of mind and creating a vicious circle. Behaviour, including learning is, however, at least as much determined by the interaction between the individual's characteristics and the situation, as by the individual's characteristics alone (Argyle et al., 1982). Many psychologists and sociologists believe that the emphasis on the individual is an unfortunate misdirection of focus. Thus rather than counselling or criticizing the 'unmotivated' student or the student who is failing to learn, it might be more fruitful on occasions to examine the organization in which he or she is placed. The clinical educator is clearly a very important influence in determining the student's environment and is therefore in a key position to influence his or her learning.

Professional socialization

'... the most forceful, professional socialization is likely to occur during clinical practice. Contact with patients, members of the health care team and exposure to clinical realities generate powerful positive and negative feelings' (Burrows, 1990).

Professional socialization can be viewed as a process whereby individuals are shaped to fit the needs of the profession. Peat (1985) believes that this process takes place mainly in the clinical environment. Professional socialization is not fully understood; concepts have been borrowed from studies of child socialization, but this is inadequate because the adult has had more experience and is subject to more diverse influences. It would be wrong to think of students as passive recipients ready to absorb the values and norms of the profession they have entered. Students both accept and reject what is delivered to them and there is usually a powerful student culture exerting far more influence than senior members of the profession.

Individuals who are selected for physiotherapy education are often similar to those already in the profession (Mercer, 1979). This ensures that the socialization process has already begun. Despite this, students often enter their professional education with preconceived and idealistic views of what the work entails. The sudden shattering of these views when clinical work is commenced has been referred to as 'reality shock' and the requirement to change rapidly from a schoolchild to a sensitive and highly responsible adult, as 'role ageing'. Atkinson (1981) found that the attitudes of medical students moved from idealism to cynicism as their education progressed.

Students are exposed to a wide variety of models as they progress through clinical education. Although the occasional model may be a 'star', Burrows (1990) points out that most serve as partial models with the students internalizing a variety of values from each. Some may serve as 'anti-models' highlighting what the student does not want to become. Many studies show, however, that professional models are not particularly influential (Atkinson, 1981).

The process of socialization encourages conformity. There is, however, considerable evidence to suggest that those with minority views are often right and can have a profound effect on the thoughts and attitudes of the majority. Burnard (1989) states that, 'the true innovators in nursing will be and always have been outsiders'. He believes that non-conformists are very valuable members of professions, as they tend to seek the truth whatever the cost, but he recognizes that they have a very difficult time and often leave the profession. It is important for clinical educators to bear this in mind in their dealings with students who do not readily conform.

Because physiotherapy is not a clear-cut scientific enterprise, students will inevitably receive varying and conflicting messages from staff both in the college and the clinical field. This not only applies to the acquisition of skills but also to learning the role of physiotherapist itself. The nature of the role has become less clearly defined over the years and there is also less agreement concerning the nature of professional values and behaviour. This can be difficult for students who are expected to fit successfully into a wide selection of departments during their education and are assessed by a variety of clinical educators. The confusion has the potential to cause anxiety and interfere with learning. It is important that the clinical educator is aware of the confusion to which students are subject and if he or she has any definite views on issues of professionalism or techniques which he or she wishes students to adopt, these should be articulated clearly. It is common for students to believe that the confusion they feel, regarding treatment techniques and behaviour, springs from within themselves rather than being an external reality.

The clinical setting provides the context in which the student engages with the real life situation and has the opportunity, not only to build upon and refine the knowledge and skills developed in the academic environment, but also to acquire new knowledge and understanding from the experience itself (Schon, 1987; Higgs, 1993). This experiential learning is central to clinical practice. Such ideas are not new; Dewey (cited in Kolb,

1984), an educationalist in the 1930s, defined experiential learning as the process that links education, work and personal development. Kolb (1984) also sees experiential learning as a process whereby knowledge is formed and reformed through experience. He developed a cyclical model to illustrate such learning: actively engaging in the experience (concrete experience) is followed by awareness of what has happened (reflective observation). Linking this with theory (abstract conceptualization) can further enhance understanding which can then be tested out in new situations (active experimentation) and so back to the experience. Time should be spent in addressing all four aspects of the cycle, not least that of reflection, which is highlighted by many writers as the key to learning (Boyd and Fales, 1983; Gibbs, 1988; Gould, 1989; Boud and Walker, 1990; Fish *et al.*, 1991–2).

This processing of experience is part of the students' own developing clinical expertise. Students are less able than experienced clinicians to recognize and elicit relevant information or to interpret written and visual data (Ryan, 1995). They therefore need to be encouraged to voice their thinking – it is insufficient for them to merely describe incidents and experiences. Drawing out the meaning students attach to their practice will facilitate their clinical reasoning abilities. Clinical teaching should take account of the emerging understanding of how expert clinicians think and act in practice (May and Dennis, 1991; Yarett Slater and Cohn, 1991; Jensen *et al.*, 1992).

Clinical reasoning studies (Barker Schwartz, 1991; Hayes Fleming, 1991; Rivet and Higgs, 1995) highlight, not only the importance of technical skills and an extensive and accessible knowledge base, but the crucial role of interpersonal skills in truly understanding the patient's illness behaviour. Davis (1990) points out that anxiety, self-doubt, prejudice and low self-esteem all work to make the student inward looking which inhibits the establishment of a therapeutic relationship. Clinical teaching should help students to know their identity and personal value and to be aware of their strengths and weaknesses. Reflection can assist in this process.

Creating a learning environment

Contemporary learning theory and teaching practice are eclectic. Griffiths (1987) views learning as 'a process of drawing out from within' and a teacher as a facilitator who is responsible for promoting or hastening the process. Brown and Atkins (1988) claim that people are 'natural decision-makers and problem-solvers'. Mason (1984) believes that the two major dimensions of successful teaching are understanding the subject matter and having the ability to create a learning environment and form relationships with students. Beard and Hartley (1984) point out that under-achievement is caused by many factors unrelated to intellect such as debilitating anxiety, emotional difficulties and a lack of security.

Mathews (1887) suggests various factors which enhance the experience of learning for nurses on the ward. These factors are also applicable to physiotherapists. They include a positive attitude from the person in charge, awareness by trained staff of their teaching responsibilities, a high morale, an emphasis on the needs of the patient rather than the needs of the ward and the encouragement of students to ask questions. Marson (1990) reaches similar conclusions. Mathews (1987) believes that most learning in the clinical situation takes place, not by formal methods but by example – the way qualified staff interact with patients and relatives, how they plan treatments and how much responsibility they give to students. Formal teaching does, however, have its place and there are many books and articles on the subject which clinical educators can consult (Beard and Hartley, 1984; Brown and Atkins, 1988; Rogers, 1989; Curzon, 1990; French et al., 1994).

Whitely (1988) gives various tips on how the ward can be used as a teaching environment, including the use of patients' notes, the display of wall posters, the availability of textbooks, participation on ward rounds and the involvement of other professionals and departments. Creating a suitable learning environment is not, however, an easy task as the clinical educator must adapt to individual needs as well as deal with clinical and administrative responsibilities.

Students' views on clinical teaching

Various studies have been conducted where physiotherapy students have been asked to give their opinions on clinical education. It appears from these studies that students view clinical educators' ability to communicate and their interpersonal skills as more important than their teaching ability and professional skills. Emery (1984) asked physical therapy students, who had completed their clinical education, to rate the importance and frequency of 43 previously identified clinical educator behaviours. These behaviours were classified as relating to communication, interpersonal relationships, professional skills and teaching skills. The students considered all the behaviours valuable but the educator's interpersonal skills and his or her ability to communicate were considered more important than his or her teaching capabilities; clinical skills were considered least important of all. It is interesting to note that the behaviours considered least important were the ones most frequently demonstrated.

Onuoho (1994) carried out a similar study with final year physiotherapy students in the UK using the same classification as Emery. Clinical educators and academic teachers were also included. His research supported the view that communication skills were deemed important but the students in his sample gave a higher rating to 'carrying out physiotherapy with competence' than to interpersonal communication which is opposite to Emery's findings. Handal and Lauvas (1987) believe that it is important to facilitate students' personal growth. They remind us that the educator's role is to 'help the student master the job … not do it for him', to allow individual style within an acceptable performance.

Concentrating entirely on the pursuit of clinical excellence can be destructive. Best (1988) states: 'Some supervisors are exacting task-masters and in their determination to produce competent clinicians often destroy the student's developing confidence so that they are unable to perform'. Orton (1984), in her study of the clinical education of student nurses, found that students rated highly considerate and understanding sisters, who treated them as learners rather than workers and who generated a team spirit. They rated highly those who spent considerable time teaching on the ward especially if they used existing ward facilities to do so.

Clinical educators' attitudes to teaching

May (1983) surveyed a large number of physical therapists in the USA by means of a questionnaire. Most believed teaching was an important aspect of their role but few thought is was a natural skill. Most of the therapists said they had learned to teach by 'trial and error'. Scully and Shepard (1983) conducted an observational study of physical therapists in the USA which included semi-structured interviews. They note that teaching activities in clinical practice are dissimilar to those used in college settings and believe that clinical teaching methods have never been adequately defined. Various advantages and disadvantages were expressed regarding working with students. Respondents commented on lack of privacy, reduced contact with patients and clients and difficulty managing time. It was necessary for the student to be a good 'guest-in-the-house' and to understand and abide by 'house rules'. Other respondents mentioned the enriching effect students had on the whole department and that the high exposure given to the work place improved staff recruitment. Sotosky (1984) found that clinical educators had very positive attitudes towards tutoring, though they were dissatisfied with the training they received and wanted to learn more about teaching. Very similar results have been found by Cupit (1988), Neville and French (1991), Cross (1992) and Maxwell (1995). Walker and Openshaw (1994) found that clinical educators wanted help in evaluating students fairly and wanted more preparation for their role.

It is clear that students have to cope with a variety of philosophies and teaching styles as they move from one department to the next. Scully and Shepard (1983) believe that they often walk a tight-rope between 'student' and 'therapist' in the way they are expected to behave and that their status among other staff depends on how they are treated by the clinical educator.

Conclusion

The role of the clinical educator is complex and multi-factorial. Greater support and education need to be developed though this is improving (Walker and Openshaw, 1994). The enhancement of teaching skills and the ability to create an environment conducive to learning will not only benefit students but also junior staff, patients and clients, in fact anyone in the department who is keen to learn. In addition many of the qualities that a clinical educator needs are those required of an effective manager or leader, thus the skills are not specific to teaching but can be generalized to other aspects of the physiotherapist's work.

References

Argyle M., Furnham A., Graham J. A. (1982) *Social Situations*. Cambridge: Cambridge University Press.

Atkinson P. (1981) *The Clinical Experience*. London: Gower.

Barker Schwartz K. (1991) Clinical reasoning and new ideas on intelligence: implications for teaching and learning. *American Journal of Occupational Therapy*. **45**(11), 1033–1037.

Baron R. A., Byrne D. (1991) *Social Psychology: Understanding Human Interaction* (6th edn). London: Allyn and Bacon.

Beard R., Hartley J. (1984) *Teaching and Learning in Higher Education* (4th edn). London: Paul Chapman Publishing.

Bendall E. (1975) *So You Passed Nurse*. London: Royal College of Nursing.

Best D. (1988) Physiotherapy clinical supervision effectiveness and the use of models. *Australian Journal of Physiotherapy*, **34**(4), 209–214.

Booy M. J. (1986) Bridging the gap in clinical supervision. *Bulletin of the Association of Teachers of Physiotherapy*, **5**, 12–14.

Boud D., Griffin V. (1987) *Appreciating Adults Learning: From the Adult's Perspective*. London: Kogan Page.

Boud D., Walker D. (1990) Making the most of experience. *Studies in continuing education*. **12**(2), 61–80.

Boyd E. M., Fales A. W. (1983) Reflective learning: key to learning from experience. *Journal of Humanistic Psychology*, **23**(2), 99–117.

Brown G., Atkins M. (1988) *Effective Teaching in Higher Education*. London: Methuen.

Burnard P. (1989) The nurse as a non-conformist. *Nursing Standard*, **27**(4), 32–34.

Burnett C. N., Mahoney P. J., Chidley M. J., Pierson F. M. (1986) Problem-solving approach to clinical education. *Therapy Weekly*, **66**(11), 1730–1733.

Burrows E. (1990) The hidden curriculum. *Therapy Weekly*, **16**(32), 6.

Chartered Society of Physiotherapy (1994) Guidelines for good practice for the education of clinical educators. *Physiotherapy*, **80**(5), 299–300.

Child D. (1974) The physiotherapist – is there an occupational stereotype? *Physiotherapy*, **60**(10), 302–305.

Child D. (1986) *Psychology and the Teacher*. London: Cassell.

Coates F. (1986) Clinical supervision – no. Clinical teaching – yes. *Bulletin of the Association of Teachers of the Chartered Society of Physiotherapy*, **5**, 5.

Cross V. (1992) clinicians' needs in clinical education: a report on a needs analysis workshop. *Physiotherapy*, **18**(10), 758–761.

Cross V. (1994) From clinical supervisor to clinical educator: too much to ask? *Physiotherapy*, **80**(9), 609–611.

Cross V. (1995) Aspects of the quality debate in clinical education. *Physiotherapy*, **81**(9), 502–505.

Cross V. (1996) Introducing learning contracts into physiotherapy clinical education. *Physiotherapy*, **82**(1), 21–27.

Cupit R. L. (1988) Student stress: an approach to coping at the interface between preclinical and clinical education. *Australian Journal of Physiotherapy*, **34**(4), 215–219.

Curzon L. B. (1990) *Teaching in Further Education* (4th edn). London: Cassel Educational.

Davis C. M. (1990) What is empathy and can empathy be taught? *Physical Therapy*, **70**(11), 707–715.

Dewey J. (1984) Cited in Kolb D. A. (1984) *Experiential Learning: Experience as the Source of Learning and Development*. New Jersey: Prentice Hall.

Emery M. J. (1984) Effectiveness of the clinical instructor: students' perspective. *Physical Therapy*, **64**(7), 1079–1083.

Entwistle N. J. (1975) Personality and academic attainment. In *Personality and Learning 1* (Whitehead J. M., ed.). Sevenoaks: Hodder and Stoughton.

Entwistle N. J., Nisbet J. B., Entwistle D. M., Cowell M. D. (1971) The academic performance of students: 1, predictions from scales of motivation and study methods. *British Journal of Educational Psychology*, **41**(3), 258–267.

Eysenck H. J. (1967) Personality patterns in various groups of businessmen. *Occupational Psychology*, **41**, 249–250.

Fish D., Twinn S., Purr B. (1990–1991) Promoting Reflection: improving the supervision of practice in health visiting and initial teacher training (HELPP). Report Number 2. Twickenham: West London Institute of Higher Education in Association with Brunel University.

Ford K., Jones A. (1987) *Clinical Supervision*. London: Macmillan.

French S., Neville S., Laing J. (1994) *Teaching and Learning: A Guide for Therapists*. Oxford: Butterworth-Heinemann.

Gibbs G. (1988) *Learning by Doing: A Guide to Teaching and Learning Methods.* London: Further Education Unit.

Gould N. (1989) Reflective learning for social work practice. *Social Work Education*, **8**(2), 9–19.

Griffiths P. (1987) Creating a learning environment. *Physiotherapy*, **73**(7), 335–336.

Handal G., Lauvas P. (1987) *Promoting Reflective Teaching: Supervision in Action.* Milton Keynes: The Society for Research into Higher Education and the Open University Press.

Hayes Fleming M. (1991) The therapist with the three-track mind. *American Journal of Occupational Therapy*, **45**(11), 1007–1014.

Higgs J. (1992) Managing clinical education: the educator-manager and the self-directed learner. *Physiotherapy*, **78**(11), 822–828.

Higgs J. (1993) Managing clinical education: the programme. *Physiotherapy*, **79**(4), 239–246.

Honey P. (1988) You are what you learn. *Nursing Times*, **84**(36), 34–36.

Honey P., Mumford A. (1982) The manual of learning styles. Cited in Jobling M. H. (1987) Cognitive styles: some implications for teaching and learning. *Physiotherapy*, **73**(7), 335–338.

Hudson L. (1966) *Contrary Imaginations: A Psychological Study of the English Schoolboy.* London: Methuen.

Jensen G. M., Shepard K. F., Gwyer J., Hack L. M. (1992) Attribute dimensions that distinguish master and novice physical therapy clinicians in orthopaedic settings. *Physical Therapy*, **72**(10), 711–720.

Jobling M. H. (1986) An investigation of some personality characteristics of a group of undergraduate physiotherapy students: with particular reference to the occupational profile. *B. Ed. Dissertation*. Roehampton: Garnett College.

Jobling M. H. (1987) Cognitive styles: some implications for teaching and learning. *Physiotherapy*, **73**(7), 335–338.

Knowles M. S. (1983) Andragogy: an emerging technology for adult learning. In *Adult Learning and Education* (Tight M., ed.). London: Croom Helm in Association with the Open University.

Knowles M. S. (1984) *Andragogy in Action.* London: Jossey Bass.

Kolb D. A. (1984) *Experiential Learning: Experience as the Source of Learning and Development.* New Jersey: Prentice Hall.

McMillan M. A., Dwyer J. (1990) Facilitating a match between teaching and learning styles. *Nurse Education Today*, **10**, 186–192.

Marson S. (1990) Creating a climate for learning. *Nursing Times*, **86**(17), 53–55.

Maslow A. H. (1943) A theory of human motivation. *Psychological Review*, **50**, 370–396.

Mason S. N. (1984) Development the teaching role of the ward sister. *Nurse Education Today*, **4**(1), 13–16.

Mathews A. (1987) *In Charge of the Ward.* Oxford: Blackwell Scientific Publications.

Maxwell M. (1995) Problems associated with the clinical education of physiotherapy students: a Delphi survey. *Physiotherapy*, **81**(10), 582–587.

May B. J. (1983) Teaching a skill in clinical practice. *Physical Therapy*, **63**(10), 1627–1633.

May B. J., Dennis J. K. (1991) Expert decision making in physical therapy – a survey of practitioners. *Physical Therapy*, **71**(3), 190–206.

Mercer J. (1979) Aspects of professionalism in the professions supplementary to medicine. *Ph. D. Thesis*. London: University of London.

Messick S. (1978) Personality consistencies in cognition and creativity. In *Individuality in Learning* (Messick S. *et al.*, eds). London: Jossey Bass Publishers.

Mezirow J. (1985) A critical theory of self-directed learning. In *Self-directed Learning: From Theory to Practice* (Brookfield S., ed.). San Francisco: Jossey Bass.

Neville S., French S. (1991) Clinical education: students' and clinical tutors' views. *Physiotherapy*, **77**(5), 351–354.

Onuoha A. R. A. (1994) Effective clinical teaching behaviours from the perspective of students, supervisors and teachers. *Physiotherapy*, **80**(4), 208–214.

Orton H. D. (1984) Learning on the ward – how important is the climate? In *Understanding Nurses* (Skevington S., ed.). Chichester: John Wiley and Sons.

Pask G. (1976) Styles and strategies of learning. *British Journal of Educational Psychology*, **46**, 12–25.

Peat M. (1985) Enid Graham Memorial Lecture: clinical education of health professionals. *Canadian Journal of Physiotherapy*, **37**(5), 301–306.

Pickles B. (1977) Correlations between matriculation entry requirements and performance in the diploma program in physical therapy at the University of Alberta. *Canadian Journal of Physiotherapy*, **29**, 249–253.

Ramsden E. L., Davitz H. L. (1972) Clinical education: interpersonal foundations. *Therapy Weekly*, **52**, 1060–1066.

Reed Ash C. (1985) Applying principles of self-directed learning in the health professions. In *Self-directed Learning: From Theory to Practice* (Brookfield S., ed.). San Francisco: Jossey Bass.

Rheault W., Shaafernich-Coulson E. (1988) Relationship between academic achievement and clinical performance in a physical therapy education program. *Physical Therapy*, **68**(3), 378–380.

Rivett D., Higgs J. (1995) Experience and expertise in clinical reasoning. *New Zealand Journal of Physical Therapy*, April, 16–21.

Rogers J. (1989) *Adults Learning* (3rd edn). Milton Keynes: Open University Press.

Ryan S. (1995) Teaching clinical reasoning to occupational therapists during field-work education. In *Clinical Reasoning in the Health Professions* (Higgs J., Jones M., eds). Oxford: Butterworth-Heinemann.

Schon D. A. (1987) *Educating the Reflective Practitioner*. Oxford: Jossey Bass.

Scully R. M., Shepard K. F. (1983) Clinical teaching in physical therapy education. *Physical Therapy*, **63**(3), 349–358.

Sotosky J. R. (1984) Physical therapists' attitudes towards teaching. *Physical Therapy*, **64**(3), 347–349.

Stengelhofen J. (1993) *Teaching Students in Clinical Settings*. London: Chapman and Hall.

Thomas-Edding D. (1987) Clinical problem-solving in physical therapy and its implications for curriculum development. Cited in Best D. (1988) Physiotherapy clinical supervision: effectiveness and the use of models. *Australian Journal of Physiotherapy*, **34**(4), 209–214.

Vroom V. H., Deci E. L. (1970) *Management and Motivation*. Harmondsworth: Penguin Books.

Walish J. F., Schuit D., Olson R. E. (1986) Preaffiliation and postaffiliation concerns expressed by physical therapy students. *Physical Therapy*, **66**(5), 691–696.

Walker E. M., Openshaw S. (1994) Educational needs as perceived by clinical supervisors. *Physiotherapy*, **80**(7), 424–431.

Whitely A. J. (1988) Using the ward as a classroom. *Nursing Standard*, **41**(2), 31.

Yarett Slater D., Cohn E. S. (1991) Staff development through analysis of practice. *The American Journal of Occupational Therapy*, **45**(11), 1038–1044.

Yerkes-Dodson Law (1908) cited in Child D. (1973) *Psychology and the Teacher*. London: Holt Rinehart and Winston.

Section 4

Psychosocial Aspects of Physiotherapy Practice

22

Ethics and moral decision-making

Julius Sim

Introduction

This chapter is to do with the place of health care ethics within physiotherapy. It is, therefore, appropriate to start by trying to outline what is to be understood by 'health care ethics'. For the purposes of this chapter, I take this to mean the application of moral reasoning to the context of health care, so as to identify those courses of action which are morally right, and those which are morally wrong. We are dealing, therefore, with a decision-making procedure, but one which is primarily guided by moral criteria, as opposed to clinical, legal, bureaucratic, or other considerations.

A number of important points follow from this initial statement. First, ethical reasoning is applied to health care, it does not spring from within it. Consequently, there is no such thing as 'physiotherapy ethics', or for that matter 'medical ethics' or 'nursing ethics'. The particular situations with which we are dealing may 'belong' to physiotherapy, but the ethical principles that are applied to them are universal. It follows that health care practitioners can claim no specific moral authority on the basis of their professional expertise (Veatch, 1973; Kennedy, 1981). To be sure, such expertise will often be relevant when dealing with moral dilemmas, but it does not itself confer any special authority in ethical matters. Second, the ultimate end of the process is to take action. We are not engaged in abstract contemplation or philosophical speculation for its own sake; ethical reasoning in health care is an action-oriented business. Third, we are concerned with what is *morally* right. The fact that a certain course of action may be correct in terms of clinical judgement does not in itself guarantee that it is the right thing to do morally. What may seem an appropriate decision on clinical grounds may be morally objectionable, and, conversely, what may seem a dubious decision purely in terms of clinical judgement, may have much to recommend it as a moral course of action. This further reinforces the point that professional expertise does not carry with it moral expertise. It is also worth noting that, as we will see, the processes of ethical and clinical decision-making may be quite similar, even though they sometimes yield very different conclusions. Finally, it should be stressed that we are dealing with matters of ethics, not etiquette (Sim, 1983). Professional courtesies are important, but they do not necessarily raise ethical issues. The notion of 'professional ethics' has come to embrace wider concerns.

In the remainder of this chapter, I will attempt to examine health care ethics, and the specific process of moral decision-making, within the context of clinical physiotherapy. In the process, the question as to the 'objectivity' of ethics will be considered, and the role of professional codes of ethics will be addressed.

How do health care ethics concern the physiotherapist?

There has been a growing concern with the ethical issues associated with medicine and health care; numerous texts have been written in this area, and there are a number of academic journals devoted to ethical and other philosophical questions in health care. Where, then, do physiotherapists fit into this picture? With which aspects of this wide-ranging subject should they be concerned? At first sight, it may seem that many of the dramatic issues that one reads about in the newspapers, and which are the subject of television documentaries, have little to do with the practice of physiotherapy. Indeed, matters such as embryo research, organ transplantation, abortion, and *in vitro* fertilization are scarcely the everyday concern of the clinical physiotherapist. The sort of ethical questions that arise in physiotherapy tends to be of a more everyday nature:

1. Are some patients more deserving of treatment than others, and if so on what grounds?
2. How should we set treatment priorities within a caseload?
3. Should we obtain informed consent before treating a patient, and if so how 'informed' must this consent be, and what form should it take?
4. Can we justify persevering with treatment that is proving ineffective, just because continued treatment has been recommended?
5. Under what circumstances is it permissible to cause patients discomfort or pain?
6. Should we ever deliberately mislead patients as to their diagnosis, or the nature of the treatment they are being given?
7. With whom is it permissible to discuss the details of a patient's case?
8. What action should we take with respect to colleagues whom we perceive as incompetent, or whose conduct we regard as unethical?

However, the fact that these are not generally 'life and death' matters does not mean that they are not worthy of careful consideration. Some comments on ethics in nursing are equally applicable to physiotherapy:

'Moral dilemmas of the "do or die" variety help us to focus upon the moral choices we must make, and so debating ethical dilemmas is a useful exercise. We should not, however, allow the big dilemmas to detract from the more routine moral choices involved in nursing' (Melia, 1989).

The impact of these seemingly more minor issues on the patients whom they affect can easily be under-estimated, particularly by health professionals, to whom they may become somewhat 'routine' considerations. For example, practitioners may not fully appreciate the value which patients attach to the notion of truthfulness:

'... many physicians talk about such deception in a cavalier, often condescending and joking way, whereas patients often have an acute sense of injury and loss of trust at learning that they have been duped' (Bok, 1978).

This having been said, it is important to remember that there are in fact some 'high profile' ethical matters in which physiotherapists may be involved, albeit indirectly. It may be the consultant who takes the initial decision to withdraw treatment from a gravely ill patient, but the physiotherapist is very much involved in the subsequent process. As a member of the team, he or she must decide the extent to which physiotherapy treatment should also be limited or withdrawn. If antibiotics and other 'active' means of medical care have been abandoned, does this mean that chest physiotherapy should also be curtailed? Similarly, physiotherapists are rarely involved in enlisting patients' participation in potentially hazardous drug trials, but while such patients remain under their care the therapists involved may have to face associated ethical problems. For example, it may become clear that the patient was insufficiently informed as to the nature of the drug being tested, or the patient may express a desire to withdraw from the study which he or she is unwilling to voice to the physician conducting the research. In such instances, the physiotherapist, although not directly involved in the affair at the outset, may feel a moral obligation to take an active role, perhaps as an advocate for the patient.

Before turning to the specific process of reaching decisions on ethical questions in physiotherapy, it is necessary briefly to address some basic theoretical issues to do with ethics and ethical reasoning.

Theoretical issues

Ethical principles and approaches to ethics

There are a number of different ways in which philosophers have approached the business of making moral decisions. However, all of these approaches tend to have in common that they rest on certain ethical principles. An ethical principle can be regarded as the statement of a fundamental ethical value or belief. Thus, in very broad terms, the principle of *beneficence* states that one should strive to confer benefits on others, while the principle of *non-maleficence* states that one should seek to avoid inflicting harms on others. The classic expression of *non-maleficence* is the famous medical maxim *primum non nocere*, which suggests that there is a paramount prohibition in health care against causing harm. The principle of *respect for autonomy* requires us to preserve, and to promote, the self-determination or freedom of action of others, while the principle of *justice* insists that we should deal with others in a way that is fair and in accordance with their individual merit. According to this principle, we should treat everybody in the same way, unless there are morally relevant differences between individuals; it is legitimate to provide a greater level of care to some patients if their clinical needs are greater than those of others, but not on the basis of one's personal feelings towards them. The principle of *respect for persons* demands that we should deal with others with due regard for their dignity as individuals (Downie and Telfer, 1969). Given the potential for 'depersonalization' that exists in busy hospitals and other health care settings, this last principle is of considerable importance. It can be seen as grounded in ideas such as these:

> 'Respecting the patient as a person calls upon us to regard patients as unique individuals and to see them in the totality of their being, with physical, psychological, social, and spiritual dimensions alike ... it is as

persons that we are all fellow human beings, fellow members of the human community' (Corr and Corr, 1986).

From these general principles, secondary principles or duties can be derived which are somewhat more specific in their application. For example, the duty of confidentiality can be extracted from the wider principle of non-maleficence (Sim, 1996), and the principle of truthfulness, or veracity, can be derived from both the principle of respect for autonomy and the principle of respect for persons (Sim, 1986). We may, similarly, be able to identify certain rights in conjunction with secondary principles or duties; for example, if we as practitioners have a duty of veracity, patients, for their part, may be seen to have a reciprocal right to the truth.

An approach to ethics which tends to be guided ultimately by principles such as these is often referred to as a *deontological* approach. A subscriber to this way of thinking would use these principles as the final test of an ethical conflict. Accordingly, a physiotherapist working within this sort of framework would ensure that all patients were fully consulted as to the form that their rehabilitation is to take, in order to remain true to the principle of respect for autonomy, and would decline to inflict unpleasant or painful treatment on a seriously ill patient, so as not to infringe the principle of non-maleficence. Given that a number of different principles are at stake, the situation will sooner or later arise where two or more principles come into some degree of conflict; in such a case, some means of prioritizing among them will be arrived at. Thus, in the second example above, it might be felt that it is justifiable to cause the patient discomfort because this is ultimately to the individual's benefit (i.e. fulfils the principle of beneficence), and that because this benefit is likely to be enduring, whilst the discomfort is perhaps only transitory, considera-tions of non-maleficence are outweighed in this instance by those of beneficence.

An alternative approach is that of *consequentialism*. In contrast to deon-tological theories, where there are a number of ethical principles, conse-quentialism has a single supreme principle, which we could term the principle of *best outcome*. Here, courses of action are chosen not on the basis of the various ethical principles which they either fulfil or contra-vene, but strictly in terms of the consequences which they will bring about. Thus the justification for insisting that the truth be told in a certain situation would be that to do so produces better consequences for all concerned, rather than because this is required by a wider ethical prin-ciple such as respect for persons. Indeed, when deciding between two actions, the consequentialist will choose the one which produces the best consequences, even if this involves breaching certain ethical principles which the alternative course of action would have left intact. To return to an earlier example, a physiotherapist using a consequentialist framework might deliberately exclude patients from the planning of their rehabilita-tion, or withhold certain information from them, if he or she felt that more patients would be successfully rehabilitated in this way. The infringement of patients' autonomy involved would not be totally discounted, but in the final analysis it would take second place to the desirable consequences brought about.

To return briefly to deontology, we can note that precisely the opposite situation may obtain. The deontologist can insist that a certain course should be pursued because it best fulfils certain fundamental ethical principles, even if it produces less desirable consequences, on balance, than the alternative. Thus, it would be claimed that the truth should always be told to patients, even when demonstrably better consequences would flow from the telling of a lie, or that confidentiality should be upheld, even if a net balance of harm results from so doing. This is similar to the popular notion that good ends cannot justify a bad means.

Character traits

The emphasis so far has been on determining the right thing to *do* in a particular situation. However, many ethicists have also stressed the need to *be* the right sort of person. In other words, it is important to possess certain virtues or character traits, in addition to performing actions that are morally right (Purtilo, 1986; Johnstone, 1994; Nicholson, 1994). Among these morally desirable character traits are compassion, sensitivity, discretion, integrity, selflessness and courage. It is not difficult to see their importance. Unless therapists are compassionate and sensitive to the needs of patients, it is likely that they will be unaware of many situations in which the interests and welfare of their patients are under threat. If they do not possess the virtue of discretion, they may not recognize those situations in which confidentiality is called for. Unless therapists possess a certain measure of courage, they may lack the resolve to carry through morally appropriate courses of action in circumstances where doing so may make them unpopular, or place their own interests at risk.

Thus, moral virtue plays an important part both in the initial recognition of a moral situation, and in the pursuit of action which has been identified as morally appropriate.

Objectivity and ethics

It is important to address the common fallacy, identified by Gillon (1985), that ethics is 'just a matter of opinion', and that, consequently, there is no rational basis for deciding between competing views. There is indeed a subjective element in ethical reasoning, and this explains why there is not necessarily a *single* correct answer to an ethical dilemma (Purtilo, 1989). However, what we are dealing with here are certain fundamental, subjectively-held moral convictions; these must be distinguished from matters of taste or personal bias:

> 'Taste involves matters of choice which are, though value-laden, essentially morally neutral. This, indeed, is what we *mean* by a matter of mere taste – that it pertains simply to preference, to matters without moral import' (Callahan, 1988, original emphasis).

Furthermore, we are obliged to provide reasons for our decisions on moral matters in a way that we are not when deciding on questions of personal taste. In other words, morality involves us in a process of justification; but, we may ask, if there is a subjective element in ethics, how can we achieve any sort of objective process of justification? Here, it is important to realize that, although we cannot always justify our fundamental moral beliefs or principles according to any objective criteria, when we apply these principles to specific cases we are subject to certain stringent demands. If we fail to fulfil them, we can indeed be criticized. Just because ethical principles have an essential subjectivity about them, this is not to say that the whole process of ethical reasoning is subjective.

The first of these demands is that the way in which we link the particular situation to fundamental moral principles must be logically sound. In other words, when we seek to justify our decision in a certain case in terms of one or more of these principles, the steps we take in this justification must be logically defensible. Beauchamp and Childress (1994) see this as a hierarchical process (Figure 22.1). Our particular judgements and actions are logically derived from certain rules, which are themselves derived from the principles which they seek to support (and these principles may be further derived from certain wider ethical theories). The second requirement is that this process of justification should be based on an accurate assessment of the facts of the specific situation. We have to justify our decision-making process in terms of the empirical evidence.

4. Ethical theory

↑

3. Principles

↑

2. Rules

↑

1. Particular judgements

Figure 22.1 Hierarchical levels of ethical justification. Reproduced by permission of Oxford University Press, from Beauchamp T. L., Childress J. F. (1994) *Principles of Biomedical Ethics* (4th edn). New York: Oxford University Press, p. 15.

To take an example to illustrate these ideas, you may wish to justify a case of truth-telling in terms of the principle of respect for autonomy. Now, there is no conclusive way in which others can invalidate this principle (or the wider ethical theory on which it is based) as the starting point for your decision. To be sure, from their own subjective standpoint they can disagree with the moral weight which you attach to it, and relegate it in importance below certain other principles, but it cannot be dismissed out of hand on any objective grounds. The way in which you proceed to base a course of action on this principle, however, must stand up to objective scrutiny on a number of counts, and may well show itself flawed. Each of the steps in the process of justification in Figure 22.1 must be defended. If you choose to formulate a specific rule concerning truth-telling in order to uphold the principle of respect for autonomy (i.e. moving between levels 2 and 3 in Figure 22.1), you must demonstrate that this rule does indeed bear a strong relationship to the principle it is designed to fulfil; it is always open to somebody else to claim that a somewhat different rule is more appropriate. Similarly, when you enact this rule and take a specific course of action such as conveying certain information to a particular patient (i.e. moving between levels 1 and 2), the onus is once again on you to show that your action is faithful to the rule. Your critics may claim that modifications to your course of action, e.g. in its timing or the manner you presented the information, would have allowed it to conform better to your rule. Finally, your action must conform to the facts of the situation. It might be argued that you misread these. Perhaps what you took to be an apparent desire for information was in fact an implicit request to be shielded from unpleasant facts. As a result, your decision may have done more to breach the patient's autonomy than to preserve it.

Thus, whilst your adherence to the fundamental principle of autonomy cannot be refuted, nonetheless the procedure whereby you derive a moral rule from this principle, the way you translate this rule into concrete actions, and how you justify this process in terms of the external evidence, are all areas where you can potentially be accused of being mistaken. Indeed, the demands of ethical decision-making are very similar to those of such processes as clinical diagnosis and treatment planning. In both cases, there is a need for logical thought processes and close attention to the specific facts of the case in question, followed by the formulation of a systematic plan of action.

Making ethical decisions

The code of ethics: a source of help?

It is characteristic of occupational groups which have attained, or aspire to, professional status that they formulate a code of ethics (Sim, 1985). Both altruism and accountability are central to the concept of professionalism, and codes of professional ethics can often be seen to affirm these notions. An ethical code generally consists of a number of ethical principles or rules, intended to guide the practice of members of the profession. The code is also often the basis for any disciplinary actions taken by the profession against one of its members.

In what sense, it may be asked, can a code of ethics be expected to provide such guidance? What exactly can physiotherapists gain from a code, and, just as important, what can they *not* gain from it? Above all, an ethical code is a consensus document. It represents the outcome of careful deliberation, by representatives of the profession as a whole, as to the sort of conduct that is required from individual practitioners. As such, it seeks to highlight the fundamental principles upon which one's professional life as a physiotherapist should be conducted, and to alert one to possible dilemmas and areas of conflict. The question remains, however, whether codes of ethics successfully fulfil this function.

In the first instance, it is not immediately clear whether codes of ethics are specifically concerned with ethics, if by 'ethics' we mean an examination of what is morally right or wrong. In many ways, ethical codes tend not so much towards ethics in this sense, as towards a sense of ethics which has 'a specific content which refers to codified procedures, but lacks the prescriptive force of morality' (Downie, 1980). The American

Physical Therapy Association was in many ways ahead of its time when it drew up its first 'Code of Ethics and Discipline' in 1935. However, as Ruth Purtilo (1987) has argued, the Code's requirements had more to do with procedural notions of etiquette than with specifically ethical concerns. More recently, the Chartered Society of Physiotherapy's Revised Rules of Professional Conduct (CSP, 1996) have stated that 'Chartered physiotherapists shall respect the rights, dignity and individual sensibilities of every patient' (Rule II), and that they 'shall ensure the confidentiality and security of information acquired in a professional capacity' (Rule III). These strike at the heart of genuinely moral concerns. However, Rule IV in the same document requires that physiotherapists should avoid criticism of other professional staff, while Rule VI insists that advertising should be 'professionally restrained'. Meanwhile, Rule VIII reads: 'Chartered physiotherapists shall adhere at all times to personal and professional standards which reflect credit on the profession'. This is not to say that no ethical justification can be adduced for such requirements, but that they seem to reflect more of a focus on the profession's own public image than a concern for patients' welfare. The therapist who relies on a code of ethics must keep in mind a clear distinction between those aspects of the code which safeguard the interests of patients, and those which are geared towards the protection of professional interests. The former will almost invariably relate to genuinely ethical concerns, whereas the later may not necessarily do so. Hence, the guidance that can be gained from an ethical code will not be necessarily, or wholly, on strictly ethical matters, such as we have defined them.

Having identified those parts of a code of ethics which deal with areas of genuine ethical import, the physiotherapist should be aware that the help that can be derived from the code can only be of a very general nature, and will inevitably be expressed in fairly clear-cut terms. Those cases which are most ethically perplexing will be far too complex and individual to be adequately catered for by a set of rules or principles. Furthermore, the sensitive and intricate nature of the patient–practitioner relationship is ill-suited to regulation by a standard set of rules:

> 'No set of rules could encompass all the subtle complexities of even the most ordinary relationship between two persons, much less the special dimensions peculiar to the medical transaction in which one person in special need seeks the assistance of another who professes to help' (Pellegrino, 1979).

Alan Johnson suggests that ethical codes can be regarded as 'signposts on the way', but warns that it is 'easy to shelter behind a code to avoid thinking through the real issues' (Johnson, 1990). Indeed, Purtilo (1987) suggests that a 'code of ethics' is more appropriately understood as a 'code of morality'. By this she means that the code serves to highlight certain key moral concepts, such as duties and rights, but does not necessarily aid the individual in analysing these concepts, or applying them systematically and critically to concrete cases. In fact, while granting its value in drawing attention to important general ethical norms, one can see a way in which a code of ethics may actually impede an analytical approach to ethics. There is a danger that its codified nature, and the rather definitive terms in which it is expressed, may encourage the practitioner to think that 'the job has been done' and that further reflection on the issues concerned is redundant. As a result, decisions on ethical questions may become unreflective and stereotyped, and individual cases which are subtly but significantly different may be subsumed under a single category. It is vital that ethical 'rules of thumb' are re-examined, and even fundamentally questioned, every time they are invoked to deal with a specific situation.

The above should not be taken as a dismissal of codes of ethics. Rather, it is intended to draw attention to some of their shortcomings, and to suggest that they are at best a partial solution to ethical dilemmas. If we refer back to Figure 22.1, we can see that any sort of rule represents only one level in the process of ethical justification. Moving up the hierarchy, these rules must be justified in terms of overall ethical principles of autonomy, beneficence, the best outcome, etc. Meanwhile, moving in the opposite direction, we see that the general guidance afforded by an ethical code should be augmented by a more critical and individualized examination of the specific ethical demands of the case in question. In the light of these specific demands, broad guidelines must be modified and prioritized, and supplemented by the physiotherapist's own individual ethical deliberation.

Case study

A 54-year-old single woman, otherwise fit and healthy and previously employed as a clerical worker, has undergone an above-knee amputation following a road traffic accident a short distance from her bungalow. She arrives at the Rehabilitation Unit to take delivery of a temporary prosthesis and to begin walking training. The physiotherapists soon gain the impression that she is poorly motivated, and shows little interest in learning how to use the prosthetic limb. She views the prospect of life in a wheelchair with apparent equanimity. The rehabilitation team feel, however, that she has the prospect of a high level of functional independence with an artificial limb, but are unable to convince her of this. Where should they go from here?

There are two broad approaches that could be taken to this situation:

1. One approach would be essentially to ignore the patient's expressed wishes, and seek to inveigle or cajole her into taking part in a gait training programme. This could be justified in two ways. From a deontological standpoint, one could point to the principle of beneficence. In accordance with this, the therapist has a duty to act in the patient's best interests. In this case, these best interests could reasonably be understood as achieving functional independence, and this therefore becomes the goal at which the therapist should aim. If the patient seems a reluctant partner in this enterprise, the therapist must take steps to secure her participation, for her own ultimate good. Alternatively, if we adopt a consequentialist view of things, it could be argued that functional independence is a desirable – indeed the most desirable – possible outcome of the situation. Not only will it improve

the patient's future quality of life, but it will also bring benefits to others (she will, for example, be less reliant on formal or informal carers for support). In line with consequentialist thinking, the utility of this outcome more than makes up for any acts of apparent coercion performed on the way. Thus, in both variants of this approach, the focus is on the ultimate goal of rehabilitation, either because this represents the best interests of the patient herself, or because it is overall the best of all the alternative outcomes for all concerned.

2. Others, however, might raise objections to this first approach, and adopt a different strategy. An alternative line of action would be to accept the patient's view, cease gait training, and begin a programme of wheelchair rehabilitation. Such a decision could be justified, in deontological terms, by the principle of autonomy. The sort of beneficent action outlined in the first approach, it might be argued, has been carried to the point at which it violates the individual's self-determination. As such, it would be seen as an example of paternalism:

'... Physical therapists who believe that it is their *primary* duty to benefit patients and protect them from harm – including harm from patients' own choices – feel justified in acting paternalistically' (Coy, 1989, original emphasis).

In other words, paternalism would suggest that the autonomy of the patient may be overridden so as better to serve her own interests, on the basis that the therapist can judge these interests better than she. In contrast to this stance, the present option places autonomy above competing principles such as beneficence, perhaps on the grounds that freedom of self-determination is part of what it is to be a person. An individual who is rendered non-autonomous loses something of his or her personal dignity. This is not to say that no value is attached to the principle of beneficence, simply that it should be regarded as *prima facie* – that is, it can be made to yield if it is at variance with another principle, such as respect for autonomy or respect for persons, which carries more moral weight in the given situation.

It is important to realize that this second course of action might very well lead to seemingly undesirable consequences for the patient – loss of mobility, greater dependence on others, reduced social contact, and so forth. However, seeking to avoid such consequences would not necessarily justify contravening the principle of respect for autonomy. As we noted earlier, it is maintained within a classic deontological approach that an ethical principle should be upheld, even if doing so seems likely to produce worse consequences overall than an alternative action which would breach this principle. Moreover, it should be remembered that the right to choose for oneself implies the right to make unwise choices, and that full respect for autonomy may involve allowing individuals to come to some degree of harm (Loewy, 1989). In any case, therapists should be wary of assuming that the patient's view of a desirable or an undesirable outcome necessarily corresponds to their own.

So far, we have seen how these alternative approaches to the situation might be justified in terms of the various ethical principles and values at stake. However, it will be recalled that ethical decisions must also be justified empirically. It is not enough to produce ethical arguments that are internally coherent, they must also be in accordance with the external evidence of the case. We must ask, then, whether the approaches we have considered are compatible with the facts of the situation (bearing in mind, of course, that we have here only a few of the facts which would be available in the real case). The first approach, in both its deontological and consequentialist variants, relies on the value of achieving functional independence, either because this is in the patient's best interests, or because it is the most favourable set of possible consequences overall. Implicit in these arguments is the idea that, on the available evidence, functional independence is a likely outcome. Given what we know of the patient – that she is comparatively young, and otherwise fit and well – this seems to be a reasonable assumption. Additionally, the fact that she is single – and thus presumably without the constant availability of a partner as a source of help – serves to reinforce the *need* for independence. The fact that it is a demonstrable benefit lends support to any beneficent action undertaken to secure it.

On the other hand, when we consider the alternative approach that may be taken to this situation, we can find some support for the contention that the patient could attain a reasonable level of independence even if dependent on a wheelchair. It is perhaps fair to assume that she could meet the demands of her job adequately in a wheelchair, and we know that she lives in a bungalow, thus obviating the need to climb stairs. However, a much more fundamental factual question may arise within this approach. The strategy adopted is founded on the patient's expressed wish not to proceed with gait rehabilitation. It is crucial that this is indeed the correct interpretation. It could be argued that what seemed to be an unwillingness to participate in rehabilitation was in fact only an expression of apprehension as to the hurdles that she will face in the process, and mistrust of her own ability to succeed (particularly if no such reluctance had been expressed by the patient previously). Another alternative is that the patient could be undergoing a reactive depression following the loss of her leg, and is thereby unable to make fully autonomous choices. If either of these were indeed the more plausible interpretation, much of the justification for the autonomy-based approach falls away.

This case illustrates how a situation may present the physiotherapist with fundamentally different ethical alternatives. Each of these has its merits, but in each case there are also possible difficulties. The question as to which is the option to be favoured cannot be settled definitively, but will always remain an open question. What matters is that, whichever course of action is adopted, it can be justified in terms of ethical reasoning and in the light of the particular facts of the case.

Whatever approach is taken, it is clear that a full and open dialogue between therapist and patient will aid the process of ethical decision-making. In this way, a clear picture of the patient's needs and desires, and an understanding of the likely effects of various possible courses of action, will usually emerge. Basically, it is hard to respect the interests and preferences of the patient if one hasn't made the necessary effort to find out what they are.

Conclusion

In this chapter, I have endeavoured to examine the place of health care ethics in physiotherapy, and to show how ethical reasoning can be applied to the sort of situations which may arise in physiotherapy practice. Although there are often no definitive answers to ethical conflicts and dilemmas, reaching a conclusion on such matters is a rigorous process, and certainly not a mere matter of opinion. Codes of ethics may give help on the way, but ultimately it is for the individual therapist to evaluate each case on its merits, and to justify the course of action decided upon. It is crucial to realize that ethical decision-making is not an optional element in the practice of physiotherapy. Just as one cannot perform competently as a therapist if one is unwilling to assess one's patients, so there is an ethical commitment that is integral to the role of the health care worker (Sim, 1983). To undertake a patient's treatment is to enter into a 'moral transaction' (Coates, 1990), with all the ethical problems that this may entail. This is inescapable, for failing to confront these problems is itself a decision with far-reaching ethical implications.

References

Beauchamp T. L., Childress J. F. (1994) *Principles of Biomedical Ethics* (4th edn). New York: Oxford University Press

Bok S. (1978) *Lying: Moral Choice in Public and Private Life*. Hassocks: Harverster Press.

Callahan J. C. (1988) Basics and background. In *Ethical Issues in Professional Life* (Callahan J. C. , ed.). New York: Oxford University Press, pp. 3–25.

Coates R. (1990) Ethics and physiotherapy. *Australian Journal of Physiotherapy*, **36**, 84–87.

Corr C. A., Corr D. M. (1986) Developing a philosophy for caring. In *Cash's Textbook of Neurology for Physiotherapists* (4th edn) (Downie P. A., ed.). London: Faber and Faber, pp. 21–32.

Coy J. A. (1989) Autonomy-based informed consent: ethical implications for patient noncompliance. *Physical Therapy*, **69**, 826–833.

CSP (1996) Rules of professional conduct. *Physiotherapy*, **81**, 460.

Downie R. S. (1980) Ethics, morals and moral philosophy. *Journal of Medical Ethics*, **6**, 33–34.

Downie R. S., Telfer E. (1969) *Respect for Persons*. London: George Allen and Unwin.

Gillon R. (1985) 'It's all too subjective': scepticism about the possibility of use of philosophical medical ethics. *British Medical Journal*, **290**, 1574–1575.

Johnson A. G. (1990) *Pathways in Medical Ethics*. London: Edward Arnold.

Johnstone M.- J. (1994) *Bioethics: a Nursing Perspective* (2nd edn). Sydney: W. B. Saunders/Baillière Tindall.

Kennedy I. (1981) *The Unmasking of Medicine*. London: George Allen and Unwin.

Loewy E. H. (1989) *Textbook of Medical Ethics*. New York: Plenum Publishing.

Melia K. (1989) *Everyday Nursing Ethics*. London: Macmillan.

Nicholson R. H. (1994) Limitations of the four principles. In *Principles of Health Care Ethics* (Gillion R., Lloyd A., eds). Chichester: John Wiley, pp. 267–275.

Pellegrino E. D. (1979) Toward a reconstruction of medical morality: the primacy of the act of profession and the fact of illness. *Journal of Medicine and Philosophy*; **4**, 32–56.

Purtilo R. (1986) Professional responsibility in physiotherapy: old dimensions and new directions. *Physiotherapy*, **72**, 579–583.

Purtilo R. B. (1987) Codes of ethics in physiotherapy: a retrospective view and look ahead. *Physiotherapy Practice*, **3**, 28–34.

Purtilo R. B. (1989) Ethical considerations in physical therapy. In *Physical Therapy* (Scully R. M., Barnes M. R., eds). Philadelphia: J. B. Lippincott, pp. 36–40.

Sim J. (1983) Ethical considerations in physiotherapy. *Physiotherapy*, **69**, 119–120.

Sim J. (1985) Physiotherapy: a professional profile. *Physiotherapy Practice*, **1**, 14–22.

Sim. J. (1986) Truthfulness in the therapeutic relationship. *Physiotherapy Practice*, **2**, 121–127.

Sim J. (1996) Client confidentiality: ethical issues in occupational therapy. *British Journal of Occupational Therapy*, **59**, 56–61.

Veatch R. M. (1973) Generalization of expertise. *Hastings Center Studies*, **1**, 29–40.

23

Defining disability: its implications for physiotherapy practice
Sally French

There is no simple way of defining disability, it can be viewed from many perspectives. Within every society there are competing models of disability with some being more dominant than others at different times. These models, although often in conflict, gradually influence and modify each other. The models put forward by powerful groups within society, such as the medical profession and the government, tend to dominate the models of less powerful groups, such as those of disabled people themselves.

It is very important to explore the ways in which disability is defined, as well as who defines it, for attitudes and behaviour towards disabled people, professional practice, and the running of institutions, such as rehabilitation centres and hospitals, are based, at least in part, on these definitions. As Oliver (1993) points out, 'The "lack of fit" between able-bodied and disabled people's definitions is more than just a semantic quibble for it has important implications both for the provision of services and the ability to control one's life'.

The individualistic model of disability

Most models of disability are based upon the assumption that the problems and difficulties disabled people experience are a direct result of their individual physical, sensory or intellectual impairments. This position is articulated most clearly in the medical model of disability.

The medical model of disability

The medical and health and welfare professions are dominant and powerful agents in defining disability. The medical model of disability has led people to view it in terms of disease process, abnormality, and personal tragedy. Brechin and Liddiard (1981) point out that the medical model has guided and dominated clinical practice with the resulting assumption that both problems and solutions lie within disabled people rather than within society. The medical approach has been insufficiently broad to concern itself with disability from the disabled person's point of view, or the disabling effects of society itself. Oliver (1990) states, '... the medical approach produces definitions of disability which are partial and limited and which fail to take into account wider aspects of disability'.

Because the medical model lies at the heart of clinical practice it may be difficult for health and welfare professionals, including physiotherapists, to consider changing their attitudes and behaviour towards disability and disabled people. McKnight (1981) points out that the existence of many professional roles are dependent on viewing disability in terms of the medical model, and that the very tools and techniques which professionals have at their disposal serve to define and individualize problems. Oliver (1993) is of the opinion that the medical model of disability may serve the needs of professionals more than the needs of disabled people, and Ryan and Thomas (1987), talking of people with learning difficulties, state:

> 'Medical model thinking tends to support the status quo. The subnormality of the individual rather than the subnormality of the environment, tends to be blamed for any inadequacies ... Within most institutions staff have a vested interest in not questioning the quality of the patients' environment too radically, for they themselves are part of that environment'.

Ryan and Thomas also believe that although the causes of learning difficulties, if known at all, are usually related to socioeconomic conditions such as malnutrition and poverty, medicine has concerned itself mainly with the study of rare syndromes, and its emphasis on abnormality and incurability has justified the appalling conditions under which people with learning difficulties have had to live. They believe that learning difficulties provide a case study of the medicalization of a social problem.

Individualistic professional definitions, those from both inside and outside the health and welfare professions, certainly have the potential to do serious harm. The medicalization of learning difficulties, which is now being questioned, is one example. Another is oralism, the belief that deaf people should dispense with sign language and learn to rely exclusively on lip reading. The philosophy and practice of oralism has led Ladd (1990) to believe that human beings are capable of disabling each other far more profoundly than could any impairment. It is certainly most unlikely that a deaf person would ever have devised such a plan. (For further information about oralism and the backlash against it, the reader is referred to Ladd (1988), and Gregory and Hartley (1991).

Other institutions within society also take a medicalized, individualistic stance to disability. This was so, until recently, in education where children were categorized fairly rigidly in terms of their impairments. It eventually became apparent that categorizing children in this way, while paying scant attention to their other characteristics and attributes, made little sense, and in the 1981 Education Act the broader notion of 'special educational needs' emerged, as well as a resolve to educate disabled children in mainstream schools.

The concept of 'special educational needs' has itself been criticized for focusing on individual children, rather than on educational policy and practice. The criteria and assessment procedures for extra help or support are heavily based on tests of impairment. Oliver (1983) states, 'The individual model sees the problems that disabled people experience as being a direct consequence of their disability. The major task of the professional is therefore to adjust the individual to the particular disabling condition'.

Ellis (1993) found that professionals, when assessing disabled people, believed that need arose directly from impairment, and that professional interventions were aimed at enabling the disabled individual to cope safely and independently.

By individualizing disability the effect of the environment upon the lives of disabled people is not addressed. Indeed the environments imposed upon disabled people in the name of treatment, for example mental handicap hospitals and Young Disabled Units, can have detrimental effects leading to greater dependency and an increase in existing problems of function or behaviour. In addition people subjected to such environments may be the very people who are most susceptible to their adverse effects.

Health and welfare professionals have considerable control in the lives of disabled people over non-medical decisions such as housing, employment and education. This has led some disabled people to complain that although their particular impairments give rise to no medical problems and cannot be improved by medical intervention, medicine has nonetheless had a dominant influence over important decisions affecting their lives (French, 1987). Finkelstein (1991) is of the opinion that issues relating to disability would be better placed in the Department of the Environment, rather than the Department of Health, and that important new disciplines in engineering and architecture need to be developed.

It should never be assumed, however, that there is consensus regarding the definitions of disability or illness between or within the various health and welfare professions. Our perceptions of disability are shaped by a multitude of factors not least of which is professional education, socialization and specialization. The effect of this is often to produce a narrowed perception of disability which can easily give rise to conflict or ineffective communication with both disabled people and colleagues (French, 1994a). (For information on the attitudes of health professionals towards disabled people, the reader is referred to Chapter 7).

Administrative models of disability

Administrative models of disability tend to be rigid and dichotomous and are often written into legislation and acts of parliament with legal implications. These models usually relate to specific areas of life such as education and employment, and are used to assess whether or not people are eligible for certain benefits, or compensation. The definitions of disability which arise from these models, as well as the measurements and criteria used for assessment, almost always relate to people's impairments rather than the physical and social environments in which they are obliged to live. One of the problems with rigid definitions such as these, is that, owing to the complexity of disability, disabled people rarely fit into the neat boxes administrators provide. For this reason administrative definitions are often viewed as unfair and divisive. It is not uncommon for severely disabled people to be denied benefits because their impairments or disabilities do not fit the rigid criteria demanded. It was not until 1990, for example, that people who are both deaf and blind were eligible for the mobility allowance.

Rigid definitions of disability can be harmful in other ways. As noted above, until recent times children with a given impairment, such as blindness or partial hearing, were educated in special schools regardless of their other characteristics and attributes, the decision being based largely on tests of impairment. Similarly until 1971 children whose IQ scores fell below a certain level were said to be 'ineducable', but it is now known that an individual's IQ score is a less than perfect predictor of ability and social capacity, and that children with learning difficulties need more, rather than less, education.

This having been said, loose administrative definitions can be even more dangerous than rigid ones because large numbers of people can be readily labelled 'disabled' and treated accordingly. Under the Mental Deficiency Acts of 1913 and 1927, for example, people could be categorized as 'mentally deficient' without any reference to their personal circumstances or intellect, and many were detained merely because of socially disapproved behaviour, such as becoming pregnant, having emotional problems, or failing to give the right answers to a series of questions (Laing and McQuarrie, 1989; Potts and Fido, 1991; Humphries and Gordon, 1992).

Finkelstein (1991) uses the term 'administrative model' in a rather different way. He views it as an over-arching model which encompasses those models of disability where disabled people are thought to be in need of care and ministration by others; he refers to it as the 'cure or care' approach. For Finkelstein the medical model is merely a variant of the administrative model; thus if the medical profession were to lose its power, the work of ministering to disabled people would be taken over by some other agency. This is happening, to some extent, as a result of 'care in the community' policies.

The philanthropic model of disability

Charities have tended to portray disabled people as helpless, sad, courageous and in need of care and protection (Scott-Parker, 1989; Barnes, 1992). Such images, presumably believed to be the most effective means of raising money, are now thought to have caused considerable harm to disabled people by perpetuating damaging stereotypes and misconceptions. Charities frequently mislead the public in the type of client they portray. Organizations for visually impaired people, for example, have tended to depict a disproportionate number of blind children with no additional impairments, whereas in reality the majority of their clients are elderly, partially sighted, or multiply disabled: people who are, perhaps, less likely to arouse emotion, public sympathy, and support.

Many disabled people find images presented by charities offensive, as their demonstrations against 'telethon' and 'red nose day' illustrate. Disabled people have complained that these and similar events serve to give publicity to companies and to provide entertainment for non-disabled people, as well as boosting their egos as they publicly donate large sums of money (*Disability Now*, 1990). Organizations such as the Campaign to Stop Patronage, and the British Council of Organization of Disabled people, believe the funds given to charities would be far better used by disabled people directly to campaign politically for their rights.

In recent years the portrayal of disabled people by charities has become a little more positive. These images can, however, be just as misleading and damaging as negative ones, for they tend to concentrate on exceptional disabled people, thereby denying or minimizing the considerable problems that the majority face, they underline the message, that society expects disabled people to overcome what are viewed as *their* problems, to be 'normal' or even superhuman.

Lay models of disability

Lay models of disability are diverse and constantly changing, they are influenced by other models such as those presented by charities and the medical profession. Models from the past, from religion, and from other cultures, such as the association between disability and sin, and disability and virtue, may still linger and are sometimes reinforced in novels and plays (Karph, 1986; Barnes, 1992). Negative images of disabled people depicting them as sad, pathetic and dangerous, are also frequently represented in the arts of today.

Disability of a family member will be defined according to the interests and beliefs of that person and his or her family, which in turn will be influenced by prevailing cultural beliefs, attitudes and practices. A child with a physical impairment may be considered very disabled in a family whose main interest is sport, but hardly disabled at all in a family with more sedentary interests. Likewise a child who finds difficulty reading may be seen as very disabled in a highly intellectual family but not in a family with little interest in academic success. What is and what is not regarded as a disability is also reflected in social structures and values. Learning difficulties, for example, have become more disabling over the course of this century as the ability to read and cope with complex situations has become more important (French, 1994b). Humphries and Gordon (1992) in their book about disability in the first half of the twentieth century, showed how, for many families, disability was a taboo subject causing shame and disappointment. These feelings were often internalized by disabled children who could not talk about their disabilities within the family or outside.

Age can influence how a disability is viewed by both the disabled person and others. Impairment or illness may be considered 'normal' or less tragic in old age depending on the particular family and culture. Disability in girls may be accepted and tolerated more readily than disability in boys, because the traditional role of the female has tended towards greater dependency. Thus ideas and perceptions of disability cannot be divorced from wider attitudes and beliefs about age and gender.

Self-definitions of disability

The social model

In the past it has been considered unnecessary to discover how disabled people view their situation. Like most under-privileged minority groups their views have been disregarded and suppressed. Disabled people have been traditionally considered dependent and in need of care. This attitude has led to the models of non-disabled people being thrust upon them. With the growing disability movement this situation has started to change. Oliver (1990) states:

'From the 1950s onwards ... there was a growing realisation that if particular social problems were to be resolved or at least ameliorated, then nothing more or less than a fundamental redefinition of the problem was necessary'.

Although it should be borne in mind that disabled people form a heterogeneous group, with widely differing attitudes, there is growing evidence that their views of disability are thoroughly out of tune with those of professional workers. Oliver (1990) believes that whereas professionals view disability as stemming from the functional limitations of impaired individuals, disabled people believe that they stem from the failure of the social and physical environment to take account of their needs. Davis (1993) points out that alternative solutions and innovative plans presented by disabled people, have often been regarded as unrealistic by professional 'experts' who tend to view disabled people within the confines of a stereotyped role.

The following definitions of impairment and disability are based upon those of the former organization The Union of the Physically Impaired Against Segregation (UPIAS) (1976):

Impairment
'Impairment is the lack of part or all of a limb, or having a defective limb, organ or mechanism of the body.'

Disability
'The disadvantage or restriction of activity caused by a contemporary social organisation which takes no or little account of people who have physical impairments and thus excludes them from the mainstream of social activities.'   (UPIAS, 1976)

These and similar definitions have been adopted by politically active organizations of disabled people. Stevens (1992) defines a disabled person as 'someone who as a consequence of their impairment experiences social oppression of whatever kind' and disablism as 'a form of social oppression towards disabled people.' Thus disability results from an interaction between impairment and the physical and social world.

Oliver (1990) regards disabled people's views as constituting a social model of disability, where the problems are seen, not within the individual disabled person, but within society. Thus the person who uses a wheelchair is not disabled by paraplegia but by building design, lack of lifts, rigid work practices, and the attitudes of others. Similarly the visually impaired person is not disabled by lack of sight, but by lack of braille, cluttered pavements, and stereotypical ideas about blindness. Finkelstein (1981) has argued that non-disabled people would be equally disabled if the environment was not designed with their needs in mind. Oliver (1990) contends that as the debate has occurred against a backdrop of discrimination and the struggle of disabled people against it, the neutral term 'social model' could just as well be replaced by the more politically laden term 'social oppression model.'

In recent years a number of disabled people, particularly women, have sought to extend the social model of disability to include impairment. Crow (1992) and French (1993a) believe that it has been necessary for disabled people to provide a clear, unambiguous definition of disability to bring about political change. Admitting that there may be a negative side to disability, or highlighting problems which cannot be readily solved by social or environmental manipulation, may undermine the campaign. This has led to disabled activists ignoring impairment which has become something of a taboo subject. Yet as Crow (1992) points out '... an impairment such as pain or chronic illness may curtail an individual's activities so much that the restriction of the outside world becomes irrelevant'. She points out that disability is not always insignificant or positive, and believes that when disabled people ignore impairment they do so at considerable cost to themselves. Shakespeare (1993) agrees, he states 'It is important not to ignore differences between impairments, despite the tendency of writers to gloss over differences in favour of the totalising and unifying role of oppression'.

These criticisms of the social model in no way invalidate it. Most of the disabled critics are merely aiming to increase its usefulness and power. As Crow (1991) explains:

> 'Integrating all the external and internal factors into the social model is vital if we are to understand fully the disability impairment equation. This does not in any way undermine the social model, nor should it weaken our resolve for change ... Disability is still socially created, still unacceptable, and still there to be changed, but integrating impairment into the equation gives us the best route to creating a world that includes us all'.

Classifying disability

The International Classification of Disease (ICD)

The International Classification of Disease (ICD) classifies disease in terms of its aetiology, pathology and manifestations, but does not consider the effects of these on the individual; it is a classification system based entirely upon the medical model of disease. The system works reasonably well when considering acute illness, such as pneumonia, but is unsatisfactory when attempting to describe or understand chronic illness or disability. For this reason a new and broader system was adopted by the World Health Organization in 1980.

The International Classification of Impairments, Disabilities and Handicaps (ICIDH)

This classification system takes a broader view of disease and impairment than the ICD by considering the consequences of it from the affected individual's point of view. The increase in chronic, long-term disease, and the decrease in acute disease, has made the ICD less and less useful. The ICIDH also attempts to classify and describe the consequences of impairments, such as absence of an eye or a limb, which cannot be described in terms of disease. 'Impairment', 'disability', and 'handicap' are defined as follows:

1. *Impairment* – Any loss or abnormality of psychological, physiological or anatomical structure or function. Thus an impairment could range from a scar on the skin to the malfunction of the liver or the heart.
2. *Disability* – Any restriction or lack of ability to perform an activity, as a result of impairment, in a manner or within the range considered

normal for a human being, for example the ability to climb the stairs or walk to the shops.

3. *Handicap* – A disadvantage for a given individual, resulting from an impairment or a disability, that limits or prevents the fulfilment of a role for that individual (depending on age, sex, and social and cultural factors). Handicap refers to the disadvantage the individual encounters, as a result of the impairment and/or the disability, when compared with his or her peers.

This scheme illustrates that the concepts of 'impairment', 'disability', and 'handicap' are independent of each other, though they can also coexist. Take, for example, a person with a facial deformity or skin disease which, using this system, would be classed as impairments. People with impairments such as these will probably experience no disability, as independent living is unlikely to be impeded. Nevertheless, they may experience considerable handicap, being denied employment in certain occupations, or full social integration. A person with a facial deformity or a skin disorder may very well experience more handicap than someone with a substantial disability, and a person with a mild disability may experience more handicap than a person with a severe disability.

The concepts of 'illness' and 'disease' are also independent of 'impairment', 'disability' and 'handicap'. For example, a person with rheumatoid arthritis, has a disease, may well feel ill, and is also likely to be disabled. On the other hand, someone who loses a limb as a result of an accident, or is partially sighted as a result of albinism, can hardly be described as ill or diseased, such people may, in fact, be extremely fit and healthy. It is unfortunate that disability is so often equated with disease and illness automatically. Harrison (1987) complains that the term 'chronically sick' is often used synonymously with disability even though those with the most profound disabilities can be quite free of disease. The Chronically Sick and Disabled Person's Act encouraged these often erroneous connections.

The ICIDH has come under severe criticism by organizations controlled by disabled people, and has been rejected by the organization 'Disabled People's International' (IDP). Although the system moves away from a narrow medical definition and acknowledges that disability has social dimensions, both disability and handicap are viewed as *arising* from impairment rather than from social and environmental sources, and the social and physical environment is taken for granted and assumed to be fixed. The system also fails to address issues of central importance to disabled people, such as their education, employment and housing, and the concept of 'normality' is accepted uncritically with little recognition of its cultural and temporal determinants.

Conflict between the medical and social models of disability

In discussing the conflict between the medical and social models of disability, the concepts of 'independence', 'normality', 'acceptance' and 'adjustment' will be briefly examined, for these are concepts on which disabled people and health professionals tend to disagree.

Independence

Physical independence, such as cooking, washing and dressing, is generally considered to be something disabled people desire above all else. In many ways this is so, for if a person is excessively dependent on others, then he or she must fit in with their schedules and plans with a subsequent loss of freedom and autonomy. In addition it is all too easy for the relationship to develop into an unequal one, with the helper having undue power and the disabled person being compelled constantly to express gratitude, or at best never to complain. This oppression is difficult to challenge because many disabled people need some assistance and its continuance may depend on expressing a sufficient degree of appreciation. The obligation is based on the often false assumption that disabled people are unable to reciprocate the help they receive.

Physiotherapists and other health professionals usually regard physical independence as a central aim of the rehabilitation process. But is it always in the best interests of disabled people to strive for independence of this type? A disabled woman featured in Campling's book, thinks not, she explains, 'I can sew but so slowly that it bores me to do it'. (Campling, 1981). Similarly, a person with a physical impairment may seek assistance in cleaning, cooking and dressing, as so many non-disabled people do, in order to save time and energy to lead a full and satisfying life. Morris (1989) found that many of the women with spinal cord injuries she interviewed chose to rely on personal assistance so that they could concentrate on other things, such as community work or involvement in political activity.

The pressures placed upon disabled people to achieve physical independence can be regarded as a form of oppression. Sutherland (1981) quotes a disabled person as saying:

> 'I've known a few people who, as adults, have refused to walk even though they could because its just not worth the effort. And people have often got angry with them, often. They've been labelled lazy and all sorts of things. They're definitely considered odd if they choose to be in a wheelchair, in the same way as you're considered odd if you don't struggle to do something that you can actually do even though it takes you six hours'.

Disabled people define independence, not in physical terms, but in terms of control. People who are almost totally dependent on others, in a physical sense, can still have independence of thought and action, enabling them to take full and active charge of their lives.

It is frequently the case that non-disabled people are dependent on disabled people in some way, perhaps as those with time to help or listen or, in the case of health professionals, as a way of earning their living! There is a huge commercial industry around disability providing lucrative work for many people. There is often an erroneous assumption that disabled people are unable to reciprocate the help they receive, whereas in reality people who require assistance are often carers themselves (Morris, 1991; Potts and Fido, 1991; Parker, 1993; Walmsley, 1993).

We are, of course, all dependent on each other to a large extent, and we all use aids, such as, washing machines, scissors, motor cars, aeroplanes, eating utensils, and computers, to save time and to overcome physical limitations such as our inability to move fast or to fly. We are also dependent on other people to produce and repair these aids. As Oliver (1993) points out, the dependency of disabled people '… is not a feature that marks them out as different in kind from the rest of the population but as different in degree'. Despite the interdependency of us all, the dependency of disabled people tends to be regarded as special and qualitatively different.

The problems disabled people face and the equipment they need, such as wheelchairs, visual aids and hoists, are also regarded as exceptional. This creates beliefs among physiotherapists and others that disabled people should 'manage' in as 'normal' a way as possible and that 'unnecessary' aids may harm them by reducing the amount of exercise they take or by making them lazy and dependent. These beliefs, and the control of professionals over resources, exacerbate the considerable practical difficulties disabled people face in acquiring the aids and equipment they need (Davis, 1993).

The physical and psychological stress involved in gaining independence in basic tasks, as well as the wasted time and reduced social opportunities incurred, are rarely given much attention by anyone other than disabled people themselves. Yet we do not insist that people walk 6 miles or even one rather than using their motor cars, or that they dispense with labour saving devices in case they become lazy, or dependent on the people who produce or repair them. Indeed, to attempt to enforce such a plan would be considered extremely patronizing and a serious breach of human rights, even if it were motivated in terms of the person's 'own good.'

Normality

Closely associated with the concept of independence is that of normality. The pressures placed upon disabled people to appear 'normal' can give rise to enormous inefficiency and stress, yet many disabled people are well into adulthood before they realize what is happening or before they find the courage to abandon such attempts (Campling, 1981; French, 1993b).

The pressure to be 'normal' is often at the expense of the disabled person's needs and rights. For example, if a person with a motor impairment who can walk short distances is denied a wheelchair, he or she may become isolated or unsuitable for certain types of education or employment. Mason (1992) believes that, 'Almost every activity of daily living can take on the dimension of trying to make you less like yourself and more like the able-bodied', and Ryan and Thomas (1987) contend that the conventional and conformist lifestyles forced upon disabled people can be an exaggeration of normality. Munro and Elder-Woodward (1992) state:

'Service users should not have to conform to the standards and values of the majority of society, nor to the expectations of service providers, they should have access to the full range of possibilities so that they can make choices using their own values and interests'.

The goal of 'normality' can also be physically dangerous, as when the person with a severe visual impairment avoids using a white stick. The use of crutches over many years can put excessive strain on upper limb joints, and rendering an impairment less visible can create social problems which are equally or more difficult to manage than when the impairment is exposed. As a disabled woman in Sutherland's book explains, 'I'm happier with something that isn't a deception than with something that is'. (Sutherland, 1981). Sutherland (1981), drawing heavily on the experiences of disabled people in encounters with health professionals, talks at length of this. He states:

> 'There's a tremendous emphasis on a child who's had polio or whatever to walk, to be as able-bodied as possible. It's like standing up is infinitely better than sitting down, even if you're standing up in a total frame – metal straps and God knows what – that weighs a ton, that you can't move in, which hurts, takes hours to get on and off and looks ugly. It's assumed that that's what you want and that's what is best for you'.

Because of the negative attitudes towards disability which prevail in society, disabled people and those who live and work with them, may come to the conclusion that attempting to be 'normal' is the only way to succeed; the goal of normality is thus justified in terms of social acceptance. For example, it can be argued that one of the objectives of deaf people learning to talk, blind people learning to use facial expression appropriately, and people with Down's syndrome having plastic surgery, is that they will be more socially acceptable, less isolated, and better able to compete with non-disabled people.

Although these ideas contain some truth, the problem with this approach is that disabled people must carry the entire burden of disability themselves, while society learns nothing of its true nature. These expectations lead many disabled people to try and become 'superhuman' so as to avoid the negative stereotypes of helplessness and inadequacy. Morris (1991) contends that those who play the role of 'honorary non-disabled person' do little to further the interests of disabled people as a whole. This type of behaviour is, however, often rewarded by health professionals and encouraged in the professional literature (Swaffield, 1986).

Morris (1991) believes that the assumption that disabled people want to be 'normal', rather than just as they are, is one of the most oppressive experiences to which they are subjected. She rejects the view that it is progressive and liberating to ignore difference believing that disabled people have a right to be both equal and different. She states, '... I do not want to have to try to emulate what a non-disabled woman looks like in order to assert positive things about myself. I want to be able to celebrate my difference, not hide from it'. (Morris, 1991).

Acceptance and adjustment

Physiotherapists and other health professionals have viewed their roles as one of helping disabled people *accept* their disabilities and *adjust* to them. Disabled people have been urged to *overcome* what are viewed as *their* problems, to learn to live with them and never to complain. Any anger or depression concerning lack of access, negative attitudes, inappropriate rehabilitation, poor housing, or non-existent educational or job prospects, have been viewed as evidence of maladjustment, denial, and 'chips on their shoulders'.

As well as making a physical adjustment it is assumed that the disabled person must also make a psychological adjustment. There has certainly been a growing trend towards counselling by health professionals indicating a developing psychological orientation. It is thought that becoming disabled is inevitably psychologically devastating, a personal tragedy. Although some people may experience disability in this way it is the experience of many disabled people that becoming disabled opens up new and satisfying opportunities (British Psychological Society, 1989). Even people who do mourn may be mourning the loss of their independence rather than the loss of bodily function or appearance, a situation which could to a large extent be eliminated by social and environmental change.

The notion that disabled people should accept their situation and adjust to it, thus arises from an individualistic model of disability where it is conceptualized as a relatively unchangeable, internal state of the individual, rather than the result of physical and social barriers which could be removed if the political will to do so was there. Individualistic conceptions of disability have been severely criticized by disabled people who have concluded that they serve the interests, not of themselves, but of the non-disabled majority. It is very convenient for society that disabled people should accept what are viewed as *their* problems and adjust to them, for in that way the status quo is maintained.

Conclusion

The relationship between disabled people and health professionals has never been an easy one, for it is an unequal relationship with the professional holding most of the power. Traditionally the professional worker has defined, planned and delivered the services while the disabled person has been a passive recipient with little if any opportunity to exercise control. Disabled people's definitions of the problems they face, and the appropriate solutions to them, are generally given insufficient weight thereby seriously hampering the rehabilitation process, for if there is no consensus little real progress can be made.

Over the last 20 years or so disabled people have become increasingly organized and politically active, Centres of Integrated Living, coalitions of disabled people and international disability organizations, run and controlled by disabled people themselves, now flourish. There are radio and television programmes promoting the views of disabled people and an increasing number of conferences, courses, journals and books on disability issues organized and produced by disabled academics. All of this amounts to a Disabled People's Movement as disabled people press for control in decision-making and for their perspectives and rights to be acknowledged and acted upon. Though still young, the movement has brought about considerable change in attitudes and practices. The pace of change has no doubt been helped by similar social movements such as those promoting 'gender equality' and 'racical equality'.

Professionals understandably tend to find these developments threatening as their status, power, role and even their jobs no longer seem secure. It has to be admitted that there are many disabled people who, disillusioned with the help they have received in the past, reject any professional involvement in the services they are developing. However, many believe that partnership and collaboration with professional workers is important, and professionals are already assisting disabled people in developing services appropriate to their needs as they define them (see Silburn *et al.*, 1994). Professionals in such a situation serve as a resource to disabled people as they strive to reach their own goals. They do not attempt to dominate, to take control, or to 'manage' disabled people but rather to act as 'supportive enablers' actively sharing their expertise and knowledge while recognizing and learning from their disabled associates – the term 'patient' is no longer appropriate.

Disabled people define their situation not in terms of individual impairment but in terms of social oppression. By doing so they are not implying that medical intervention is wrong, or that it cannot be sensible, helpful or vital. What disabled people are demanding of professional workers is a broadening of their perspective on disability and a relinquishing of their power.

Disabled people's definitions of the problems they encounter, and the appropriate solutions to them, are generally given insufficient weight in the education and practice of professional health and welfare workers. This situation has given rise to countless examples of inappropriate, oppressive, and damaging practices and policies. Physiotherapists must be accountable to disabled people and organize their services and resources flexibly. They need to extend their view point well beyond the medical model of disability but in doing so must take care not to exercise even greater power and control over the lives of disabled people.

References

Barnes C. (1992) *Disabling Imagery and the Media*. Halifax: The British Council of Organisations of Disabled People and Ryburn Publishing Limited.

Brechin A., Liddiard P. (1981) *Look at it This Way – New Perspectives in Rehabilitation*. Sevenoaks: Hodder and Stoughton.

British Psychological Society (1989) *Psychology and Physical Disability in the National Health Service. Report of the Professional Affairs Board of the British Psychological Society*. Leicester.

Campling J. (1981) (ed.) *Images of Ourselves: Women with Disabilities Talking*. London: Routledge and Kegan Paul.

Crow L. (1992) Renewing the Social Model of Disability. Greater Manchester Coalition of Disabled People. *Coalition*, July, 5–9.

Davis K. (1993) The Crafting of Good Clients. In *Disabling Barriers – Enabling Environments*. (Swain J., Finkelstein V., French S., Oliver M., eds). London: Sage.

Disability Now (1990) Telethon is a Modern Day Freak Show. July 3rd.

Ellis K. (1993) *Squaring the Circle: user and carer participation in needs assessment*. London: Joseph Rowntree Foundation.

Finkelstein V. (1981) To deny or not to deny disability. In *Handicap in a Social World* (Brechin A., Liddiard P., Swain J., eds). Sevenoaks: Hodder and Stoughton.

Finkelstein V. (1991) Disability: an administrative challenge. In *Social Work, Disabled People and Disabling Environments* (Oliver M., ed.). London: Jessica Kingsley.

Finkelstein V., French S. (1993) Towards a psychology of disability. *Disabling Barriers – Enabling Environments* (Swain J., Finkelstein V., French S., Oliver M., eds). London: Sage

French S. (1987) The medicine epidemic. *Therapy Weekly*, **11**(34), 4.

French S. (1993a) Disability, impairment or something in between? In *Disabling Barriers – Enabling Environments* (Swain J., Finkelstein V., French S., Oliver M., eds). London: Sage.

French S. (1993b) 'Can you see the rainbow?' The roots of denial. In *Disabling Barriers – Enabling Environments* (Swain J., Finkelstein V., French S., Oliver M. eds). London: Sage.

French S. (1994a) Disabled people and professional practice. In *On Equal Terms: Working with Disabled People* (French S., ed.) Oxford: Butterworth-Heinemann.

French S. (1994b) In whose service? – A review of the development of services for disabled people. *Physiotherapy*, **80**(4), 200–204.

Harrison J. (1987) *Severe Physical Disability*. London: Cassell.

Humphries S., and Gordon P. (1992) *Out of Sight: The Experience of Disability 1900–1950*. Plymouth: Northcote House.

International Classification of Impairments, Disabilities and Handicaps (1980) Geneva: World Health Organization.

Karph A. (1986) *Doctoring the Media*. London: Routledge.

Ladd P. (1988) The modern deaf community. In *British Sign Language* (Miles D., ed.). London: BBC Books.

Ladd P. (1990) Language oppression and hearing impairment. In the book of readings of the disability equality pack *Disability – Changing Practice* (k665x). Milton Keynes: Open University.

Laing J., McQuarrie D. (1989) *50 Years in the System*. Edinburgh: Mainstream Publishing Company.

McKnight J. (1981) Professionalised service and disabling help. In *Handicap in a Social World*. (Brechin A., Liddiard P., Swain J., eds). Sevenoaks: Hodder and Stoughton.

Mason M. (1992) Internalised oppression. In *Disability Equality in the Classroom: A Human Rights* Issue (2nd edn.) (Rieser R., Mason M., eds). London: Disability Equality in Education.

Morris J. (1989) *Able Lives*. London: The Women's Press.

Morris J. (1991) *Pride Against Prejudice*. London: The Women's Press.

Munro K., Elder-Woodward J. (1992) *Independent Living*. Edinburgh: Churchill Livingstone.

Oliver M. (1983) *Social Work and Disabled People*. London: Macmillan.

Oliver M. (1990) *The Politics of Disablement*. London: Macmillan.

Oliver M. (1993) Disability and dependency: a creation industrial societies? In *Disabling Barriers – Enabling Environments* (Swain J., Finkelstein V., French S., Oliver M., eds). London: Sage.

Parker G. (1993) *With this Body: Caring and Disability in Marriage*. Buckingham: Open University Press.

Potts M., and Fido R. (1991) *A Fit Person to be Removed. Personal Accounts of Life in a Mental Deficiency Institution*. Plymouth: Northcote House.

Ryan J., Thomas F. (1987) *The Politics of Mental Handicap*. London: Free Association Books.

Scott-Parker S. (1989) *They Aren't in the Brief*. London: King's Fund Centre.

Shakespeare T. (1993) Disabled People's Self-Organization: a new social movement? *Disability and Society*. **8**(3), 249–264.

Silburn L., Dookum D., and Jones C. (1994) Innovative practice. In *On Equal Terms: Working with Disabled People* (French S., ed). Oxford: Butterworth-Heinemann.

Stevens A. (1992) *Disability Issues. Developing Anti-discriminatory Practice*. London: Central Council for Education and Training in Social Work.

Sutherland A. T. (1981) *Disabled We Stand*. London: Souvenir Press.

Swaffield L. (1986) Every day a miracle. *Therapy Weekly*, **13**(17), 4.

UPIAS (1976) *Fundamental Principles of Disability*. London: Union of the Physically Impaired Against Segregation.

Walmsley J. (1993) Contradictions in caring: reciprocity and interdependence. *Disability, Handicap and Society*, **8**(2), 129–141.

24   Learning difficulties: changing roles for physiotherapists

Jan Walmsley

This chapter introduces some salient issues in learning disability, considers the role of the physiotherapist in relation to people with learning difficulties, and the implications for practice carried by different beliefs and theoretical frameworks. In the first edition of this book there was no specific information about learning disability in relation to the work of physiotherapists. Since then, the Chartered Society of Physiotherapists has established a Learning Disability Special Interest group to promote good practice and research in relation to people with learning difficulties. Julie Waring, a member of this group, assisted in the writing of this chapter.

On the face of it, there is no particular reason for physiotherapists to know about or specialize in learning disability. It is easy, but erroneous, to assume that people with learning difficulties have similar needs to the majority of the population. This is the case for two reasons: first, there is a growing body of research evidence to show that people with learning difficulties have a higher than average set of health care needs sometimes, but not always, related to their disability (RCGP, 1990: Greenhalgh, 1994). Second, the health professional who comes into contact with people with learning difficulties and those who care for them faces particular challenges in providing high quality service because of basic problems of access and communication (Rodgers and Russell, 1995). Obtaining informed consent is particularly problematic. Therefore, an introduction to some salient issues in learning disability is important, both for physiotherapists who intend to specialize in this area, and for others who, as integration and community living become more common, are likely to encounter people with learning difficulties in their day-to-day practice.

Definitions

In a field bedevilled by terminological debate it is important to clarify from the outset the choice of terms. 'Learning difficulties' is the term preferred by service users for the condition once known as 'mental handicap'. As two people with learning difficulties put it to a researcher, 'mental handicap' is rejected because 'it means we can't do anything for ourselves and we need support all the time which we don't' and 'it makes people outside see us as children to pity' (Simons, 1992). Accepting that people with learning difficulties should be able to determine for themselves the label that is applied to them makes sense in a context of community care where the emphasis is on choice and self-determination, ideas already familiar to readers of this volume. However, the term 'learning disability' is also current, and is the term used by the Department of Health and the Chartered Society of Physiotherapists.

Defining learning difficulties is, however, an area which is fraught with imprecision. First of all we must exclude people with specific *learning* difficulties, such as dyslexia, from our group. This leaves roughly 2–3% of the population in western societies who are labelled as having learning difficulties. Fewer than a third of these have an identifiable organic pathology such as Down's syndrome (Jenkins, 1993). Various attempts have been made to define intellectual incapacity. For example, the 1913 Mental Deficiency Act defined mental deficiency as 'a condition of arrested or incomplete development of mind existing before the age of 18 years'. (Lyons and Heaton Ward, 1955). Like many other attempts to define the condition, this is vague, and there is no clear dividing line between normal and abnormal. Over time different attempts have been made to identify distinguishing and measurable characteristics. For example, in the late nineteenth century it was believed that mental defect was discernible in an individual's physical features, so-called 'stigmata', of which the distinctive facial characteristics of people with Down's syndrome are the best known (Sutherland, 1984). The introduction of intelligence testing in the early twentieth century held out the possibility of scientific measurement of intelligence, and today an IQ below 70 and the 'mental age of a child' are commonly accepted as indicators of learning difficulties. The Health of the Nation's definition incorporates three related factors: reduced ability to understand new or complex information, to learn new skills: and reduced ability to cope independently (impaired social functioning); which started before adulthood with a lasting effect on development (Department of Health, 1995). However, most authorities recognize that it is not possible to make a completely objective judgment about what does, and what does not constitute a learning difficulty.

The absence of scientific definitions alerts us to a key issue in learning difficulties, namely that it is in part a 'social construct', not only an objective property of individuals. The environment can make a difference to who is labelled as having a learning difficulty. A glance back in time demonstrates this. During and shortly after the Second World War numerous disabled people, including residents of mental deficiency hospitals, found employment due to a labour shortage (Humphries and Gordon, 1992: Annual Reports on Bromham Hospital, 1943-1946). As service personnel returned to civilian life, disabled people, like women, resumed their positions on the margins of the labour market.

This suggests that the social model of disability (see Chapter 23) can also be applied to learning disability, though it is hard to imagine a society where the social barriers which people with learning difficulties face would disappear. As Fiona Williams (1989) writes, 'A society which valued people with learning difficulties would have to question seriously the primacy it gives to cognitive skills at the expense of other attributes such as emotional wisdom, insight and imagination. In turn, it would have to examine the institutions of education, paid work and financial rewards which sustain these priorities'. Most of us would agree that this represents an enormous challenge!

Whilst the social environment can influence the labelling process, and the life experiences of people with learning difficulties, many do have above average incidence of certain illness and physical conditions, requiring particular attention from health professionals. The tension between treating people with learning difficulties as human beings above all, at the same time as recognizing that they have particular needs, is a key theme of this chapter. The 'social model' cannot explain all.

Hospital to Community: A Changing Context

The ways in which people with learning difficulties have been viewed have changed radically during the twentieth century, and are in a continuing state of revision. The conceptual framework adopted by the practitioner will influence their approach, as will the way services for people with learning difficulties are structured and provided. I therefore outline some of the major shifts in attitude and policy.

People with learning difficulties came to be seen as a major social problem around the turn of the twentieth century. Known as 'mental defectives' or 'feeble-minded', they were seen both as people who needed protection for their own good, and as the cause of numerous social evils such as petty crime, promiscuity and illegitimacy. The preferred solution came to be seen as institutional care in specialist long stay homes, hospitals or colonies, and the 1913 Mental Deficiency Act urged local authorities to identify and supervise mental defectives in their areas, and to build institutions to house them. Under the Act, many people were certified and spent many years in institutions, shut away from the world (Potts and Fido, 1991). The National Health Service took over the running of these institutions in 1948, though few inmates were ill in the conventional sense of the word (Stainton, 1992). By no means everyone who was certified as mentally deficient was institutionalized – many continued to live with their families – but if no family carer was available, hospital was, in most areas, the only option. Physiotherapists found their way into these institutions, and worked with large numbers and limited aims – to keep patients mobile, to perform passive movements, to encourage good positioning, and to facilitate chest care.

From the early 1950s the assumption that institutional care was the optimum way to treat people with learning difficulties began to be challenged, initially on civil liberties grounds (NCCL, 1951). A Royal Commission which sat from 1954 to 1957 found that there was 'shortage of beds, shortage of building, shortage of staff and shortage of money' (Jones, 1972) and the 1959 Mental Health Act which followed sought to re-orientate the mental health services away from institutional care towards care in the community (Jones, 1972). There has been much speculation as to the motivation for the switch to community care as a preferred option (Dalley, 1989). Justified as morally superior, especially after a series of scandals about the abusive practices in hospitals in the sixties and seventies (Donges, 1982), it has also been urged that the motive is financial, community care being seen as cheaper.

The switch from hospital to community took many years. Even as late as 1993 15% of adults with learning difficulties (20 000 people) were living in hospitals (Mental Health Foundation, 1993). However, by far the majority of people now live in what is conventionally called the community, in hostels, group homes, family homes, their own flats and houses, and with foster families. This means that the context in which health professionals who provide services to people with learning difficulties operate has also changed. Whereas at one time rudimentary health care was provided on site to the inmates of large institutions, now the professional will operate in a variety of settings, often with multidisciplinary teams and access may well be problematic, both for service provider and service user. For example, in 1995, of an estimated 750 people with learning difficulties in Tower Hamlets, London, 250 were known to the Community Learning Disability Team, and 55 received physiotherapy (Waring, 1995). We return to this below. (For further information on institutional and community living, the reader is referred to Chapter 3.).

Integration and normalization: a Framework for action

The shift to community care was accompanied by a set of theories which can be grouped under the broad title of 'normalization'. The argument is that people with learning difficulties had, because of their label, been deprived of opportunities to enjoy normal patterns of life. The job of services, therefore, becomes to reverse the devaluation of people with learning difficulties by ensuring that they are given every opportunity to enjoy normal patterns of life (Nirje, 1969) and to relate to people without disabilities. 'An Ordinary Life' was the slogan coined by the King's Fund in the early 1980s to describe the sorts of service provision that would foster inclusion in community life: ordinary homes in ordinary streets with every opportunity to become integrated in the community through participation in work, in volunteering, and in leisure activities. Services were to be sited in valued areas, and service users encouraged to adopt life styles which enable them to participate in activities enjoyed by the majority of the population.

Within the normalization paradigm service interventions are influenced by the need to assist people in becoming acceptable to a wider society. For example, psychologists devise behavioural programmes which aim to eradicate inappropriate or abnormal behaviours such as carrying soft toys, or embracing people on first meeting them (Felce and Toogood, 1988). In this context, the job of the physiotherapist becomes one of assisting the person with learning difficulties to increase independence, and to have access to activities like dance and sport which are valued by a wider society. This implies a holistic approach from services rather than one which focuses on a person's disability in isolation from the rest of his or her life. Case study one illustrates that this is not as straightforward as it may seem.

Case study one: 'Sarah' [1]

Sarah is a young woman, small in stature, who has no speech. She communicates by movement, such as turning her head. She has difficulty in walking, and in drinking from a cup. Her mother, Carole, describes her experience of services:

> 'I think the response to Sarah's needs shows that services find it very difficult to cater for an individual. The way they've been set up is to cater for a group of people and they find it hard to come back to the individual. I think they've tried in lots of ways and one of these ways is through assessments. They first started this with Individual Programme Plans which we went along with and thought they might be a good idea. And we had four years of meetings and we've got a stack of reports that high, where it starts off with Sarah's strengths and needs. And it seemed to be a list of disabilities, you know, things like "Sarah needs to maintain eye contact," "Sarah needs to eat properly", "Sarah needs to strengthen her arms", "Sarah needs to suck through a straw". But Sarah has learnt all the skills she needs through going to the pub with friends, you know. We tried for a long time to get Sarah to hold a glass or a cup, she wouldn't do it. When she's in the pub with friends she'll hold a glass because all her friends are doing it, and it's got alcohol in it which is a bit of a bonus ...
>
> 'They saw a need for a walking frame which I disagree with. Sarah doesn't need to walk and it had castors on which was quite dangerous, you know, sort of whizzing about the Day Centre. It never arrived, you know, they said Sarah needs physiotherapy, but it never arrived so to me the whole thing was a waste of time'.

Carole argues that it was opportunity and motivation that was missing from Sarah's life, and providing opportunities and motivations was far more effective than a professional focus on her various disabilities. Furthermore, she was in her interview critical both of the analysis of Sarah's needs, and the failure to provide the services which could make good those needs as stated. Not only did Carole think that Sarah's needs had been misinterpreted, insult was added to injury when the service Sarah was deemed to need was not made available.

In terms of normalization it is clear that there were at work in Sarah's case two conflicting interpretations. Carole's interpretation was that enjoyment of an ordinary life is best fostered by creating relationships which enable Sarah to go out with people of her own age and enjoy some of the activities other young people take for granted. From Carole's account service personnel took a narrower view of Sarah's needs based on medical diagnoses of her physical deficiencies. This may lead us to question the process of assessment. Was the physiotherapist actually involved in the assessment, or was the walking frame summoned by others who had limited knowledge of different options? Did Sarah have an opportunity to contribute her own views, or did her mother speak for her? The case highlights the fact that if joint, practical and meaningful goals are not set interventions will fail, and a situation of non-compliance may be set up between professional, client and carer. Carole had become disillusioned by the mechanistic approach to Sarah's needs, yet sensitive

---

[1] Names have been changed. The Case Study is adapted from information recorded in a taped interview with 'Carole', at which 'Sarah' was present.

physiotherapy interventions may have been of considerable benefit, as shown in Case study two.

Case study two 'Theresa' [2]

Theresa is 36 years old and has severe learning difficulties, associated physical disabilities and epilepsy. She lives at home with her mother and was initially referred to physiotherapists in the Community Learning Disabilities Team because when she went into respite care for brief periods carers found it hard to manage Theresa's physical needs, and to get her to move about. On examination, it was found that Teresa was kyphotic, her hips were beginning to wind-sweep, her knees were flexed, and she had swollen ankles and feet. She was, in short, becoming chair-shaped, and it was hard for anyone to move her. Physiotherapy interventions included an improved seating system in her wheelchair, a Spa chair to use at home, exercises to stretch her limbs, weekly hydrotherapy sessions, and programmed periods in a standing frame daily at the Day Centre. It resulted in Theresa being able to get in and out of bed without help, to walk for short distances, and to get on and off the toilet.

Attention was also paid to Theresa's home. A through floor lift was installed, and a hoist to get her in and out of the bath. Day Centre staff were also involved in the programme. They were encouraged to prompt her to move, and trained in appropriate lifting techniques. She used the Snoezelen (Multi-sensory) room at the centre regularly, which enabled her to come out of her wheelchair and experience different positions, and to enjoy massage. Staff noticed that as Theresa became more mobile she communicated more, being able to make eye contact more readily.

However, her severe epilepsy caused a deterioration in Theresa's condition. She became barely able to stand, and sometimes could not move without assistance. Day Centre staff noticed that her personal hygiene suffered. Her mother was no longer able to change her incontinence pads, or bath her. At a review meeting an independent advocate was engaged to represent Theresa, a recognition that Theresa and her mother had different needs which had to be addressed. The review resulted in the appointment of three helpers to go in daily on a rota basis to help her mother bath Theresa, to toilet her, and to assist her to bed.

This still did not resolve all the difficulties. It was hard to bathe Theresa because of the need to bend over the bath. The need to move Theresa onto and off the toilet was a heavy burden on Day Centre staff, as it required three people. The physiotherapist decided to reassess the situation, both at the hydrotherapy pool and at home, and these sessions were videoed for use with others who were involved in Theresa's care, so they could see what Theresa's abilities were, and how to handle and move her.

Funding was also sought for an adjustable bed, and a shower unit at home, to make it easier to care for her when she was unable, through seizures, to move herself.

---

[2] This case study was provided by Julie Waring, Tower Hamlets Community Team for People with Learning Disabilities, Isle of Dogs, London.

The case study shows the potential of physiotherapy input in a multi-disciplinary team to address some needs fundamental to an ordinary life. Theresa's life is still far from 'normal', but her quality of life has been improved, and a semblance of dignity retained. The case study also shows the importance of paying attention to the large network of people involved with Teresa – her mother, Day Centre staff, the Social Services employees who were employed to help bathe Theresa, the occupational therapists who provided necessary amendments to the home: all needed to be included in Theresa's programme, and this was not a once and for all training, but needed to be renewed and revised in the light of her changing condition. The physiotherapist was a key figure in this, whilst maintaining links with specialists in the multi-disciplinary team, including occupational therapists, speech therapists, community nurses, and doctors. Theresa will never 'get better', but imaginative and skilled physiotherapy interventions are important to her quality of life.

Self-advocacy: a challenge to services

In neither of our case studies has the voice of the person at centre stage been heard. In Sarah's case, her mother spoke on her behalf. Theresa's situation was described by the physiotherapist who treated her. But a major development in learning disability since the mid 1980s has been the development of self-advocacy or speaking out. To people new to the area of learning disability it may or may not come as a surprise that until then it was generally assumed that people with learning difficulties could not speak up for themselves. Their interests were represented by professionals or by organizations such as Mencap which began as an organization for the parents of backward children, not the disabled people themselves. The interests of parents and their offspring were assumed to be identical.

Crawley (1988) described the beginning of self-advocacy: 'for the first time opportunity has been generated for individuals to speak out and confer with peers in an environment of support'. Self-advocacy is a term which encompasses both personal development – learning to be assertive, to make choices, to have self-respect – and organizations like People First which are run by and for people with learning difficulties (Simons, 1992). Many self-advocacy organizations run conferences, offer training to professionals, market services such as advice on how to create information intelligible to people with learning difficulties, and promote their interests through activities such as the 1994 Civil Rights campaign. Self-advocacy has drawn attention to the fact that some people with learning difficulties can speak for themselves, and their interests are sometimes in conflict with those of their carers and service providers. This potential conflict of interest was acknowledged in our second case study where Theresa, who could not speak for herself, was represented by an independent advocate. Ideally, Theresa would have articulated her own wishes and desires. An independent advocate was the next best thing.

Assessments influenced by the principles of self-advocacy will ensure that the service user is at the centre of the process: approaches which seek to achieve this include Shared Action Planning (Brechin and Swain, 1986) and Personal Futures Planning (Mount and Zwernik, 1988). Such approaches challenge traditional professional–client relationships – for example it should be up to the user to decide who is present at his or her assessment meeting, and this may well exclude specialists such as physiotherapists from a direct input. Instead, written reports may be sought to be included in the agenda, follow up may include specialist input. Our third case study illustrates how this worked for one client, Pat.

Case study 3: Pat[3]

Pat is 30 years old, and has spent most of her life in residential care, and has close contact with her family who live nearby. When her placement broke down an assessment meeting was held to assist Pat in deciding where she would like to live. At the meeting it became clear that some of Pat's difficulties stemmed from a painful hip and back which limited her mobility and generally left her feeling uncomfortable. One of the results of the assessment was a referral to the Community Learning Disability Team. Pat was unwilling to take part, arguing that she had no pain, but her wishes were overridden, and on examination it was found she had a shortening of the right leg of 8 cm. She showed the physiotherapists two pairs of shoes with a 7.5 cm external raise, but insisted she would not wear them, and preferred to endure the pain rather than draw attention to herself in this way. After a discussion, Pat agreed that she would wear trainers, and discussed this with the orthotist. She now has a pair of trainers on order with a smaller raise, part of it on the sole.

Pat's case study shows the importance of a sensitivity to the wishes of the client. Her reluctance to discuss her footware with the physiotherapists was overridden on the grounds that she did not have enough information to make a real choice. Having the opportunity to influence the way her physical disability was managed led to a compromise which respected her wishes without abandoning principles of self-advocacy and normalization. It also means, we hope, that she will use the trainers, and benefit from the professional expertise. It's interesting to compare the approach in this case study with the approach to Theresa's treatment in case study 2. What would Theresa have said if she could have done – and would she readily have accepted the treatment she was offered? Informed consent is a consistent dilemma for professionals working with people with learning difficulties.

Self-advocacy may well lead to a more radical reappraisal of the type of medical interventions which are appropriate for people with learning difficulties. This is well illustrated by reference to debates on conductive education and plastic surgery for people with Down's syndrome.

Whilst parents have been demanding the provision of conductive education as a means of enabling children with limited mobility to achieve a greater normality (Beardshaw, 1993), disabled people have been vehemently critical of an approach which seeks to normalize them. This

---

[3] This case study was kindly provided by Aase D. Walker, Superintendent Physiotherapist with the Newham Community Learning Disabilities Team.

partly explains Carol's objections to the assessment that Sarah needed to learn to walk with a frame, though we do not know Sarah's own views on the subject. An analogous normalizing intervention is plastic surgery for people with Down's syndrome. Participants at 'Not Just Painted On', a Conference for people with Down's syndrome questioned this:

> 'Usually it is other people who make the decision to have plastic surgery, not us. We feel that if you need plastic surgery for medical reasons, that's OK. But it should not happen just to make us look like other people. Our faces are not just painted on. We can't just take them on and off. They are ours and we should be proud of them ... Differences should be fun' (People First, 1995).

The quotation highlights an important factor for physiotherapists to bear in mind when working with people with learning difficulties. There are perhaps going to be conflicts between carers, professionals and the client as to whose views prevail. Being made more 'normal' is not necessarily what clients want, though, as Pat's case study shows, its very important for some people to have the opportunity to exercise a truly informed choice and to have access to equipment and aids which are aesthetically pleasing, and do not draw attention to their impairment.

Access and integration

As the emphasis in service philosophy has switched from specialist treatment offered in institutions where people with learning difficulties are congregated to inclusion and integration in ordinary communities, problems of access to health care have become paramount. Special services provided in residential and day centres have the advantage of being on tap, so to speak. The physiotherapist can visit a hospital ward and readily treat a group of patients. If those former patients are now citizens living in a variety of settings scattered across a wide geographical area, can they be expected to take the necessary steps to locate a dentist or GP, to arrange transport for themselves, and to make appointments when they need them? From another point of view, will mainstream health professionals have the necessary skills and empathy to communicate with people with learning difficulties: indeed, will they be prepared to accept them onto their lists at all, when it is likely they will make higher than average demands on health services?

The National Health Service Management Executive identified three main ways in which health care may be problematic for people with learning difficulties: higher than average incidence of ill health and physical disability; difficulty in diagnosis; and low health care expectations (NHSME, 1993). We examine these in turn.

Ill health and physical disability

People with learning difficulties are likely to experience additional ill health related to any particular syndrome, such as diabetes associated with Prader Willi syndrome or respiratory infections associated with Down's syndrome: (Howells, 1986; RCGP, 1990). One case study estimated the incidence of epilepsy amongst people with learning difficulties at 26% (RCGP, 1990).

In addition, the kinds of ill health and disability which affect everyone also affect people with learning difficulties, but are often overlooked and attributed to the learning difficulty. Deafness or partial hearing, and sight problems are particularly likely to be overlooked (Howells, 1986 CHANGE, 1994), and standard tests used on the general population are often inappropriate because of communication or speech problems. Many people with learning difficulties are obese. One study found that 27.5% of men and 58.5% of women were overweight, and the authors comment: 'These numbers are alarming, not only a serious concern from a medical standpoint but from the standpoint of integration in the community' (Rimmer *et al.*, 1993). Problems such as obesity are exacerbated by poor diet, due both to poverty and to lack of knowledge about healthy eating (Rodgers and Russell, 1995).

Is is hard to over-estimate the impact of the alarmingly high rates of undetected medical conditions which one study put as high as 66% (Rodgers, 1993). Physical difficulties may actually be more limiting than the learning difficulty.

Difficulty in diagnosis

If someone with a severe learning disability is in pain how do they communicate this? Theresa relied on carers to be alert to changes in her physical or mental condition, and it was the day centre staff who drew attention to difficulties, both in handling Theresa, and in her personal hygiene. It wasn't Theresa's learning disability that caused her problems, though it exacerbated them because she was unable to make her medical needs known to others. The term 'diagnostic overshadowing' has been coined to describe the tendency to attribute problems to a learning disability rather than other causes. In some pioneering work on psychotherapy, undertaken at the Tavistock Institute, Valarie Sinason found that challenging behaviours previously associated with the patient's learning difficulty were often due to uncommunicated trauma from abuse or emotional damage (Sinason, 1992). But lesser conditions can be equally hard to detect. Howells (1986) found that only 29 of 72 people attending a day centre in Wales could give a coherent account of experiences. Even those who could communicate fluently were unable to describe symptoms.

Assumptions about the ability of people with learning difficulties to understand instructions are often erroneous. Greenhalgh (1994) quotes one woman who had been told to avoid spicy food, but did not know what 'spicy' meant. Her favourite food was chilli con carne. Routine optician's tests rely on the ability to read letters but many people with learning difficulties cannot read.

Low expectations

A number of studies have indicated that people with learning difficulties, their carers and health care personnel have low expectations of their general state of health, Howells (1986) comments:

> 'Common treatable complaints were often seen by the carers as relatively trivial when compared with the major handicaps which were untreatable and for this reason medical advice was not sought'.

Langan *et al.* (1993) found the primary health care teams often did not offer cervical smear tests to women with learning difficulties, and were not aware that many women were unable to examine their own breasts for lumps. They also found that less than 25% of GPs had any specialist training in awareness of the specific health needs of people with learning difficulties, though almost a half recognized they may benefit from such training.

The tendency for service personnel to attribute common symptoms of ill health such as lethargy, depression, eating disorders and anti-social or, in the jargon, 'challenging' behaviour to the disability rather than to other conditions is sometimes alarming. A woman aged 72 left hospital to settle in a residential home. At the same time she began to show symptoms of anorexia, followed by a relentless clinical decline resulting in her re-admission to the hospital. The initial diagnosis was that she had behavioural problems associated with the move and other life changes. Only after the insistence of the medical team at the hospital was she given an endoscopy, and found to have an annular constricting cancer of the oesophagus, the classic symptoms of which had been present but explained away because she had learning difficulties (Bird, 1995).

Poor information, difficulties with transport, and embarrassment on the part of carers also contribute to poor uptake of generic health services by people with learning difficulties. The well known correlation of low social class and poverty with poor health standards is compounded by the existence of a disability, for, whilst not all people with learning difficulties live in poverty, the disability imposes extra costs (Mencap Campaigns Department, 1994), and the likelihood that people with learning difficulties and their families rely on state benefits means they are often downwardly mobile in terms of social class (Jenkins, 1991).

Dilemmas and solutions

The philosophy of normalization and community integration presents dilemmas when it comes to health care for people with learning difficulties. In a research project into providing better health information for a group of women with learning difficulties living independently in Milton Keynes, Greenhalgh found that normalization was misinterpreted by care staff as meaning 'we can't interfere' (Greenhalgh, 1994). Members of the group had a number of previously undetected and therefore untreated health problems, including back pain, stress, and menstrual irregularity or pains. Greenhalgh concludes that 'No one had a pro-active role as regards either monitoring people's health or in enabling them to become better skilled or better informed'. She attributes this to poor training, and lack of interest from managers.

What are the solutions? We can look at solutions from two angles: first, steps to empower users of services, and second, the way health services are supplied.

Empowerment of users

Fundamental is the need to develop an awareness of health and information about where and how to get treatment among the people themselves, and their carers. The development of self-advocacy and advocacy services will contribute to this, but it is a slow process. In my own research, undertaken in 1991–1992, I found that only 6 out of 22 relatively able people with learning difficulties even knew the meaning of the terms. Ideally, people with learning difficulties will become active and assertive consumers of health, ready and willing to demand treatment. There are signs that self-advocacy groups are taking health onto their agenda, particularly in relation to women's issues (Open University, 1996). However, none of the research undertaken so far suggests that this will happen in the foreseeable future for anything other than a small minority of service users, and for people, like Theresa, with more severe disabilities it is almost unimaginable.

The provision of accessible information which is relevant to people with learning difficulties is also an identifiable goal. The Department of Health has taken a lead in this, commissioning a translation of the Patients' Charter into symbols, and funding research into people's health information needs (Greenhalgh, 1994). This needs to be seen in context, however. Translating existing information into plain English with illustrations or symbols should be seen as a way to provide resources for service providers to use, rather than a solution in itself. Case study 3 shows it is the relationships which are key to success. Information by itself would not have been helpful to Pat.

The involvement of users and carers in service planning and training of health professionals is a promising area. The Mid Downs Project is an example of a sustained and fully resourced attempt to enable people with learning difficulties, and users of mental health services, to influence the provision of health care to people with learning difficulties in one health authority. The process is a slow one, but shows the importance of including service users in the very fabric of the organization, rather than, as is so often the case, holding one-off consultations.

The provision of services

How far health care should be provided by mainstream services, and how far by specialists is a key area of debate. For many in the learning disability field, full integration of services to people with learning difficulties in mainstream services is an ideal, commensurate with the principle of normalization. However, as Greenhalgh's research shows, simplistic interpretations of normalization can be damaging. Few would argue for the return of the long stay hospital, but a recognition that people with learning difficulties will not necessarily be able to get the best out of the health services unaided is absolutely crucial. One day centre in Scotland reintroduced dentist's visits to the centre for its users after finding that its scattered rural population were making little use of dental services.

The learning disability register can be a key resource for targeting improved health care for people with learning difficulties (Dobson, 1995), offering a route of access to people via the community learning disability teams (CLDTs). At the conference held to launch The Health of the Nation Strategy for People with Learning Disabilities in 1995 it was recommended that CLDTs act as catalysts for alerting their clients and those who work with them to health care issues. Rather than assume other members of the team have a remit for health care and education it should be seen as the responsibility of each team member as he or she comes into contact with individuals. Theresa's case study illustrates how this team approach works.

A register-based approach, however, does have limitations, other than the moral one of tying a label even more firmly around people's necks. One GP reported that rudimentary research into her practice registers revealed 22 people with learning difficulties, fewer than half of whom were known to the CLDT. For this reason some projects have turned to referral rather than register-based systems (Rose, 1995), though this appears to carry huge implications for education of both consumers and providers of health care.

Conclusion

There is a tension in combining a concern for the health and well-being of adults with learning difficulties with respect for their rights to a normal life. Structural inequalities combined with the effects of the disability on powers of communication mean that they are peculiarly disadvantaged as consumers of health care, and there is an emerging consensus that furnishing the preconditions for an ordinary life means there needs to be extraordinary vigilance in ensuring that the health care they need is available. It is hard to guarantee informed consent when clients have very limited access to even rudimentary knowledge about basic health yet efforts need to be made to respect the citizenship of adults with learning difficulties when assessments are made and treatments delivered. The importance of a team approach, where workers and carers in day-to-day contact with potential clients feel that health care is within their remit, and know how to access specialist help when needed, appears to offer the best hope of effecting improvements. But the message from conferences like 'Not Just Painted On' is a warning that paternalistic assumptions that mum, dad, or the professional know best need to be constantly challenged if people with learning difficulties are to be genuinely empowered in accessing the health care that they require.

References

Atkinson D., Bytheway B. (1996) Speaking out for equal rights: In *Learning Disability: Working as Equal People*. Bucks: Open University.

Beardshaw V. (1993) Conductive education: A rejoinder: In *Disabling Barriers – Enabling Environments* (Swain J., Finkelstein V., French S., Oliver M. eds). London: Sage, pp. 166–169.

Bird J. (1995) Pitfalls in diagnosis: Does the diagnosis get in the way? In *Enabling People with Learning Disabilities to use the Health Service Conference Proceedings*. St George's Hospital Medical School.

Board of Control (1943, 1944, 1945, 1946) *Bromham Hospital: Annual Report*. Board of Control.

Brechin A., Swain J., (1986) *Changing Relationships*. London: Chapman and Hall.

Crawley B. (1982) The feasibility of trainee committees as a means of self advocacy in adult training centres. *Unpublished Phd Thesis*, Manchester.

Dalley G. (1989) Community care: the ideal and the reality: In *Making Connections* (Brechin A., Walmsley J. eds). Hodder and Stoughton, pp. 199–208.

Department of Health (1995) *Health of the Nation: A Strategy for People with Learning Disabilities*. HMSO.

Dobson H. (1995) Commissioning services which promote health for people with learning disabilities. Paper given at the Launch Conference for *The Health of the Nation: A Strategy for People with Learning Disabilities*.

Donges P. (1982) *Policy Making for the Mentally Handicapped.* Aldershot: Gower.

Elwell L., Platts H., Rees G. (1995) Putting people first. Assessment and care management. In *Values and Visions* (Philpot T., Ward L. eds). Butterworth-Heinemann, 123–139.

Felce D., Toogood S. (1988) *Close to Home.* British Institute of Learning Disabilities.

Gold M. (1976) A new definition of mental retardation. Unpublished paper quoted in McConkey R. (1994) An ordinary life for special people in *Taking Control: Enabling People with Learning Difficulties* (Coupe O'Kane J., Smith B., eds). David Fulton.

Greenhalgh L. (1994) *Well Aware: Improving Access to Health Information for People with Learning Difficulties.* NHS Executive Anglia and Oxford.

Howells G. (1986) Are the medical needs of mentally handicapped adults being met? *Journal of the Royal College of General Practitioners,* **36**, 449–453.

Humphries S., Gordon P. (1992) *Out of Sight: The Experience of Disability 1900–1950.* Northcote House/Channel 4.

Hurt J. (1988) *Outside the Mainstream: A History of Special Education.* Batsford.

Jenkins R. (1991) Disability and social stratification. *British Journal of Sociology,* **42**(4), 557–580.

Jenkins R. (1993) Incompetence and learning difficulties: anthropological perspectives. *Anthropology Today,* **9**(3), 16–20.

Jones K. (1972) *A History of the Mental Health Services.* Routledge, Kegan and Paul.

King's Fund Centre (1980) *An Ordinary Life.* King's Fund Centre.

Langan J., Russell O., Whitfield M. (1993) Community care and the general practitioner: primary health care for people with learning difficulties: Norah Fry Research Centre. *Unpublished Report to the Department of Health.*

Lyons J. F., Heaton Ward W. A. (1955) *Notes on Mental Deficiency.* John Wright and Sons.

Mencap (1994) *Strategic Framework.* Mencap.

Mental Health Foundation (1993) *Learning Disability: The Fundamental Facts.* Mental Health Foundation.

Mount B., Zwernik K. (1988) *It's Never too Early, It's Never too Late.* St Paul, Minnesota: Governor's Planning Council.

National Council for Civil Liberties (1951) *50,000 outside the law.* NCCL.

National Health Service Management Executive (1993) *Learning Disabilities.* National Health Service Management Executive.

Nirje B. (1976) The normalisation principle. In *Changing Patterns in Residential Services for the Mentally Retarded* (Kugel R., Shearer A., eds) President's Committee on Mental Retardation.

Oliver M. (1993) Conductive education: if it wasn't so sad it would be funny: In *Disabling Barriers – Enabling Environments* (Swain J., Finkelstein V., French S., Oliver M. eds). London: Sage, pp. 163–166.

Open University (1996) *Learning Disability: Working as Equal People.* Open University.

People First (1994) *Oi! It's My Assessment.* People First.

People First (1995) *Not just Painted On: A Report of the First Ever Conference run by and for people with Down's Syndrome.* People First.

Potts M., Fido R. (1991) *A Fit Person to be Removed.* Northcote House.

Rimmer J., Bradock D., Fujira G. (1993) Prevalence of obesity in adults with mental retardation: implications for health promotion and disease prevention: *Mental Retardation* **31**(2).

Rodgers J. (1994) *Primary Health Care Provision for People with Learning Difficulties.* Norah Fry Research Centre.

Rodgers J., Russell O. (1995) Healthy lives: the health needs of people with learning difficulties: In *Values and Visions* (Philpot T., Ward L., eds). Oxford: Butterworth-Heinemann, pp. 304–319.

Rose S. (1995) Supporting access to primary and secondary health care. Paper given at the Launch Conference for *The Health of the Nation: A Strategy for People with Learning Disabilities.*

Royal College of General Practitioners (1990) *Primary Care for People with a Mental Handicap*. Occasional paper No. 47 RCGP.

Ryan J., Thomas E. (1987) *The Politics of Mental Handicap*. Free Association Books.

Shennan V. (1980) *Our Concern: The Story of the National Association for Mentally Handicapped Children and Adults*. National Association for Mentally Handicapped Children and Adults.

Simons K. (1992) *Sticking Up for Yourself Self Advocacy and People with Learning Difficulties*. Joseph Rowntree Foundation.

Sinason V. (1992) *Mental Handicap and the Human Condition*. London: Tavistock.

Stainton T. (1992) *Community Living*. London: Tavistock.

Sutherland G. (1984) *Ability, Merit and Measurement*. Clarendon Press.

Waring J. (1995) Personal Communication.

Williams F. (1989) Mental handicap and oppression. In *Making Connections* (Brechin A., Walmsley J. eds). Hodder and Stoughton, pp. 253–260.

25

Sexuality and disability

Paul Lawrence and John Swain

'The thread of sexuality is woven densely into the fabric of human existence. There are few people for whom sex has not been important at some
time and many for whom it has played a dominant part in their lives'
(Bancroft, 1989).

Discussion concerning sexuality has always been problematic even more
so when this discussion is in relation to the sexuality of disabled people,
and yet if we accept the perspective offered by Bancroft then it is right to
ask why this is so. Why does the recognition and acknowledgement of
the sexuality of disabled people and support in the expression of sexuality appear so controversial? The starting point for this chapter is the
denial and suppression of the sexuality of disabled people and thus the
denial of common humanity. We argue that sexuality is socially conferred
and constructed rather than being biologically defined. It is from this
vantage point that we explore the key role that sexuality has played and
continues to play in the oppression of disabled people. We turn next to
the barriers that disabled people face in their functioning and identity as
sexual beings concentrating particularly on the experiences and views of
disabled people themselves. Finally, we focus specifically on the role that
physiotherapists can play in acknowledging and supporting the sexuality of disabled people.

This is an awareness-raising chapter. References are provided for
physiotherapists seeking specific information and resources for direct
practical purposes. Our main aim, however, is to promote and facilitate
understanding and discussion in the profession around issues relating to
disability, sexuality and identity.

Defining sexuality

Any discussion concerning sexuality invariably comes face to face with
the problem of definitions. Kempton (1983) suggests that the term
'sexuality' can be defined as the integration of the biological, physiological, sociological and psychological aspects of an individual's
personality which expresses his or her maleness or femaleness. Rosen
and Hall (1984) talks in terms of sexuality being a blend of imperative
elements of gender, that is to say the physical differences between male
and female, and optional elements of gender or the social and psychological aspects of gender. Craft and Craft (1983) use the term 'psycho-
sexual' to mean sexual development in its widest sense including gender,
role and a sense of identity. Christiaens (1985) distinguishes between two
meanings of sexuality, sexuality as a means of experiencing 'desire' and
sexuality as a medium for forming relationships. Christiaens goes on to

argue that although these two dimensions can be distinguished they are so 'intricately interwoven' they cannot be separated. Other writers have, if not provided us with a definition, suggested that human 'sexuality' needs to be seen in terms of both the biological/physiological and psychological development of individuals. However, like Brown (1994), we would argue that the importance of 'defining sexuality' does not lie in the building of academic theory and models. Sexuality is defined through lived experiences which are constructed and shaped by social position, resources and ideology. Questioning assumption about the sexuality of people with learning difficulties, Brown quotes from the more recent analyses of concepts of sexuality:

> '… instead of seeing sexuality as a unified whole, we have to recognise that there are in fact many sexualities, there are race sexualities and there are sexualities of struggle and choice. The invention of sexuality was not a single event, now lost in the past. It is a continuous process in which we are simultaneously acted upon and actors, objects of change and its subjects' (Weeks, 1989).

From this viewpoint, sexuality is not a biological imperative, but rather 'a property which is largely ascribed, a current through which social status and group membership is conferred and regulated' (Brown, 1994). From this view point, too, we all, including physiotherapists, inevitably play a role in constructing the sexuality of disabled people. For instance, insofar as an asexual role is prescribed to disabled people it is instrumental in shaping an asexual identity. Sexuality, like disability, is a social concept and cannot be defined in terms of the individual's behaviour, physical attributes or even psychological identity. Indeed, sexuality and disability are closely intertwined.

Oppression: through history

Goethe wrote, 'He who cannot draw on three thousand years is living from hand to mouth' (quoted in Gaarder, 1995). The gist of this quote certainly applies to sexuality and disability. Present day negative attitudes and discrimination draw on a history of the oppression of disabled people in which the denial and suppression of sexuality and sexual abuse have played crucial roles. There is a danger in looking back in that it is tempting to see history as the story of progress. However, if there has been progress it has been painfully slow (Brown, 1994) and the prejudgments within present day society have evolved and been passed down from the prejudgments over the centuries, if not thousands of years (Wolfensberger, 1975). The Greek philosophers Plato and Aristotle argued that only people with desirable physical and mental qualities should be allowed to have children in the ideal city state, which would presumably have excluded disabled people. However the direct link between sexuality and the perceived undesirable qualities of disabled people was not fully developed until the mid-nineteenth century (see Wolfensberger, 1975: Haller, 1984, Ryan and Thomas, 1987). It was the publication of Darwin's *Origin of Species* in 1859 that inspired his cousin Francis Galton to devote much of his life to establishing a 'scientific' understanding of heredity and variation in humankind. For Galton the answer to the question 'what controls individual difference?' lay in tracing the 'pedigrees' of families in order to demonstrate that inheritance was the key factor in both physical traits and intellectual ability. Galton and his followers claimed that some families were not only biologically 'unfit' but were actually the cause of many of society's ills such as crime, poverty and prostitution. They argued that such families, if permitted to reproduce, would lead to the physical degeneracy of the race and the downward spiral to eventual 'feeble-mindedness'. This belief led Galton's followers to launch the Eugenics Education Society (see Mazumdar, 1992). The Society's aims were first to broadcast the view that the manifestly 'unfit' were at large in society and free to propagate their kind which would inevitably lead to national tragedy as their numbers increased to the point where they outnumbered those from 'good stock', then to argue for a legislative solution to the problem of 'defectives'. The Eugenics Education Society was successful in these aims as in 1913 the Mental Deficiency Act was passed. Following this act there was a massive increase in the building of asylums to house those identified as defective. As Ryan and Thomas (1987) demonstrate

> '... between 1918 and 1931 the number of places in institutions registered under the Mental Deficiency Act nearly tripled. In the eight years that followed it nearly doubled again, to reach 32 000 by 1939'.

Although the 1913 Act also allowed for supervision within the community in the form of guardianships the numbers of people being placed in long-term institutions grew. As the numbers rose it was the increasing financial burden to the tax payer that fuelled the argument that segregation was no longer the solution to the problem of the 'unfit'. A new solution was advocated, mass sterilization. Although the focus on this new solution was people with learning difficulties housed in the long stay institutions some argued for an ever wider casting of the legislative net in an attempt to stem the tide into national degeneracy. In his book, *The Sterilisation of the Unfit*, Gallichan (1929) asked the question, who are the unfit in our society? Gallichan suggested that the unfit are not only the feeble-minded and physically defective, but by definition should include militant anarchists, prostitutes, arsonists and even those found guilty of 'train derailment'. Once again the eugenics movement lobbied for a change in the law.

The Brock Committee (set up to investigate the question of legal sterilization) published its report in 1934 suggesting that legislation should be used to allow for voluntary sterilization. The focus of the debate was who should be included on the list. The Brock Report concluded that consideration should be given to the physically impaired, the blind, the deaf, individuals with haemophilia and brachydactly and according to Trombley (1988), the Committee's estimations would have included 3.5 million people.

Fortunately for disabled people in Britain legislation was never passed. In Germany, however, not only were sterilization operations performed on disabled people in large numbers but the elimination of disabled people on the grounds of 'Lebensunwertes Leben' (life unworthy of life) became policy. Lifton (1986) and Burleigh (1994) have documented the process of the elimination of disabled people under the Nazi regime.

With the end of the war and the liberation of those who had survived the Nazi hygiene policy, the full horror of what took place came to light. The evidence presented at the Nuremberg trials and the news reels of the death camps helped to discredit many of the ideas of the eugenists. However the immediate post-war provision for many disabled people remained one of 'out of sight, out of mind'. It was with the growing anti-institutional movement of the 1960s and the publication of works which critically analysed the effects of institutional life on individuals such as that by Goffman (1962), Cartwright (1964) and Morris (1969) which called into question the appropriateness of this provision. Since then the debate has been around the question of 'care in the community' and yet there are still some who would argue for selective abortion and infanticide based on the notion of 'life unworthy of life' (Fletcher, 1972). More recently advances in genetic knowledge has again enabled those who would advocate the elimination of disabled children to cloak themselves in scientific respectability (Stanworth, 1989). Writing about the struggle for one person with Down's syndrome for access to health care in the USA, Peters (1995), reminds us:

'There is also a growing debate among ethicists about intelligence as a determinant of quality of life. One argument states that parents should have 28 days after childbirth to decide on infanticide if the new baby qualifies as a "life that has begun very badly".'

The importance of understanding this history of oppression lies not merely in an appreciation of history for its own sake but to help sustain an awareness that although the 'eugenic ideal' has been discredited many of the concepts on which it was based hide just beneath the surface of much of today's medical ethics, research and practice.

Oppression: present day

Nosek *et al.* (1994) write:

'Women with physical disabilities face long-standing, substantial barriers to expressing their sexuality. Sources of these barriers include the physical environment, the attitudes of society, and the abusive behaviours of people close to them'.

It is a widely held belief that attitudes towards disabled people are generally improving. Whilst this may be so in certain respects, prejudice against disabled people lies scarcely below the surface of present day society and becomes clearly apparent whenever questions of sexuality and sexual relationships arise. In a survey of the press and media coverage of the sterilization of a young woman with learning difficulties, Werthiemer (1988) found that much of the news coverage was based on inaccurate and conflicting information and beliefs:

'At times the newspaper reader must have found it hard to decide whether "Jeanette" was a teenage vamp looking for sexual adventure or a little girl who needed protection from the rest of the world ... despite the fact that she was neither of these'.

Abuse is the clearest manifestation of the continued oppression of disabled people. Many disabled children and adults are subject to sexual abuse and exploitation, and the statistics are shocking. Turk and Brown (1992), for instance, recorded 120 new cases of sexual abuse of adults with learning difficulties over a 2 year period in one regional health authority. Doucette (1986) reported that disabled women with various impairments were one and a half times as likely to have been sexually abused as children as non-disabled women. In many general reviews of research, such as Sobsey (1994), it is commonly accepted that disabled people face an increasing risk of sexual abuse, and many more cases go unreported. It is interesting to note that in the case of people with learning difficulties access to sex education may contribute to safeguarding them from abuse. Brown and Craft (1992), when reporting one study into the sexual abuse of adults conclude that:

'Significantly, those individuals who had received prior sex education were less likely to have been abused that those who had not. This was particularly so for women'.

Experiencing barriers: impact of impairment

Denial and suppression of sexuality, prejudice and abuse can be understood, then, at a societal level. The complex and diverse picture of sexuality and disability is, however, multi-faceted. Another level of understanding focuses on the experiences of individuals. This, in itself, can be viewed from different standpoints or models (see Chapter 23). Pursuing a social model of disability our discussion here is orientated towards the barriers that disabled people face and the strategies they adopt in expressing their sexuality, establishing a sexual identity and functioning as a sexual being.

Davis, et al. (1982) suggest that the physiological impact of impairment on sexual functioning can be identified under two headings: the direct effect of the impairment and the indirect effect of the impairment. The nature of the effect will be determined by the nature of the impairment.

The impact on those who have a spinal cord injury is dependent on the site and extent of the lesion but people with a spinal cord injury are likely to have no sensation or incomplete feeling from as high as below the shoulders. There may be the loss of erection and ability to ejaculate, there may be lack of vaginal and clitoral sensation as well as difficulties with vaginal lubrication which generally accompanies sexual arousal. As Rosen and Hall (1984) explains,

'... when a man's spine is injured so that signals cannot travel down the spinal cord from the brain, he will not have an erection, no matter how exciting he finds sights, sounds, thoughts or other psychogenic stimuli'.

Lack of physical sensation may also be a difficulty faced by those with spina bifida. Men sometimes experience retrograde ejaculation (where the sperm is directed into the bladder). Although with most people with cerebral palsy there are no difficulties relating to sensation and feeling in the genital area, like some people with other neurological conditions, control of spasms can have an inhibitory effect on sexual relationships.

Despite these potential difficulties many disabled people report that a fulfilling sex life is enjoyed and even orgasm reached by concentrating on sensations from other areas of the body. For example,

> 'I felt asexual for a long time because a man's sex was supposed to be in his penis, and I couldn't feel my penis ... it didn't occur to me that it felt good to have the back of my neck licked, or that it felt good to have my arms stroked lightly. Stroking the wrists, then to the arms, then up the arms, is a sequence that I've since learned can be very exciting' (Smith, 1981).

Morris (1989) provides a number of examples of women who found similar experiences.

> '... gradually I found that though without vaginal or clitoral sensation, other erogenous zones compensate and that if the relationship is good it is possible to reach orgasm'.

and

> 'We get a great deal of pleasure from the sex I can manage. I am fairly sure I get what are called 'phantom orgasms' and we are always game to try new experiences and positions. It is definitely true to say that we get far more enjoyment from sex then we ever thought possible. We use mouth and nose and facial stroking a great deal, with back tickling as well. We both get thoroughly turned on by these things and we culminate by my husband entering me. I am very ticklish in certain places and I can get an orgasm from being stroked there (for example under my arms)'.

Areas of the body can be explored as potential sites of pleasure, with an individual telling a partner what feels best. However it would be wrong to suggest that the solution is merely to find other stimulation techniques. Clearly some disabled people do find it difficult to come to terms with lack of sensation. As Gina, another contributor to Morris' book on the experiences of disabled women, states:

> 'It's a big strain on top of all the other problems – to get it right ... I felt terribly frustrated at not having the sensitivity that I had before and I think my boyfriend found it hard. I think I became too over eager to make things alright again'.

Indirect effects of spinal injury on sexuality are related to negative body image combined with paralysis, spasticity and the presence of catheters. Again as Morris (1989) documents, a number of the contributors felt that incontinence was inhibiting when developing a sexual relationship. However, Alan and Margaret, a married couple who are both 'doubly incontinent' felt that although urinary appliances in themselves were not a problem, developing tolerance was the key to the relationship (Newman, 1983).

Pain associated with conditions such as arthritis can have an effect on sexual activity where finding positions for love making may pose problems. Restricted movement can also create difficulties. Fifty-four percent of women and fifty-six percent of men with arthritis, in a study by Ferguson and Figley (1979), reported sexual difficulties relating to pain, weakness and movement. Drugs such as anti-hypertensives and anti-spasmodics can also affect sexual activity.

Experiencing barriers: impact of the social environment

Sexual self-concept

This is a broad theme encompassing concepts of self, body image, sexual identity and self-esteem. It is inevitably a social theme which incorporates the influence of family, friends and, of course, professionals. Embarrassment and loss of self-esteem along with feelings of unattractiveness have all been reported by disabled people. Experiences of being seen as an object when encountering the medical profession can only contribute to the loss of self-esteem. As one disabled woman relates:

'I remember a humiliating experience I had when I was twelve. It was in the physiotherapy room. I was seeing the doctor who came from the local hospital on weekly visits. On this particular day he had brought five male student doctors with him, and I was made to walk naked in front of them and then lie on a mat while in turn they examined my body, opening and closing my legs, poking and prodding here and there and making comments. I was at the age when I was developing from a child into a woman and they made me feel so embarrassed. I used to cry on these visits. Then I started to lose respect for my body but it wasn't so embarrassing for me. There was no one I could talk to mainly because I was too young to understand what was happening. I had learned how to defend myself from an early age. I had to be strong-minded and strong-willed and by the age of fourteen I started to respect my body again. It took a long time and even today I sometimes find it difficult'. (Anderson and Ricci, 1990).

There are a number of different elements to this theme of self-concept. Bancroft (1989), for instance, suggests that the psychological impact of impairment on disabled people can affect sexuality in a number of ways. From their interviews, Nosek et al. (1994) found that disabled women seek to restrict or limit the implications of impairment. They state:

'The sexually well woman is able to isolate functional impairment to the body function impaired, even if that is related to sexual activity, without perceiving her entire sexual being as impaired'.

There is also a social dimension to self-concept and self-esteem in particular. We become the people we are in our relationships with others and as a reflection of the society in which we live (Swain, 1995). In a society where we are surrounded by images which conform to a limited view of physical attractiveness, those of us who do not conform to this image can find ourselves oppressed by this very notion of what is 'acceptable'. Literature, films and visual art have helped construct the concept of what is desirable and the more deviant one is perceived from a 'norm' the more likely one will experience anxiety about oneself as a sexual being. The media, for instance, consistently depict a restricted range of physical characteristics which define the norm of physical attractiveness. It is this norm which individuals strive to attain. As Hahn (1990) writes:

'... for decades, non-disabled viewers have been bombarded with almost unattainable media images of physical "perfection" that most of them could never possibly approximate'.

Sexual information

The past 20 years or so has seen a burgeoning of available literature, developing sex education programmes and increasing sources of advice on sexuality for disabled people. In general these developments tend to be directed more towards people with learning difficulties and people with acquired impairments, rather than people disabled from birth or early childhood. Nevertheless, the literature has consistently documented the lack of information accessible to disabled people, and particularly specific groups of disabled people. O'Toole and Bregante (1992), for instance, highlighted the dearth of information for disabled lesbians. They write:

'Whilst many disabled lesbians have active sexual lives, they have very limited access to services, information and support'.

Kempton (1972), Edmonson and Wish (1975) and Watson and Rogers (1980) have all suggested that people with learning difficulties, both institutionalized and non-institutionalized have sexual knowledge which involves serious errors. This would imply that the 'vehicles' for gaining knowledge are not available for people with learning difficulties. Although Wertheimer (1988) found that some patients do take a stance which denies the sexuality of their son or daughter, Shepperdson (1988) in his study of people with Down's syndrome suggests that many parents do acknowledge their child's emerging interest in sex during adolescence, but that sex education was usually limited to warnings rather than explanations. Explanations concerning sexual intercourse, pregnancy or birth were rarely attempted by parents as this example from Shepperdson (1988) illustrates:

'One mother simply said "boys make babies and girls have babies", but was at a loss as to how to elaborate on this since she said, "it's like talking to a 5-year-old".'

Possibly because of the difficulties of making explanations understood over one-third of parents in this study felt it was not possible to provide sex education. Of the remaining parents most felt that such education should be left to the school. One parent had even approached the GP and was told 'Tell her if she goes with anyone she'll have a baby'.

Craft and Cromby (1991) in a survey of parental involvement in sex education for people with learning difficulties undertaken as part of the Nottingham Sex Education Project found that, once informed, parents were often relieved that the issues were being addressed. Although there are a number of teaching packages available specifically designed to meet the needs of people with learning difficulties (see Craft, 1991: McCarthy and Thompson, 1992; O'Sullivan and Gillies, 1993), educational and residential and day service staff are understandably reluctant to undertake any 'hands on' education because guidelines and policy statements limit this. If an individual with learning difficulties needs help to learn to masturbate for example who should undertake this role? For some people with learning difficulties the use of visual materials alone may not be sufficient.

Sexual relationships

Anderson and Clark (1982) undertook a study, part of which looked at the fears and aspiration of disabled adolescents. Using semi-structured interviews they compared the responses of disabled adolescents to a control group of non-disabled adolescents. When asking about relationships the data revealed a striking difference between the two groups:

> 'Nearly half the control group currently had or had once had a steady boy- or girlfriend, while over one quarter went out with one sometimes. In contrast, the great majority of the handicapped pupils (80 per cent) reported that they had little or no experience of dating'.

When asked about their worries about relationships the most frequently cited worry was that they would never find a boy- or girlfriend because they would be seen as unattractive.

For many disabled people merely gaining access to the social world of their peers can be a major problem. Physical barriers which ensure a segregated life style deny disabled people the opportunity to meet with others, to share experiences and develop relationships.

A major barrier that people with learning difficulties face is the attitudes of others towards them as sexual beings. The notion that people with learning difficulties are and always will be children has obvious implications on their ability to achieve and maintain adult status and all that is conferred on that role by society including opportunities to develop sexual relationships. The lack of privacy experienced by many people with learning difficulties due to the perceived need for constant supervision ensures that any overt display of sexuality is often seen as a problem of self-control over 'sexual urges' rather than as a consequence of restricted life opportunities. For many people with learning difficulties their struggle for others to acknowledge them as sexual beings can bring them into conflict with carers. As the example provided by Atkinson and Williams (1990) in their book *Know me as I am*, an anthology of work by people with learning difficulties, discloses:

> 'I want to be with my boyfriend because I love him very much. My mum and dad don't want me to be like that, but my life is more important. I'm different to my mum and dad. My relationship with my boyfriend is important to me'.

A positive role for therapists

So far we have been exploring the role of sexuality in the history and continuing oppression of disabled people and the experiences of disabled people as sexual beings. Overall, we have attempted to develop a picture which does not depict sexuality and disability as a self-contained, clearly defined set of issues, but rather as a diverse topic which draws in social, psychological and biological aspects which are crucial to the lives and lived experiences of disabled people.

Our search of the literature which directly addresses this focus has unearthed much of relevance but little which is specifically aimed at physiotherapists. There has been research which clearly demonstrates that sexual concerns are manifest in the therapist–client relationship. It is, however, negative in orientation as that research suggests that a high percentage of physiotherapists experience inappropriate sexual behaviours from their patients and clients (McCombes *et al.*, 1993). Though this in itself is clearly unacceptable and has direct implications, for education for example, it is beyond the remit of this chapter. In terms of our present discussion, the research highlights from a different angle the relevance of sexual issues to physiotherapy practice.

Starting points for a positive role for physiotherapists are found in their attitudes towards both sexuality *per se* and their role in intervention. The Plissit Model is a conceptual scheme of use to physiotherapists. Plissit is an acronym for four stages of intervention: permission (P), limited information (LI) (i.e. limited in the sense of being specific to a particular impairment), specific suggestions (SS), and intensive therapy (IT). In relation to day-to-day physiotherapy practice, permission is most immediately relevant to developing clients' positive self-concepts. Keller and Buchanan (1990) state:

> 'Permission implies that many patients merely need to have reassurance that their behaviour, coping strategies, fantasies and ideas are normal and acceptable. Such permission often removes sexual anxieties and barriers to sexual expression'.

There are also more positive aspects to the physiotherapists' role. As we stated above, research has begun to identify the wide-spread incidence of the sexual abuse of disabled children and adults and the physiotherapist has a role to play in safeguarding against this form of oppression. Brown and Craft (1992) have developed training materials for those working with people with learning difficulties, yet the key questions which they suggest need to be asked by service providers are applicable whatever the context. These key questions concern the recognition of abuse, the development of skills and systems to respond to sexual abuse, protecting individuals and supporting service users. For some disabled people the physiotherapist may be the only contact felt appropriate for disclosure.

Another aspect of a positive role for physiotherapists is in providing information. It can be argued that there is now such a wealth of possible sources of support, including literature and national and local groups, that lack of access to literature for disabled people is inexcusable. It may be that the most effective approach is to provide disabled people with both knowledge and skills in this area, the therapist, as part of a multidisciplinary team, has an important role to play.

When working with disabled people with a physical impairment the therapist may be the most appropriate person to offer information concerning the impact of impairment on sexual activity as access to adequate information can be a major barrier which confronts disabled adults. By taking the role of 'sexual ally' and helping disabled people challenge the negative views that many have concerning their sexuality, therapists will begin to see their task as empowering disabled individuals. Physiotherapists can be both a direct source of information themselves and, perhaps more importantly, they may provide access to further sources of information.[1]

There are also a number of dimensions to a positive role for physiotherapists in the development of positive and productive relationships with disabled people.

1. The first is the organization, management and provision of physiotherapy. This needs to be planned and evaluated with a view to the experiences of disabled people in terms of their developing sexuality. For instance, privacy is an important consideration here.
2. The second is physiotherapy practice as a form of communication, with messages of both sexuality and asexuality. Consideration needs to be given, for instance, to processes of touch and proximity.
3. Physiotherapy can also involve members of the families of disabled people such as partners in the case of adults and parents of younger disabled clients. The general awareness of sexual concerns is important and, again, there is the possibility of the physiotherapist providing information.
4. Finally, at a more general level of thinking, consideration of sexuality in physiotherapy practice requires a 'holistic' approach with clients. This does *not* mean that physiotherapists have either the responsibility or the right to delve into and open up everything about the client and his or her life for the sake of therapy. The control that the client has over the situation is of paramount importance. Indeed, in this context this is the crux of a 'holistic' approach: physiotherapy practice which is open and flexible in responding to the client's concerns as defined by the client.

Physiotherapists are, of course, not sex therapists or sex educationalists. They do, however, work with people who are sexual beings and who experience many barriers to the realization of their sexual identity and functioning. They inevitably have a significant role to play which requires careful reflection if it is to contribute positively rather than negatively to the sexuality of disabled people.

References

Atkinson D., Williams F. (1990) *Know me as I am*. London: Hodder and Stoughton.
Anderson E., Clark L. (1982) *Disability in Adolescence*. London: Methuen.
Anderson J., Ricci M. (eds) (1990) *Society and Social Science*. Milton Keynes: The Open University

---

[1] There are a number of sources of information to which the physiotherapist may turn. We would recommend *The Directory for Disabled People: A handbook of information and opportunities for disabled and handicapped people* compiled by A. Darnbrough and D. Kinrade (Woodhead-Faulkner in association with The Royal Association for Disability and Rehabilitation) which is frequently updated. *Practical Issues in Sexuality and Learning Disabilities* (1994) edited by A. Craft (Routledge). SPOD (Association to Aid the Sexual and Personal Relationships of Disabled People), 286 Camden Road, London N7 0BJ.

Bancroft J. (1989) *Human Sexuality and it's Problems*. London: Churchill Livingstone.

Brown H., Craft C. (1992) *Working with the Unthinkable*. London: FPA Education Unit.

Brown H. (1994) An ordinary sexual life? A review of the normalisation principle as it applies to the sexual options of people with learning disabilities. *Disability and Sexuality*, **9**(2) 123–143.

Burleigh M. (1994) *Death and Deliverance*. Cambridge: Cambridge University Press.

Cartwright A. (1964) *Human Relations and Hospital Care*. London: Routledge and Kegan Paul.

Christiaens M. (1985) We do it normally, just like other people. In *Sexuality & Handicap* (Deschesne B. H. H. D. *et al.*, eds). Cambridge: Woodhead-Faulkner.

Craft A., Craft M. (eds) (1983) *Sex Education and Counselling for Mentally Handicapped People*. Tunbridge Wells: Costello.

Craft A. (1991) *Living Your Life: A Sex Education and Personal Development Programme for Students with Learning Difficulties*. London: LDA.

Craft A., Cromby J. (1991) *Parental Involvement in the Sex Education of Students with Severe Learning Difficulties*. Nottingham: University of Nottingham Medical School.

Craft A. (ed.) (1994) *Practical Issues in Sexuality and Learning Disabilities*. London: Routledge.

Darnbrough J., Kinrade D. (1988) *Directory for Disabled People* (5th edn). Cambridge: Woodhead-Faulkner.

Davis M., *et al.* (1982) *Sexuality and the Physically Disabled*. London: SPOD.

Dechesne, B. H. H. D., *et al.* (eds) (1981) *Sexuality & Handicap*. Cambridge: Woodhead-Faulkner.

Doucette J. (1986) *Violent Acts Against Disabled Women*. Toronto: DAWN (Disabled Women's Network).

Edmonson B., Wish J. (1985) Sex knowledge and attitudes of moderately retarded males. *American Journal of Mental Deficiency*, **80**(2).

Ferguson K., Figley B. (1979) Sexuality and rheumatic disease. A prospective study. In *Sexuality and Disability*, **2**, 130–138.

Fletcher J. (1972) *Indicators of Humanhood: A Tentative Profile of Man*. In Hastings Centre Report, Vol. 2, No. 5. November 1972.

Gaarder J. (1985) *Sophie's World*. London: Phoenix House.

Gallichan W. (1929) *The Sterilization of the Unfit*. London: T. Werner Laurie.

Goffman E. (1962) *Asylums*. London: Anchor Books, Doubleday & Co.

Hahn H. (1990) Can disability be beautiful. In *Perspectives on Disability* (Nagler M. ed.). Palo Alto: Health Markets Research.

Haller M. (1984) *Eugenics*. New Jersey: Rutgers University Press.

Keller S., Buchanan D. C. (1990) Sexuality and disability: an overview. In *Perspectives on Disability* (Nagler M., ed.) Palo Alto: Health Markets Research.

Kempton W. (1972) *Guidelines for Planning a Training Course on Human Sexuality and the Retarded*. Philadelphia: Planned Parenthood Association of South Eastern Pennsylvania.

Kempton W. (1983) Sexuality training for professionals who work with mentally handicapped persons. In *Sex Education and Counselling for Mentally Handicapped People* (Craft. A., Craft. M., eds) Tunbridge Wells: Costello.

Lifton R. (1986) *The Nazi Doctors*. Basingstoke: MacMillan.

McCarthy M., Thompson D. (1992) *Sex and the 3R's*. Brighton: Pavilion.

McCombes J., Hebert C., Glacomin C. *et al.* (1993) Experience of students and practising physical therapists with inappropriate patient sexual behaviour. *Physical Therapy*, **73**(11) 762–769.

Mazumdar P. (1992) *Eugenics, Human Genetics and Human Failings*. London: Routledge.

Morris J. (1989) *Able Lives*. London: The Women's Press.

Morris P. (1969) *Put Away*. London: Routledge and Kegan Paul.

Newman B. (1983) *Sex for Young People with Spina Bifida or Cerebral Palsy*. London: Association for Spina Bifida and Hydrocephalus.

Nosek M. A., Howard C. A., Young M. E. *et al.* (1994) Wellness models and sexuality among women and physical disabilities. *Journal of Applied Rehabilitation Counselling*, **22**(1) 50–58.

O'Sullivan A., Giles P. (1993) *You, Me and HIV*. Cambridge: Daniels.

O'Toole C. J. Bregantes J. L. (1992) Lesbians with disabilities. *Sexuality and Disability*, **10**(3) 163–172.

Peters N. (1995) *America agonises over disabled patient doctor's won't treat. Sunday Times*, 5th November.

Rosen R., Hall E. (1984) *Sexuality*. New York: Random House.

Ryan J., Thomas F. (1987) *The Politics of Mental Handicap*. London: Free Associated Press.

Shepperdson B. (1988) *Down's Syndrome*. London: Cassells.

Smith D. (1981) Spinal cord injury. In *Sexuality and Physical Disability: Personal Perspectives*. St Louis: Mosby.

Sobsey D. (1994) Sexual abuse of individuals with intellectual disability. In *Practice Issues in Sexuality and Learning Disabilities* (Craft A., ed.). London: Routledge.

Stanworth M (1989) The new eugenics. In *Making Connections* (Brechin A., Walmsley J., eds). London: Hodder and Stoughton.

Swain J. (1995) *The Use of Counselling Skills: A Guide for Therapists*. Oxford: Butterworth-Heinemann.

Trombley S. (1988) *The Right to Reproduce*. London: Weidenfield and Nicholson.

Turk V., Brown H. (1992) Sexual abuse and adults with learning difficulties. *Mental Handicap*, **20**(2) 56–58.

Watson G., Rogers R. (1980) Sexual instruction for the mildly retarded and normal adolescents: a comparison of educational approaches, parental expectations and pupil knowledge and attitude. *Health Education Journal*, **39**(3) 88–95.

Weeks J. (1989) *Sexuality*. London: Routledge.

Wertheimer A. (1988) *According to the Papers*. London: CMH.

Wolfensberger W. (1975) *The Origin and Nature of our Institutional Models*. New York: Human Policy Press.

26

Key issues in the psychological development of the child: implications for physiotherapy practice

Christopher A. Whittaker

Introduction

In 1787 Tiedemann published what is generally regarded as the first scientific account of the behaviour of a young child (Tiedemann, 1787). He carefully charted the ages at which specific behaviours occurred and emphasized the variability to be seen in development:

> 'I grant that what has here been observed cannot be taken as a general law, since children ... progress variously, the one with speed the other more slowly'.

In the last century, in particular, innumerable detailed attempts have been made to describe the behaviour of a wide range of children in naturalistic and experimental settings. Tiedemann believed that when sufficient data had been collected then:

> 'it will be possible by means of comparison to strike an average for the common order of nature'.

Two centuries later his goal remains unrealized. There is no widely accepted notion of which invariant factors control child development. Part of the problem lies in the interface between theory, observation and interpretation – what we believe determines what we look for, what we see, and what we do about it. The particular theoretical orientation which we were trained to take, or which has emerged from our clinical practice, determines the sort of research questions we ask, the methodology we adopt, the instruments we use to record our observations and the theories we apply to the interpretation of our findings about children. Broader cultural and sociopolitical issues related to gender, race, disability and power are also seen as influencing these processes of decision-making (Barton and Tomlinson, 1984; Ribbens, 1994).

Any overview of the psychology of child development, confined to a chapter, can only be highly selective. In my selectivity I have been guided by the need to provide a brief synopsis of some current major themes in the psychology of child development, with a focus on research relevant to the physiotherapist's clinical practice. Quite extensive use will be made of references to key readings as a guide to in-depth treatment of the themes raised here.

Developmental milestones or theoretical orientations?

The concept of 'developmental milestones' is one familiar to physiotherapists, for many of the major traditional texts in this field have that orientation. More recent texts, for example Bedford (1993), while outlining Piagetian theory, also emphasize the developmental milestone approach. These accounts of childhood attempts to record, in more or less detail, what children actually *do* at different ages. Developmental milestones are key factors typically grouped under concepts such as language, motor development and play.

Perhaps the most accessible text is Mary Sheridan's *Spontaneous Play in Early Childhood* (1992) which has influenced a generation of professionals in the field of health and education. An equally seminal work, at a more complex and detailed level, is K. S. Holt's (1991) *Child Development: Diagnosis and Assessment*. The focus is on paediatric assessment but it gives an in-depth insight into the pattern of child development. A third key work, also in the paediatric literature, is R. S. Illingworth's (1987) *The Development of the Infant and the Young Child.*

Sheridan, Holt and Illingworth all give recognition to the pioneering work of Gesell (Gesell and Amatruda, 1947). Four major fields are covered in Gesell's Scales: motor development, adaptive behaviour, language and personal-social behaviour. Gesell's developmental theory is essentially one of the uniform unfolding of biological mechanisms through the maturation of the nervous system.

'A behaviour pattern is simply a defined response of the neuro-motor system to a specific situation' (Gesell and Amatruda, 1947).

Such 'norm-referenced scales' have the advantage of: familiarity through long usage in clinical settings; ease of application without complex equipment; and intrinsic interest for many children. It might be argued that a detailed understanding of developmental milestones is a sufficient grounding for physiotherapists, given the other demands and constraints on their time during initial and post-graduate education and clinical practice. It will be argued that this is not the case. In particular, it is suggested that the differing theoretical positions outlined here can radically alter our perception of the relative importance of given aspects of the development of the child, and that these can lead to very different clinical outcomes.

Clarke and Clarke (1974) indicated that norm referenced tests had their origins in the application of the concepts of normal distribution and correlation analysis to the field of intelligence at the turn of the century. An examination of scales such as the Gesell, or Griffiths (1970) shows their *empirical, and observational foundation*. They were devised to compare individual children with an identified pattern of development common to a supposedly *representative population* of children of the same age. Yet some were validated a generation or more ago, on cross-sectional samples, not longitudinal ones. So different groups at each age band were tested, rather than the same group of children being monitored as they developed. Samples generally over-represented middle class white populations from western countries.

The empirical basis of test construction often leads to conceptually unrelated items being grouped together under broad headings as indicators of a particular developmental level. On the Cattell Scale (Catell, 1940) items such as patting a mirror and taking two cubes, are seen as indicative of a 7-month level. Kiernan (1974) pointed out that this empirical orientation means that items are only included if they highlight differences between age levels, that is they occur at one age level not another. Yet a third item, excluded for spanning both ages, might be a vital conceptual link, which could be used in an intervention programme with a child with atypical development.

In an important early study Stott and Ball (1965) sought to explain the poor predictive validity of norm-referenced infant scales that show only low correlations with later intelligence test scores. They found inconsistent factor content at different levels indicating that the same abilities are not being measured at each stage. On the Gesell Scale the distribution of items by factor analysis, a powerful statistical technique for identifying relationships in data, is totally different from the format laid down by its authors: the items are measuring different abilities from those intended. Stott and Ball (1965) suggested that a Piagetian theory-based scale should prove of value with infants. Subsequent research, reviewed below, has supported this perception.

A recurring criticism of norm-referenced scales is that they concentrate on perceptual motor items while ostensibly measuring cognitive development (Jones, 1972; Gaussen, 1984). The Bayley Mental Scale (Bayley, 1969) for instance, has six items which require the same cognitive object performance skill of retrieving a totally hidden object, but some items demand significantly more complex motor skills. Such tests will clearly disadvantage motor impaired children.

Practitioners need to examine the range of empirically based norm-referenced scales which they routinely employ and consider if these need to be supplemented by theory based instruments in order to gain a more complete picture of the children they are assessing. To assist this process theoretical issues in child development and the implications raised for clinical practice will be examined.

Piaget and his legacy

Developmental theory is dominated by the work of Jean Piaget, and a great deal of research which followed him was predicated on supporting or refuting his claims (Boden, 1985). His output of research was prodigious and the depth and complexity of his argument along with its uncompromising style, makes reading Piaget hard, even for specialists in the field. These difficulties spawned a plethora of 'Guides to Piaget' of which Ruth Beard's (Beard, 1969) is still one of the most accessible and Flavell's (Flavell, 1963) one of the most comprehensive. It is vital however to place Piaget's work in the context of more recent research and a very readable review is provided by Mitchell (1992). Ignorance of the subtle insights to be found in the original work, may have blunted our perceptions of important aspects of Piaget's theory: however difficult, it rewards patient scrutiny.

Piaget believed that there are distinct stages in the child's development of understanding of the world, each qualitatively different from the preceding one. He did not mean by this the commonsense notion that older children had acquired more facts because they had lived longer. Rather that a child's developing view of the world is radically different from an adult one. His stages are:

1. Sensorimotor stage – birth to 2 years.
2. Pre-operational stage – 2 to 7 years.
3. Concrete operations stage – 7 to 12 years.
4. Formal operations stage – 12 years onwards.

Research of relevance to physiotherapists has mainly occurred in the first two of these stages, and it is these which will now be considered.

Research into the sensorimotor stage

Piaget believed that babies develop by means of 'action schemas' which they generalized to different aspects of the environment: a process he called 'assimilation'. At the same time the action schemas themselves become modified, so extending the range of behaviours the infant could employ. This process he called 'accommodation'. Optimal development comes when assimilation and accommodation work in unison.

Piaget identified six hierarchical substages in the sensorimotor period, with gradual differentiation of action schemas into areas such as problem solving, causality, imitation and object permanence. His sensorimotor theory (Piaget, 1953, 1955) was developed by meticulous observation of only three children, his own – which by any reckoning is not a very representative sample.

Researchers were quick to see the potential of devising theory-based assessment procedures based on how infants think. By far the most widely used are the Ordinal Scales of Psychological Development (OSPD) (Uzgiris and Hunt, 1989). Standardized on a sample of approximately 200 infants in the USA, they generally confirmed the order and stages of concept development identified by Piaget. In 1980 Carl Dunst produced a useful clinical manual to supplement the OSPD which contained an excellent profiling procedure, additional scale items, age norms and advice on educational programming. The OSPD have been used extensively with typically developing children (Uzgiris and Hunt, 1987), children with severe and profound learning disabilities (see reviews by Kahn, 1976; Hogg, 1988), children with multiple impairment (Sharpe, 1990) and those with cerebral palsy (Cioni et al., 1993) An IBM PC expert system version of the OSPD incorporating profiling and educational advice with additional coverage of prelinguistic, early language and play measures to cover the transitional period into early pre-operational thinking has been developed and is undergoing clinical trials (Whittaker, et al., 1995). Procedures which could be used to measure cognitive development using physiological rather than motor responses with both very young and motor impaired children were reviewed by Gaussen (1984, 1985), although additional problems such as epilepsy may affect the reliability of such data.

Although Piaget examined a wide range of concepts at the sensorimotor level, one in particular has been put under a great deal of scrutiny – the concept of 'object permanence'. This is probably because of the intriguing nature of the observations made by Piaget, and the novelty of his explanations. Piaget believed that very young babies did not have an understanding that a world of permanent objects existed outside themselves and perceived it instead as a series of transitory images. A wide range of ingenious experiments has challenged his view (see Bower, 1974; Baillargeon *et al.*, 1985; Baillargeon, 1987).

Research into pre-operational thought

The development of the use of 'mental imagery' or 'foresight' in solving problems, marks the transition to pre-operational thinking. An example is searching for a causal mechanism to activate a novel wind-up toy without demonstration. Piaget (1951) and Werner and Kaplan (1963) contend that the child's idiosyncratic symbolic system, manifest, for example in deferred imitation and pretend play, is a precursor of the shared symbolic function of language. Normative data on the development of symbolic play in young children have been presented by Lowe and Costello (1988), McCune-Nicholich (1975), Rosenblatt (1977) and Largo and Howard (1979a,b) and all give general support to Piaget's formulations. The pretend play of children with autism (Wing, *et al.*, 1977; Jarrold *et al.*, 1993), severe learning difficulties (Jefree and McConkey, 1976; McConkey and Martin, 1980) and profound learning difficulties (Whittaker, 1980) have all been reported to follow a broadly similar, although attenuated, sequence of development.

A serious and persistent criticism of Piaget is that he took too little account of the social dimension in development. This will be examined more closely when considering the social context of communication, below.

As well as underestimating the social dimension in his theory, Piaget stands accused of largely ignoring it as a researcher. His claim that the pre-operational child is egocentric has been seriously challenged in Donaldson's (1978) *Children's Minds*. Her thesis is that Piaget underestimated children's abilities because they did not understand what was required in the tasks that he set them. In a well known experiment Piaget showed children a model of three mountains, each one of which had a distinctive feature at its summit. The child's task was to select a photograph of the scene representing the view of a doll which was sitting on the opposite side of the model. Children under seven tended to chose a view of the model from their own rather than the doll's perspective, and Piaget interpreted this as egocentric – a failure to perceive another's view of the world. Donaldson claimed that in fact because the task was outside their experience and the questions were linguistically complex, the children had difficulty in working out what the experimenter wanted them to say. To illustrate this interpretation, Hughes (1975) devised a hide and seek game with toys in which the children had to hide a robber from a policeman in a model partitioned into four 'rooms'. Essentially in the correct solution the robber could be seen by the child but not by the policeman. Ninety percent of children between 3 and 5 years solved the problem, disproving, according to Hughes and Donaldson, that they were egocentric. They did this, so it was claimed, because the story was more within their compass of knowledge and made 'human sense'.

Mitchell (1992) challenged their interpretation. He suggested that the policeman scenario was a simpler problem than the mountain task and invoked Flavell's theory of Level One and Level Two perspective taking (Flavell *et al.*, 1981) in explanation. This proposed that children as young as 3 can understand that someone does not share their perspective, but it is only 4 year olds who can imagine what that person *can* see. Mitchell (1992) equated Level One perspective taking to the policeman task and a Level Two perspective to the mountain situation, providing a partial vindication of Piaget's position.

A rapidly growing body of evidence has examined another aspect of the difference between 3 and 4 year olds, one which focuses even more on their developing social awareness – the so-called 'Theory of Mind'.

Theory of mind

'Do you gossip?' is a question asked in some personality inventories. If you say 'no' they score it as a lie, the assumption being that we all indulge in, and enjoy, this form of social interchange. We talk and think not just about what people do, but also speculate on the motives behind their actions. This understanding that other people have needs, thoughts and beliefs seems a natural part of being a person, it is called a Theory of Mind (ToM) but when does it develop? And what would we be like if we didn't possess it? Over almost two decades a burgeoning range of research has sought to answer these questions. The response to the first appears to be by about 4 years of age. The answer to the second, some authorities (see Frith, 1989) would have us believe, is that we would be labelled as having autism.

One aspect of ToM which has figured largely in this research is the attribution of a 'false belief' to someone else, where we have to suspend our own knowledge of a situation and imagine how someone else thinks about it. In a series of apparently simple experiments it has been claimed that many 4 year olds can attribute a false belief to others while most 3 year olds fail to do so (Perner *et al.*, 1987). In one version, 'The Sally-Anne Experiment', a doll leaves her marble in one location then exits the room, the second doll moves it. The child is asked where the first doll will look for the marble when she returns. Younger children are said to fail because they do not conceptualize that someone can have a false belief, when they (the children) know the truth. How far this finding will stand up to systematic variation in the language used, the use of multiple hiding places, or to non-verbal versions of the task remains unclear. Astington (1994) provided an excellent introduction to ToM and its links with pretend play. More complex literature reviews are given in Astington *et al.* (1988) and Baron-Cohen *et al.* (1993).

Autism and theory of mind

Physiotherapists may encounter less able children with autism through sensory integrative therapy, reviewed below. Additionally motor problems are common in 'Asperger's syndrome', a form of autism seen in more able individuals, and it is possible that physiotherapists may be increasingly involved in working in this field.

Autism is characterized by problems with reciprocal interaction, non-verbal/verbal communication and imaginative activity; as well as a markedly restricted repertoire of activities and interests (Frith, 1989). Particular difficulty in understanding the subtleties of social interaction and taking language on a literal level, is very common, no matter how high the person's intelligence. I was sitting with Ben, a ten year old, who has autism, and genuinely admiring his dexterity on the *Lion King* video game. Rather naïvely I inquired: 'Are you the Lion?', *'I'm* not a lion!' he retorted with a mixture of scornful disdain and incredulity. However amusing examples such as this are, they point to the sort of problems that people with autism face in a world which is less tolerant and more exploitative than we would wish.

Jones (1995) outlined the difficulties faced by someone without a theory of mind: predicting what others will do; failing to understand what people will find interesting; difficulty in appreciating hidden meanings as in teasing or sarcasm; an inability to realize that a factual statement of truth can be hurtful. Comprehension of the reasons behind these difficulties, which are ones often shown by people with autism, could aid tolerance, and help professionals and others to develop more effective social skills training programmes. While physiotherapists new to working with people with autism need to familiarize themselves with effective methods of interacting and communicating with them.

Persuasive though these arguments on ToM are, there are increasing doubts about aspects of the methodology underlying these experiments. In order to demonstrate that ToM problems are specific to autism then careful 'mental age matching' needs to take place between the experimental group of children with autism and control groups of typically developing children and youngsters with learning disabilities (Frith, 1989). Many of the studies in this area, reviewed by Happé (1995), use a simple vocabulary measure, the British Picture Vocabulary scale (BPVS) (Dunn *et al.*, 1982), to compute the verbal mental age of the participants in order to match groups. Given the well-reported language difficulties in semantics and pragmatics that people with autism have, and the verbal bias of the ToM tests, the use of BPVS seems somewhat surprising. When a much more robust measure of verbal mental age, the Wechsler Intelligence Scale for Children – Revised (WISC-R) (Wechsler, 1974), was used by Yirmiya and Shulman (1995) no significant differences were found between individuals with autism and those with severe learning disabilities on the false belief task, thus calling into question the view that failure in ToM tasks is specific to autism, and not a function of learning disability. Yirmiya and Schulman argue persuasively for studies which examine a broad spectrum of cognitive, linguistic and social-emotional factors alongside a wider range of ToM tasks.

Piaget's influence

Piaget's greatest impact has been on education, particularly in the 1960s and 1970s when his followers were influential in the child-centred approach to primary education (Plowden, 1967). Criticisms of his stage theory, and the lack of control of the social dimensions in his experiments, meant that his influence waned considerably after his death. Indirectly however, the influence of both Bruner (Bruner *et al.*, 1976) and Piaget can be seen in the play-orientated curriculum in nursery schools and in cognitive approaches to learning (Furth and Wachs, 1972; Forman and Kuschner, 1977; Feurstein, 1979; Floyd, 1979).

Physiotherapists are primarily concerned with the motor system and movement, yet most of their treatment with children is through play, so an understanding of recent advances in cognitive psychology is essential in appreciating the child's perspective. Children under seven are clearly more capable of logical thought than was believed a generation ago, and the 3 to 4 year olds are less egocentric. But there is perhaps more evidence that they struggle to make sense of the complex social encounters that adults draw them into. Clinicians, as well as cognitive researchers, would do well to think carefully about the context of their social encounters with children – to be wary of the language employed, and the level of comprehension assumed, in these often unnatural settings.

The social context of communication

Many of the children referred to physiotherapists have language and communication difficulties in addition to motor impairments, and it is important to keep informed about developments in this complex area.

Until the 1960s the intriguing question of how children acquired language was dominated by the 'operant conditioning theory' of B. F. Skinner (Skinner, 1957). He believed that care-givers unknowingly 'shaped' the infant's production of sounds, reacting very positively to new ones that the child made. As the parents became used to this sound their response would diminish, so that the child would have to work harder to get a positive reaction. By chance the infant would emit a different sound: the parent would again react positively and the process would continue. Words would be shaped in the same way and so would the expansion of the child's vocabulary. It is important to realize, particularly in the light of recent research, that 'external reinforcement' in this case the care giver's positive response, was seen as the controlling process, with the child having a largely 'passive' role.

Where Skinner's theory collapsed as an overall explanation of language acquisition was in its inability to explain the 'grammatical' development of the child. When children come to put words together they do so in a particular, grammatical way, and by the age of six they have mastered the use of most of the syntactical rules of their native tongue. This rapid expansion of ability could not be accounted for by external reinforcement, but it was seen by many to be explained by the 'psycholinguistic theories' of Naom Chomsky. In 1959 Chomsky published his famous rebuttal of Skinner and his own theory followed in 1965. Chomsky came to believe that we are born with an inherited 'Language Acquisition Device' (LAD) which is able to identify the particular 'surface structure' of the grammar of the language we are brought up in, and convert this into an innate 'deep structure'. This deep structure has a universal grammar which he claimed was possessed by all human beings. In this way he sought to explain the rapid growth in the child's understanding of the rules by which words can be linked to make acceptable utterances. His theories dominated language research for well over a decade.

Those of us working with children with complex learning disabilities during the 1970s, when Chomsky's influence was at its height, did not find his theories particularly helpful in practice. We came across an unaccountably large number of children who rather carelessly seemed to have mislaid their innate LAD, and were particularly resistant to finding it. What did help us were views which emphasized the 'reciprocity of the communication process' within an understanding of the child's cognitive development (Whittaker, 1984, 1996).

Donaldson (1978), reviewing the Chomskian revolution of the previous decade, placed importance not on grammatical structure but on the child's development of meaning:

> 'it is the child's ability to interpret situations which makes it possible for him through active processes of hypothesis testing and inference, to arrive at a knowledge of language'.

The search to determine how this process of 'construction of meaning' works, and how it affects children's thinking is on-going. We examined aspects of it when considering Donaldson's work and Theory of Mind earlier in the chapter. Mitchell (1992) gives an important review of research on the developing skills of children in the task of understanding that messages give clues to meaning. This suggests that young children's comprehension of the distinction between what is *said* and what is *meant* emerges gradually between the ages of three and six. It has significant ramifications for the way professionals interact with children in this age group, the nature of the settings in which this takes place, and our appreciation of the child's actual understanding.

The child's construction of meaning, then, is a long drawn out process, but when does it begin? The answer seems unequivocally to be in infancy, perhaps in the neonatal period itself. This research has its theoretical foundations in concepts of 'attachment' (Ainsworth, 1964; Bowlby, 1971), 'joint reference' (Bruner, 1975), and 'reciprocity' (Schaffer, 1977), all of which relate to the interactive nature of the child–care-giver relationship.

Meltzoff and Moore (1985) outlined a series of sophisticated and apparently well controlled experiments in which neonates appeared to be capable of facial imitation, indulging in tongue/lip protrusion and mouth opening following the presentation of these gestures by an adult. Given that neonates produce these movements anyway, Meltzoff and Moore's task was to demonstrate that they occurred at a greater than chance level, which they do report. They believed that their remarkable results can be explained by either an 'Innate Releasing Mechanism' (IRM) or by 'Active Intermodal Mapping (AIM). The latter is essentially imitation – the infant taking in the information visually and mirroring a motor response. If AIM were true then existing theories concerning the development of imitation (Piaget, 1951) would need radical revision, IRM, by contrast, is posited as an innate package of responses triggered by a particular visual display, analogous to the patterning seen in gulls (Tinbergen, 1951).

Meltzoff and Moore favour the more radical AIM explanation and suggest research strategies to differentiate the two explanations. It would be interesting to see these results replicated in another laboratory, and to compare the neonates 'imitation' responses to other face-like objects as in the early smiling experiments (see Schaffer, 1971).

Recent research has examined the interactional patterns between mothers and their premature babies in neonatal units. Henriksen (1994) described the 'helplessness response' of these infants and the dangers in mothers modelling their behaviour on the professionally detached 'efficient' pattern of care seen as necessary by staff in these high dependency units. The extremely specialized role of the physiotherapist within the neonatal intensive care unit is covered in a detailed and informative overview by Sheahan and Brockway (1992).

A wide range of prelinguistic communication with infants has been investigated including: modified adult facial/vocal behaviour; gaze; the use of motherese (the speech of adults to young children); touch; variation in rhythm and pace of the interaction and turn taking. An excellent review is given in Nind and Hewett (1994) which also details how these approaches can be used with older disabled children. At the core of these interactions is the adult's belief in the infant's 'intentionality', for early interactions:

'are sustained only through the mothers initiative in replying to the infant's responses as if they had communicative significance'. (Schaffer, 1977)

The baby is not the passive organism envisaged by Skinner, but an active partner engaging in a reciprocal relationship.

Bowlby (1965) believed that attachment had to be with a single person and that maternal deprivation in infancy would lead to later delinquency. Cross-cultural studies on Kibbutzim and in Africa, along with studies of children who had survived extensive social trauma have demonstrated that this view is unduly pessimistic. Rutter (1972) suggested that it is the child who has never bonded with a care giver rather than one who has been separated afterwards, who is most at risk of later emotional disturbance.

In a series of experiments it has been demonstrated that generally between 8 and 12 months of age children show both separation anxiety and fear of strangers when left by their care-giver. This transient behaviour is probably a key factor in the child's development, for as Bowlby (1971) pointed out, exploration of the environment and play are antithetical to physical attachment to the care giver. Schaffer (1971) indicated that we do not know what enables the child to leave the care giver, but suggested:

'it seems likely ... that this is dependent on his growing ability to represent the other person to himself in her absence, so that the internalized image provides him with the security which formerly only her physical presence provided'.

Replication of this separation anxiety research, with both typically developing children and disabled children using the OSPD scales as a cognitive measure could aid clarification of this issue.

Physiotherapists need to be aware that very young babies appear to have a greater awareness of their social and material environment than was thought a generation ago. By focussing only on their motor behaviour, rather than their sensory and perceptual abilities, there is a risk of under-estimating their competence.

Assessment of motor development

A comprehensive overview of the field of paediatric physiotherapy, emphasizing a 'whole child' approach, has recently been edited by Eckersley (1993). Here we will examine some current protocols and tests related to the process of motor development in typically progressing children and disabled children.

Van Sant (1994) provided a useful summary of gross-motor development in infancy with suggestions for further reading. An extensive overview of eye–hand coordination in infancy was given by Erhardt (1992); while Exner (1992) examined in-hand manipulation skills and the *Erhardt Developmental Prehension Assessment* (Erhardt, 1982) outlined in detail manipulative activity from the neonatal period until 6 years.

Physiotherapists often need a method of rapidly screening the motor behaviour of a young child to decide if formal treatment procedures are required. The Milani-Comparetti Screening Tests first described by Milani-Comparetti and Gidoni (1967) has undergone extensive revision. In its current form (Stuberg, 1992) it can be administered in less than 10 minutes by an experienced observer. The test allows the recording of both spontaneous and evoked responses from the child with an emphasis on functional motor behaviour and the reflexes underlying it. Results are presented graphically on an accessible and well-designed scoring chart which provides a useful overview of the normative timescale expected for the reflexes of early childhood.

The Bruininks-Oseretsky Test of Motor Proficiency (Bruininks, 1978) can be used to give separate and combined scores for fine and gross motor skills with typically progressing, and developmentally disabled youngsters from the age of 4½ to 14½ years. Although it has excellent test – retest reliability the standardization is based upon USA norms from the 1970s.

The Pediatric Evaluation of Disability Inventory (Haley, 1992) has a different premise from the Bruininks-Oseretsky, based instead upon an assessment of functional skill in children from 6 months to 7½ years. The areas covered are self-care, mobility and social function. An important distinction is made between capability and functional performance.

Sensory integration and psychomotor approaches

In the USA in particular, there is a long history of psychomotor work with children with varying degrees of learning difficulties. Building on the theories of Strauss in the 1940s (Strauss and Lehtinen, 1947), Frostig (1966), Cruickshank (1967), Kephart (1971) and Cratty (1974) all produced detailed programmes for working with children labelled as brain-injured, attention-deficit disordered, or having learning disabilities. British approaches of the same era are summarized by Haskell *et al.*

(1977). The most enduring body of work in this field, is the neurobehavioural approaches to Sensory Integrative Therapy (SIT) of Jean Ayres. Her Southern California Sensory Integration Tests included scales which examined space visualization, figure–ground perception, position in space, kinesthesia, manual form perception, finger identification, graphesthesia, localization of tactile stimuli and double tactile stimuli perception (Ayres, 1978, 1989). Highly detailed therapy programmes are presented based upon the tests, language measures and clinical observations (Ayres, 1973). In a recent exhaustive review however, Hoehn and Baumeister (1994) declared unequivocally that SIT was 'not merely an unproven, but a demonstrably ineffective' remedial treatment for its target populations.

Smyth (1992) provided an important review of the literature on so-called 'clumsy' children and stressed that secondary emotional problems are common in the mildly and moderately affected members of this group. Clumsiness has also been associated with Asperger's syndrome, a form of autism (American Psychiatric Association, 1994), and with dyslexia in some children (Tansley and Panckhurst, 1981). There is an important and largely unfilled role for physiotherapists in the identification and remediation of these subtle difficulties, in conjunction with other members of the interdisciplinary team.

Conclusion

The nature of physiotherapists' work means that they are often in close and prolonged contact with children and their families. They need a broad grasp of changing perceptions of development, and to be able to communicate these easily and effectively to parents and care-givers over a period of time. Useful guides to the professional skills of working with parents are McConkey (1985), Cunningham and Davis (1985) and Hartley (1993).

The importance of subtle prelinguistic communication in the social interaction between children and adults has been examined. This is particularly true when the youngster is operating at a sensorimotor level, whether as a baby or as an older child with learning disabilities. Touch and movement are subtle and powerful communicators, and it may be precisely because of the intimacy of contact that some physiotherapists believe that a brisk professional detachment is best adopted. The child is the likely loser in such an exchange. Obviously professionals who wish to use a more intensive interactional approach need to do so within clearly defined and agreed ethical parameters (Nind and Hewett, 1994). Therapists need to be aware also of the context of social encounters when working with older children who have language – and to monitor carefully their own style of communication.

The child develops within the primary ecosystem of the family, and the secondary ecosystem of the culture. For it is now generally recognized that social cognition is an essentially reciprocal process which takes place between the child and the socially mediated environment. The parents' role has long been acknowledged, but the part played by siblings and culture in this process remains relatively unexplored (Borstein et al., 1992; Azmitia and Hesser, 1993; Farver and Wimbarti, 1995). Yet despite a growing acceptance of the reciprocal nature of development, concepts of disability and typicality are still often located 'within the child' (see Chapter 23). It is particularly difficult for us as professionals to accept that we may be involved, however unwittingly, in the construction of the very disability that our vocation has drawn us to ameliorate.

Almost invariably physiotherapists practise in interdisciplinary teams drawn from professions with different training, cultures and power structures. In this situation efficient communication, always a crucial element in any workgroup, is vital. A key element has to be that members strive to understand and appreciate the professional orientation of colleagues. A sharing of knowledge on different perspectives of child development is not an undermining of professional expertise, but a way of strengthening bonds, and a recognition of the rich complexity and fascination of children.

References

Ainsworth M. D. S. (1964) Patterns of attachment behaviour shown by the infant in interaction with his mother. *Merrill-Palmer Quarterly*, **10**, 51–58.

American Psychiatric Association (1994) *Diagnostic and Statistical Manual of Mental Disorders* (4th edn). (DSM-IV). Washington: American Psychiatric Association.

Astington J. W. (1994) *The Child's Discovery of the Mind*. London: Fontana.

Astington J. W., Harris P. L., Olson D. R. (1988) *Developing Theories of the Mind*. Cambridge: Cambridge University Press.

Ayres A. J. (1973) *Sensory Integration and Learning Disorders*. Los Angeles: Western Psychological Services.

Ayres A. J. (1978) *Southern California Sensory Integration Tests*. Los Angeles: Western Psychological Services.

Ayres A. J. (1989) *Sensory Integration and Praxis Test*. Los Angeles: Western Psychological Services.

Azmitia M., Hesser J. (1993) Why siblings are important agents of cognitive development: a comparison of siblings and peers. *Child Development*, **64**, 430–444.

Baillargeon R. (1987) Object permanence in 3½ and 4½-month-old infants. *Developmental Psychology*, **23**, 655–664.

Baillargeon R., Spelke E. S., Wassermann S. (1985) Object permanence in 5-month-old infants. *Cognition*, **20**, 191–208.

Baron-Cohen S., Tager-Flusberg H., Cohen D. J. (eds) (1993) *Understanding other Minds: Perspectives from Autism*. Oxford: Oxford University Press.

Barton L., Tomlinson S. (1984) *Special Education and Social Interests*. London: Croom Helm.

Bayley N. (1969) *Manual for the Bayley Scales of Infant Development*. New York: Psychological Corporation.

Beard R. (1969) *An outline of Piaget's Developmental Psychology*. London: Routledge and Kegan Paul.

Bedford S. (1993) The developing child. In *Elements of Paediatric Physiotherapy* (Eckersley P. M., ed.) Edinburgh: Churchill Livingstone.

Boden M. A. (1985) *Piaget*. London: Fontana.

Borstein M. H., Tamis-LeMonds C. S., Tal J., *et al.* (1992) Maternal responsiveness to infants in three societies: the United States, France, and Japan. *Child Development*, **63**, 808–821.

Bower T. G. R. (1974) *Development in Infancy*. San Francisco: Freeman.

Bowlby J. (1965) *Child Care and the Growth of Love* (2nd edn) Harmondsworth: Penguin.

Bowlby J. (1971) *Attachment and Loss. Volume 1: Attachment*. Harmondsworth: Penguin.

Bruininks R. H. (1978) *Bruininks-Oseretsky Test of Motor Proficiency: Examiner's Manual*. Circle Pines, MI: American Guidance Services.

Bruner J. S. (1975) The ontogenesis of speech acts. *Journal of Child Language*, **2**, 1–19.

Bruner J. S., Jolly A., Sylva K. (1976) *Play – It's Role in Development and Evolution*. Harmondsworth: Penguin.

Cattell P. (1940) *The Measurement of Intelligence of Infants and Young Children*. New York: Psychological Corporation.

Chomsky N. (1959) Review of *Verbal Behaviour* by B. F. Skinner. *Language* **35**: 26–58.

Chomsky N. (1965) *Aspects of Theory of Syntax*. Cambridge, Massachusetts: MIT Press.

Cioni G., Paolicelli P. B., Sorti C., Vinter A. (1993) Sensori-motor development in cerebral-palsied infants assessed with the Uzgiris–Hunt Scales. *Developmental Medicine and Child Neurology*, **35**, 1055–1066.

Clark A. D. B., Clarke A. M. (1974) The changing concept of intelligence: a selective historical review. In *Mental Deficiency: The Changing Outlook* (2nd edn) (Clarke A. D. B., Clarke A. M., eds). London: Methuen.

Cratty B. J. (1974) *Motor Activity and the Education of Retardates*. Philadelphia: Lea and Febiger.

Cruickshank W. M. (1967) *The Brain-Injured Child in Home, School and Community*. New York: Syracuse University Press.

Cunningham C., Davis H. (1985) *Working with Parents: Frameworks for Collaboration*. Milton Keynes: Open University Press.

Donaldson M. (1978) *Children's Minds*. London: Fontana.

Dunn L. M., Dunn L. M., Whetton C., Pintilie D. (1982) *British Picture Vocabulary Scale*. Windsor: NFER-Nelson.

Dunst C. J. (1980) *A Clinical and Educational Manual for use with the Uzgiris and Hunt Scales of Infant Psychological Development*. Baltimore: University Park Press.

Eckersley P. M. (ed) (1993) *Elements of Paediatric Physiotherapy*. Edinburgh: Churchill Livingstone.

Erhardt R. P. (1982) *The Erhardt Developmental Prehension Assessment* (EDPA). Tucson, AZ: Therapy Skill Builders.

Erhardt R. P. (1992) Eye–hand coordination. In *Development of Hand Skills in the Child* (Case-Smith J., Pehoski C., eds). Rockville: American Occupational Therapy Association.

Exner C. E. (1992) In-hand manipulation skills. In *Development of Hand Skills in the Child* (Case-Smith J., Pehoski C., eds). Rockville: American Occupational Therapy Association.

Farver J. A., Wimbarti S. (1995) Indonesian children's play with their mothers and older siblings. *Child Development*, **66**, 1493–1503.

Feurstein R. (1979) *The Dynamic Assessment of Retarded Performers*. Baltimore: University Park Press.

Flavell J. H. (1963) *The Developmental Psychology of Jean Piaget*. New York: Van Nostrand.

Flavell J. H., Everett B. A., Croft K., Flavell E. R. (1981) Young children's knowledge about visual perception: further evidence for the Level 1–Level 2 distinction. *Developmental Psychology*, **17**, 99–103.

Floyd A. (1989) *Cognitive Development in the School Years*. London: Croom Helm.

Forman G. E., Kuschner D. S. (1977) *The Child's Construction of Knowledge. Piaget for Teaching Children*. Monterey: Brooks/Cole Publishing.

Frith U. (1989) *Autism – explaining the enigma*. Oxford: Blackwell.

Frostig M. (1966) *Marianne Frostig Developmental Test of Visual Perception*. Palo Alto: Consulting Psychologists Press.

Furth H. G., Wachs H. (1972) *Thinking Goes to School. Piaget's Theory in Practice*. London: Oxford University Press.

Gaussen T. (1984) Developmental milestones or conceptual millstones? Some practical and theoretical limitations in infant assessment procedures. *Child: Care, Health and Development*, **10**, 99–115.

Gaussen T. (1985) Beyond the milestone model – a system framework for alternative infant assessment procedures. *Child: Care, Health and Development*, **11**, 131–150.

Gesell A., Amatruda C. S. (1947) *Developmental Diagnosis*. New York: Hoeber/Hamish Hamilton.

Griffiths R. (1954) *The Abilities of Babies*. London: University of London Press.

Haley S. M. (1992) *Pediatric Evaluation of Disability Inventory (PEDI): Development, Standardization and Administration Manual*. Boston: New England Medical Centre Hospitals and PEDI Research Group.

Happé F. G. E. (1995) The role of age and verbal ability in the theory of mind task performance of subjects with autism. *Child Development*, **66**, 843-855.

Hartley P. (1993) Parents and children. In *Elements of Paediatric Physiotherapy* (Eckersley P. M., ed.) Edinburgh: Churchill Livingstone.

Haskell S. H., Barrett K., Taylor H. (1977) *The Education of Motor and Neurologically Handicapped Children*. London: Croom Helm.

Henriksen M. (1994) A reflective look at the use of comforting touch on infants receiving high dependency care in the neonatal unit, and the importance of parental participation. *Unpublished Dissertation*. Newcastle: University of Northumbria.

Hoehn T. P., Baumeister A. A. (1994) A critique of the application of Sensory Integration Therapy to children with learning difficulties. *Journal of Learning Disabilities*, **27**(6) 338–350.

Hogg J. (1988) Early development and Piagetian tests. In *Assessment in Mental Handicap* (Hogg J., Raynes N. V., eds). London: Croom Helm.

Holt K. S. (1991) *Child Development: Diagnosis and Assessment*. London: Butterworth-Heinemann.

Hughes M. (1975) Ego-centrism in pre-school children. *Unpublished Doctoral Dissertation*: Edinburgh University.

Illingworth R. S. (1987) *The Development of the Infant and Young Child: Normal and Abnormal*. Edinburgh: Churchill Livingstone.

Jarrold C., Boucher J., Smith P. (1993) Symbolic Play in Autism: A review. *Journal of Autism and Developmental Disorders*. **23**(2) 281–307.

Jefree D., McConkey R. (1976) An observational scheme for recording children's imaginative doll play. *Journal of Child Psychology and Psychiatry and Allied disciplines*, **17**, 189–197.

Jones G. E. (1995) Enhancing provision for children with autism: What can we learn from current approaches and practice? *Unpublished Manuscript*. University of Birmingham.

Jones M. (1972) A developmental schedule based on Piaget's sensori-motor writings: an examination of the schedule's potential value as an instrument for assessing severe and profoundly subnormal children. *Unpublished M.Sc. Thesis*. University of London.

Kahn J. (1976) Utility of the Uzgiris and Hunt scales of sensori-motor development with severely and profoundly retarded children. *American Journal of Mental Deficiency*, **80**, 663–665.

Kephart N. C. (1971) *The Slow Learner in the Classroom*, (2nd edn). Columbus: Merrill.

Kiernan C. C. (1974) Behaviour modification. In *Mental Deficiency: The Changing Outlook* (2nd edn) (Clarke A. M., Clarke A. D. B., eds). London: Methuen.

Largo R. H., Howard J. A. (1979a) Developmental progression in play behaviour of children between nine and thirty months. I. Spontaneous play and imitation. *Developmental Medicine and Child Neurology*, **21**, 299–310.

Largo R. H., Howard J. A. (1979b) Developmental progression in play behaviour of children between nine and thirty months. II. Spontaneous play and language development. *Developmental Medicine and Child Neurology*, **21**, 492–503.

Lowe M., Costello A. J. (1988) *Manual for the Symbolic Play Test*. Windsor: NFER.

McConkey R. (1985) *Working with Parents. A Practical Guide for Teachers and Therapists*. London: Croom Helm.

McConkey R., Martin H. (1980) *The Development of Pretend Play in Down's Syndrome Infants: A Longitudinal Study*. Dublin: St Michael's House.

McCune-Nicholich L. (1977) Beyond sensori-motor intelligence: assessment of symbolic maturity through analysis of pretend play. *Merrill-Palmer Quarterly*, **23**(2), 88–99.

Meltzoff A. N., Moore M. K. (1985) Cognitive foundations and social functions of imitation and intermodal representation in infancy. In *Neonate Cognition, Beyond the Blooming Buzzing Confusion* (Mehler J., Fox R., eds) Hillsdale: Lawrence Earlbaum.

Milani-Comparetti A., Gidoni E. A. (1967) Routine developmental examination in normal and retarded children. *Developmental Medicine and Child Neurology*, **9**, 631–638.

Mitchell P. (1992) *The Psychology of Childhood*. London: Falmer Press.

Nind M., Hewett D. (1994) *Access to Communication*. London: Fulton.

Perner J., Leekham S. R., Winner M. (1987) Three-year-olds' difficulty with false belief: the case for a conceptual deficit. *British Journal of Developmental Psychology*, **5**, 125–137.

Piaget J. (1951) *Play, Dreams and Imitation in Childhood*. London: Routledge and Kegan Paul.

Piaget J. (1953) *The Origin of Intelligence in the Child*. London: Routledge and Kegan Paul.

Paiget J. (1955) *The Child's Construction of Reality*. London: Routledge and Kegan Paul.

Plowden B. H. (1967) *Children and Their Primary Schools. A Report of the Central Advisory Council. Vol 1: The Report*. London: HMSO.

Ribbens J. (1994) *Mothers and Their Children. A Feminist Sociology of Childrearing*. London: Stage.

Rosenblatt D. (1977) Developmental trends in infant play. In *Biology of Play*. (Clinics in Dev Med. No. 62) London: Heinemann.

Rutter M. (1972) *Maternal Depreciation Reassessed*. Harmondsworth: Penguin.

Schaffer H. R. (1971) *The Growth of Sociability*. Harmondsworth: Penguin

Schaffer H. R. (1977) *Studies in Mother–Infant Interaction*. London: Academic Press.

Sharpe P. (1990) An Assessment of the cognitive abilities of multiply handicapped children: adaptations of the Uzgiris and Hunt scales and their use with children in Britain and Singapore. *Child: Care, Health and Development*, **16**, 335–353.

Sheahan M. S., Brockway N. F. (1992) The high risk infant. In *Pediatric Physical Therapy* (2nd edn) (Tecklin J., ed.). Philadelphia: J. R. Lippincott.

Sheridan M. D. (1992) *Spontaneous Play in Early Childhood*. Windsor: NFER-Nelson.

Skinner B. F. (1957) *Verbal Behaviour*. New York: Appleton-Century-Crofts.

Smyth T. R. (1992) Impaired motor skill (clumsiness) in otherwise normal children: a review. *Child: Care, Health, and Development*, **18**, 283–300.

Stott L. H., Ball R. S. (1965) *Evaluation of infant and pre-school mental tests*. Monog. of.Soc.Res. in Child Dev.

Strauss A. A., Lehtinen L. E. (1947) *Psychopathology and Education of the Brain-injured Child*. New York: Grune and Stratton.

Stuberg W. A. (1992) *The Milani-Comparetti Motor Development Screening Test* (3rd edn rev.). Omaha, NE: University of Nebraska Medical Centre.

Tansley P., Panckhurst J. (1981) *Children with Specific Learning Difficulties*. Windsor: NFER-Nelson.

Tiedemann D. (1787) *Beobachtungen uber die Entwicklung der Seelenfahrrifkeiten bei Kindern*. Alterburg: Bonde.

Tinbergen N. (1951) *The Study of Instinct*. London: Oxford University Press.

Uzigris I., Hunt J., McV. (1987) *Infant Performance and Experience. New Findings with the Ordinal Scales of Psychological Development*. Chicago: University of Illinois Press.

Uzgiris I., Hunt J., McV. (1989) *Assessment in Infancy: Ordinal Scales of Psychological Development* (2nd edn). Chicago: University of Illinois Press.

Van Sant A. F. (1994) Motor development. In *Pediatric Physical Therapy* (2nd edn) (Tecklin J., ed). Philadelphia: J. B. Lippincott.

Wechsler D. (1974) *Wechsler Intelligence Scale for Children – Revised*. New York: Psychological Corporation.

Werner H., Kaplan B. (1963) *Symbol Formation*. New York: Wiley.

Whittaker C. A (1980) A note on developmental trends in the symbolic play of hospitalized profoundly retarded children. *Journal of Child Psychology and Psychiatry and Allied Disciplines*, **21**, 253–261.

Whittaker C. A. (1984) *Cognitive development and aspects of prelinguistic and manual communication in severely and profoundly retarded children*. Paper (by proxy) to the American Academy of Child Psychiatry, Toronto, October.

Whittaker C. A., Philipson C., Walker A. (1995) *The Early Mental Representation Profile*. Newcastle upon Tyne: University of Northumbria at Newcastle.

Whittaker C. A. (1996) Spontaneous proximal communication in children with autism and severe learning disabilities: Issues for therapeutic intervention. Paper to International Conference on *Therapeutic Interventions in Autism: Perspectives from Research and Practice*, April 1–3, 1996, College at St Hild and St Bede, University of Durham.

Wing L., Gould J., Yeats S. R., Brierley L. M. (1977) Symbolic play in severly mentally retarded and in autistic children. *Journal of Child Psychology and Psychiatry and Allied Disciplines*, **18**, 167–178.

Yirmiya N., Shulman C. (1995) Seriation, conservation and Theory of Mind abilities in individuals with autism, mental retardation and normal development. Proceedings of the International Conference on *Psychological Perspectives in Autism*. 105–116. Sunderland: Autism Research Unit.

27

Health, health education and physiotherapy practice
Jane S. Owen Hutchinson

Identifying the problem

Because of their centrality within practice, most physiotherapists will, during the course of their work, have considered the concepts of 'health' and 'health education'. Opportunities to reflect upon these subjects are amply provided within the literature of the human sciences, including that of physiotherapy, where various definitions and models of health and health education have been documented (see for example, Warren, 1985; Burkitt, 1986; Warren, 1986; Twomey, 1986; Ritchie, 1989; Sim, 1990; Condie, 1991; Parry, 1991; Roberts, 1994; Higgs and Titchen, 1995; Hills, 1995). Personal experience supported by written evidence, however, suggests that whilst many physiotherapists may be acquainted with a wide range of health models on an abstract, theoretical level, their practice is nevertheless predominantly characterized by the biomedical model (see for example, Brechin and Liddiard, 1981; McIntosh, 1989; Ritchie, 1989; Sluijs, 1991; Balfour, 1993; Sluijs *et al.* 1993; Adamson and Nordholm, 1994; Marshall and Walsh, 1994; Strachura, 1994; Jaggi and Bithell, 1995). Most therapists continue to regard members of the public to whom they give a service as 'patients'. These 'patients' are perceived as 'individuals' presenting with a physical 'diagnosis': the patient is not infrequently classified as 'a back', 'a fractured shaft of femur' or 'a ruptured tendo Achilles'. The diagnosis may refer to an acute or chronic condition: the former demands immediate 'cure', the latter requires long-term management by the 'expert'.

Research conducted by Hills (1995) indicates that physiotherapists also seem to favour a model of health education (as described by Burkitt, 1986; Coutts and Hardy, 1989; Webb, 1994; Ewles and Simnett, 1995) whose principal focus is on the individual. The aim is prophylaxis or 'prevention' (at primary, secondary and tertiary levels) of that individual's problem through the dissemination of factual information delivered by traditional teaching approaches and methods. Thus physiotherapists attending a workshop on health education organized by the Chartered Society of Physiotherapy (CSP) and the former Health Education Council (HEC) in 1985 (CSP and HEA, 1987), reported that they perceived their role 'mainly in terms of tertiary prevention on a one-to-one basis, but increasingly moving towards secondary prevention, in the form of, for example, back schools and contributing to radio programmes' with 'initiatives ... towards primary prevention, for example, working with sports coaches and keep-fit teachers' (CSP, 1988).

It is noted in the same document that physiotherapists work with individuals and groups and give specific and general 'information and advice' about selected conditions and their management and emphasize the importance of health education (associated with the 'treatment' and 'prevention' of particular conditions) for carers and other professional personnel. Other surveys confirm these findings. Leathley (1988) reports that 85% of her sample of physiotherapists considered 'back care education' to be 'the most important health education activity', whilst 47% ranked 'ante- or post-natal work' as most important. The respondents identified 'hospital staff' and 'carers, particularly those in the community' as the primary target groups for health education (see also Lilley, 1983; Lyne, 1985; Leathley and Stone, 1986; List, 1986; Lyne, 1986; MacLarity, 1986; Shore, 1986; Twomey, 1986; Hayne, 1988; Glazer-Waldman et al., 1989; McIntosh, 1989, Sluijs, 1991; Sluijs et al., 1993; Hills, 1995).

Increasingly, physiotherapists are becoming involved in health education initiatives in schools. In an article on the work of Penny Slade, a community superintendent physiotherapist, Friend (1995) reports Slade's estimate that 'half the children performed poorly in tummy exercises'. During her visits to schools, Slade has also 'encountered an "amazing" number of youngsters complaining about back pain and others with "horrendous posture and appallingly ill-fitting shoes" '. Slade addresses these problems by exhorting classes of 'unfit' children to adopt a healthier life style by learning about the structure and function of their 'bodies'. 'A knee joint from the butcher', 'a skeleton and a flexible spine' are the teaching aids used to facilitate this learning process and Slade claims that she has 'kept the attention of five-year-olds for an hour'. Children are subsequently taught a range of physical exercises including postural correction programmes in which they 'walk and sit straight and … walk and sit slouched'.

Furthermore, it appears that many physiotherapists tend to equate the role of health educator with high status and power. According to the report from the CSPs workshop (CSP and HEA, 1987), physiotherapists perceive themselves as experts capable of influencing ' "the system" at a policy/decision-making level' by educating employers, hospitals/social service managers and education authorities in the importance of appropriate staff training and good ergonomic design of the workplace (CSP, 1988). Referring to physiotherapists employed in occupational health, Creswell (1995) emphasizes the crucial role of 'This growing band of specialists' who 'are really on the frontline in dealing with injuries at work and, perhaps more importantly trying to prevent them recurring'. Physiotherapists describe how, through their involvement with ergonomic issues, they are able to influence company policy. One physiotherapist comments that her 'skills as a physiotherapist and knowledge of the body is a real help when looking at such matters as designing footwear'. Physiotherapists also influence the behaviour of employees. One practitioner 'encourages staff to think of other ways of maintaining a healthy life-style; liaises with the catering department to run events on healthy heating; and runs courses on subjects like Alexander Technique and self-defence'. Another interviewee states that: 'We can identify the problems and work on rehabilitation to get the person back to full fitness. It helps keep people at work and prevents their well-being from deteriorating'.

Unfortunately, however, this zealous (and characteristically biomedical) approach to health education has not met with unqualified success. Edmonds (1988) identifies the problem:

> 'The current debate within the National Health Service (NHS) on the approach to treatment based on the whole needs of the patient, and treating the patient as a person, is nowhere more pertinent than in the physiotherapy profession. It is unfortunate that the motivation of those who are deeply caring tends to emerge as judgmental and directive. Anecdotal evidence is embarrassingly abundant of instances where consideration of the person rather than the patient would have led to a more satisfactory outcome of consumer/practitioner interaction. Actual practice has too often resulted in the effect of "institutionalising" and "taking over" patients rather than seeking to care for them as people'.

Given this situation, an attempt to re-focus attention on the limitations of the biomedical model of 'health' and 'health education' seems to be particularly appropriate. Clearly, within the confines of a short chapter it would be impossible to do more than to introduce a selection of what many writers consider to be the crucial issues in this area. It is hoped, however, that the following discussion will stimulate further analytical and critical reflection upon the concept of 'health' and its education which will lead, subsequently, to a reappraisal of the underlying philosophy of physiotherapy, together with a re-evaluation of some of the techniques employed in its practice.

The biomedical model of health: its origins and salient features

Let us remind ourselves that the biomedical model of health evolved as a consequence of the scientific revolution which commenced in Europe in the seventeenth century. Doyal (1991) describes how 'the natural science which developed during the Renaissance transformed the Aristotelian view of the world which had dominated Western thought for 1500 years'. Doyal continues:

> 'Increasingly, science was no longer concerned with understanding the essence or teleological purpose of the natural/supernatural world. Rather, the scientist (or natural philosopher as he was called) attempted to discover and explain those regular and recurring sequences of events which could be described and codified in a quantitative and generalizable way. It was believed that this would make possible the utilisation of nature through the making of accurate predictions based on these codified generalisations. In other words, the new science increasingly equated an understanding of the natural world with a capacity to control it'.

Within the medical context, the Renaissance scientist was preoccupied with the exploration and documentation of the body's structure and function. It is important to emphasize Doyal's point that:

> 'These early investigations were largely founded upon a mechanistic view of the nature of men, and of human sickness and health. That is to say, they followed the more general pattern of Renaissance science in analyzing

living things as sets of mechanical parts – as machines rather than organically integrated wholes'.

The Aristotelian emphasis on 'the organic unity of living things' was effectively challenged by such philosophers as Thomas Hobbs and Rene Descartes, whose mechanistic conceptions of human beings is generally reflected in contemporary orthodox medical practice which sanctions the biomedical model of health. Undoubtedly, the ideological roots of this model lie in Cartesianism. Descartes believed in a particular variety of dualism with which his name has hitherto been associated. This theory holds that the (immaterial) 'Mind' and the (material) 'Body' of a given individual, although they somehow interact, are essentially distinct 'entities' (Hart, 1985; Descartes, trans. Cottingham *et al.*, 1989; Doyal, 1991; Jones, 1994; Roberts, 1994). In common with many other Renaissance thinkers, Descartes was preoccupied with the concept of knowledge, its origins and criteria. He was committed to scientific reductionism, as defined by Popper (1972), Flew (1983), Pratt (1989) and Roberts (1994), an allegiance which influenced his mechanistic approach to physiological analysis (see below). Descartes considered a body to be 'healthy' if, like a properly functioning machine, that body was in good working order; conversely, a body was classified as 'diseased' if an impairment of its function could be detected (Descartes, trans. Cottingham *et al* 1989).

Doyal (1991) points out that modern orthodox medicine has generally become regarded as being primarily concerned with the 'Body' at the expense of attending to the 'Mind' and thus continues to espouse a mechanistic concept of health. This approach is consistent with 'The scientific paradigm or empiricist model of knowledge ... (which) ... provides the basis for the medical model'. (Higgs and Titchen, 1995). Fundamentally, the paradigm 'relies on observation and experiment in the empirical world, resulting in generalizations about the content and events of the world which can be used to predict future experience. Knowledge is discovered (i.e. universal and external truths are grasped) and justified on the basis of empirical processes which are reductionist, value-neutral, quantifiable, objective, and operationalisable. Only statements publicly verifiable by sense data are valid'. (Higgs and Titchen, 1995). Beattie (in Beattie *et al.* 1993) juxtaposes the life sciences against the human sciences and provides further valuable insight into the characteristics of the biomedical perspective.

> 'Within the professions and institutions of medicine, "mechanistic" approaches to analysis are still dominant: they are seen as "hard", and in keeping with the canons of the natural science tradition. In contrast, "humanistic" approaches are given a place at the margins, but are seen as "soft", and associated with the less prestigious traditions of sociological or literary inquiry'.

(See also Jones, 1994)

In the biomedical tradition, health is 'determined secondarily to disease; if a definition of disease can be formulated, health can then be thought of as its polar opposite' (Sim, 1990). Health is thus perceived in negative terms: as the absence, or antithesis of disease. Sim (1990) suggests that 'because the two concepts are seen to lie on a single dimension' the 'variety of sophisticated means of detecting and quantifying disease processes in the patient … are equally measures of [biological] health'. Diagnosis of a disease is contingent upon the identification of a particular collection of 'signs and symptoms' presented by the individual 'sufferer' or 'victim'. The objective is, unquestionably, to 'cure' the disease or disability by medical intervention (see, for example Oliver, 1983; Oliver, 1990; Galler in Beattie *et al.* 1993; Swain *et al.*, 1993; Keith, 1994; Morris in Davey *et al.*, 1995).

The central focus of attention within biomedical ideology is upon individuals (Beattie, in Beattie *et al.*, 1993; Fatchett, 1994). Emphasis is, however, on a certain kind of 'individualism' which, as Hyland (1988) suggests, 'finds fullest expression in the writings of Descartes'. Jewson's tripartite analysis of the modes of production of scientific knowledge (Jewson in Beattie, *et al.*, 1993) is helpful in providing an historical background to the development of the biomedical model of health. Jewson suggests that scientific medicine passed through three stages: 'bedside medicine', 'hospital medicine' and 'laboratory medicine' and that this latter stage consolidated medicine as an experimental science, firmly committed to 'biological reductionism' which 'reinforced the tendency to view the patient as an object to be manipulated – a trend which has reached its apotheosis in post-war scientific medicine (Doyal, 1991).

Other significant characteristics of the biomedical model deserve mention. Jones (1994) states that 'A high value is put on the provision of specialist medical services, in mainly institutional settings' and Beattie notes that the biomedical model adopts a paternalistic, or 'top-down' approach to health and policy-making (Beattie, in Beattie, *et al.*, 1993). As Jones (1994) suggests, the objective is to return the 'patient' to 'normality' within the shortest possible time-span in order 'to get people back to productive labour'. Such an approach requires the 'patient' to submit to the authority of an omniscient and omnipotent clinical 'expert' whose dominance within the relationship is legitimized by the privileged possession of scientific 'knowledge' which is closely guarded (Collier, 1989). This empowers the clinician to restore the patient's physical health by making an accurate diagnosis of the disease whose process can subsequently be reversed or retarded by the administration of appropriate 'treatment'.

In this latter context, the clinician's role is often to 'educate' the patient in the management of a particular disorder by imparting carefully selected, 'relevant' factual information and prescriptive instruction concerning that individual's body. Risk factors are emphasized and strategies designed to minimize future problems are presented (Jones, 1994). The premise seems to be that, if facts are presented in such a way as to promote understanding, patient 'compliance' can be anticipated (see for example, Glossop *et al.*, 1982; Sluijs *et al.*, 1993). Having received this knowledge and 'advice', patients are expected to take ultimate responsibility for their subsequent actions. The biomedical approach believes that since each person has the capacity for choice in all matters, people can choose to be more or less healthy. Incontrovertibly, a rational individual would choose to be healthy, particularly when that choice is facilitated by the possession of 'correct' factual information. To ignore such information is irrational according to authoritarian clinicians, who regard their patients' lapses from obedience to the prescribed 'rules' as a serious offence. Clinicians are often irritated and affronted by what they consider to be the patient's flagrant breach of the tacitly agreed medical contract. Clinicians frequently express their 'disappointment' in the patient's conduct and 'blame' the patient for what is perceived as a failure in compliance due either to an inability to understand and learn information and instructions or to a rejection of proven – and therefore incontrovertible – 'scientific facts' (Hart, 1985; Burkitt, 1986; Currer and Stacey, 1986; Hannay, 1988; Hyland, 1987; Hyland, 1988; Morgan *et al.*, 1988; Turner, 1988; Coutts and Hardy, 1989; Sim, 1990; Doyal, 1991; Beattie *et al.*, 1993; Armstrong, 1994; Jones, 1994; Davey *et al.*, 1995; Ewles and Simnett, 1995).

Proposed method

Having outlined the characteristics of the biomedical model of health, we shall begin our discussion by considering some of its theoretical difficulties as related to metaphysical, ethical and sociological issues and show how these have implications for health education. Inevitably, this investigation will reveal some theoretical problems associated with alternative models of health and health education. Turning next to an example from contemporary practice, we shall identify the biomedical model's salient features as exemplified by the practitioner's approach and choice of language. Undertaking this analysis will enable us to appreciate the importance of theoretical consistency in the context of health-care practice. Finally, we shall propose an alternative concept of health to that offered by the biomedical model. Whilst it is acknowledged that this paradigm is not without its disadvantages, we shall suggest that it provides a more rational theoretical framework upon which to base physiotherapy practice.

Metaphysical considerations

Our first criticism of the biomedical model of health may be levelled at its Cartesian foundations. Cartesian dualism has received serious challenges from exponents of metaphysical doctrines such as alternative versions of (non-Cartesian) dualism and monism (comprising idealism and various forms of materialism including behaviourism, functionalism and physicalism) (see for example Campbell, 1970; Ryle, 1973; Teichmann, 1974; McGinn, 1982; Strawson, 1984; Williams, 1985; Smith and Jones, 1987). Of particular significance to physiotherapy practice is that Cartesian dualism fails to provide a satisfactory account of how interaction between two separate, contrasting 'entities' (mind and matter) can occur, given that, according to this theory, each possesses a different (but equal) ontological status. If the body is conceived of as a mere machine, how is it connected to the mind? (Teichman, 1974). Indeed, problems of intelligibility arise when it comes to understanding what, in fact, mind is, since it tends to be described negatively: it is *not*, for example, the brain. If mind is *not* located in space, a logical difficulty arises as to how mind–body interaction can occur. How can a causal relationship exist between a non-physical substance and a physical entity? For Descartes to 'locate' the mind in the pineal gland and then to suggest that it can cause a physical response rests upon the contradiction that immaterial substances can be 'located' anywhere in space (McGinn, 1982).

Exponents of this 'official doctrine' are guilty of making a 'category mistake' (Ryle, 1973). Cartesian dualism 'represents the facts of mental life as if they belonged to one logical type or category … when they actually belong to another'. The upshot of this is the representation of a person as a 'ghost mysteriously ensconced in a machine'. Citing Klein (1992), Fatchett (1994) notes 'that people have likened the NHS to "a garage for putting faulty human bodies back on the road again" '. Thus a health educator, having made this initial 'category mistake', predictably conceives of 'health education' as providing the 'ghost' with relevant facts about 'machine' maintenance and then supervising the repair job! It is not surprising, therefore, that many 'ghosts' find these facts meaningless, become disenchanted with the tedium of this work and frequently abandon their 'machine' when the supervisor is not watching! As Whitehead (1989) revealingly comments:

> 'In schools … there is evidence that single lesson lectures are still commonly employed with the aim of influencing social problems like illegal drug use, sexual activity in relation to AIDS, smoking and drinking habits and so on, even though any long-term behaviour change is highly unlikely with such a method'.

(See also Roberts *et al.* in Davey *et al.*, 1995).

Let us assume, then, that one of a health educator's aims is to change a person's behaviour; Ryle's objections to Cartesianism lead us to conclude that the biomedical approach to practice seems unlikely to produce these permanent alterations. Ryle's behaviourist perspective prompts him to argue that the Cartesian concept of the 'ghost' in the 'machine' has no appropriate practical application in terms of its ability to describe intelligent performance since it necessarily relies upon an infinite regress. He states that:

> 'The crucial objection to the intellectualist legend is this. The consideration of propositions is itself an operation the execution of which can be more or less intelligent, less or more stupid. But if, for any operation to be intelligently executed, a prior theoretical operation had first to be performed and performed intelligently, it would be a logical impossibility for anyone ever to break into the circle'. (Ryle, 1973).

(See also Smith and Jones, 1987).

Thus, for Ryle, the question is 'how' mental activity causes physical activity is irrelevant. He claims that 'my performance has a special procedure or manner, not special antecedents'. Thus on this account, it would seem to be necessary for a therapist to establish certain behavioural criteria of 'health' and 'disease' against which a person's physical state could be judged following an assessment of behavioural patterns. Once the problem had been identified, 'health education' would consist of various forms of behaviour modification until the individual displayed appropriate 'healthy' behaviour (Ewles and Simnett, 1995).

Health, health education and physiotherapy practice   403

As we might expect, however, behaviourism, in common with other branches of materialism, is not without its problems. In contrast to Cartesianism, behaviourism classifies persons as merely physical bodies: mental processes are reduced to brain processes. It is a serious objection to behaviourism that because 'mind' is identified with 'brain', the theory fails to provide a satisfactory explanation of the subjectivity of human experiences, for example, those of pain, or 'feeling unwell'. Thus, in the context of general health care management, behaviourism may fail to acknowledge such subjective feelings because its primary focus would be on the person's observable behaviour. In view of this inadequacy, therefore, behaviourism seems to be only marginally superior to Cartesianism in terms of its ability to provide a satisfactory metaphysical basis for physiotherapy practice.

Sociological and ethical considerations

Turning now from the metaphysical to considerations of a more sociological and ethical nature, Sim (1990) identifies other 'limitations' of the biomedical model of health. He observes that 'its stamp of objectivity rests upon a "realist" view of diseases – i.e. they have an independent existence, which is unaffected by both the fact and the mode of their perception by the observer'. That 'the very identification of disease' is inextricably linked with the making of 'certain value judgments' implies that diseases 'become social constructs': 'they are developed within, and therefore embody, specific social values and processes'.

We have noted above that the biomedical model owes much to a certain kind of individualism. Because its orientation is in terms of 'individual physiology, this model tends to seek only biological causes of disease' (Sim, 1990). Clearly, this perspective ignores the undeniable socio-economic and cultural determinants of disease as identified by numerous writers (see for example Hart, 1985; Frank and Maguire, 1988; Hannay, 1988; Morgan *et al.*, 1988; Turner, 1988; Beattie *et al.*, 1993; Armstrong, 1994; Bond and Bond, 1994; Wilkinson and Kitzinger, 1994; Benzeval *et al.*, 1995; Davey *et al.*, 1995; Ewles and Simnett, 1995). In their study of the former Health Education Council's campaign against coronary heart disease, Farrant and Russell (1986) examined the HEC's literature *Beating Heart Disease*. Their research exposes similar weaknesses of the biomedical model. In contrast to Downie (1988) they remain unimpressed by science and highlight the inadequacy of the 'explanatory power of the conventional risk factors' utilized by the HEC to 'educate' the general public about how to avoid chronic heart disease. Underlying Farrant and Russell's specific criticism of the biomedical approach is the important, general point to which we have earlier alluded: that a practitioner's concept of a person will necessarily determine how he or she conceives 'health'; this in turn will influence his or her ideas about how such persons are to be 'educated' and which methods are most suitable. Given the biomedical model's individualistic conception of persons, and given the HEC's allegiance to this ideology, it is not surprising that Farrant and Russell discover that the booklet 'focuses on the personal risk factors' of CHD and that 'the responsibility for reducing risk factors is placed firmly upon the individual'. They highlight the HEC's reluctance to view the person as existing within a socio-economic framework, reflected in the booklet's failure to mention other contributory factors to CHD prevalence such as:

> 'the role of the food industry and tobacco industry in maintaining unhealthy consumption patterns, or ... the social and economic factors (poverty, stress associated with adverse living and working conditions ...) that are related to social inequalities in diet, smoking etc., and that militate against attempts at individual risk factor reduction'.

As these authors emphasize, 'a model of CHD aetiology has been hypothesized that locates the primary cause of CHD (and therefore the appropriate point for intervention) in the wider social and economic environment' which 'utilizes the concept of chronic psychosocial stress as the major linking factor between an individual's environment and his or her cardiovascular system'. Thus, 'Exhortations to stop smoking, eat less fat, take more exercise, etc.' sound hollow and insincere when delivered by the 'expert'. Health education that ignores social influences and whose style is prescriptive and patronizing is thus doomed to failure as indicated in Farrant and Russell's chapter, *Lay Perspectives on Beating Heart Disease.*

Significantly, however, Farrant and Russell report that this failure in health education is not solely associated with the HEC's disregard of social issues. The bourgeois attitude often adopted by orthodox health professionals towards their patients is also considered to contribute to communication breakdown. Farrant and Russell identify misconceptions in professionals' beliefs that the prevalence of 'lay ignorance of orthodox medical "facts" about disease aetiology' justifies the corrective role of health education. Their findings suggest that 'it is not ignorance of "the facts" so much as the credibility the individual accords to these facts, as presented in health education literature, vis-a-vis personal "proof" that has been built up over years of observation and experience'. Thus, when confronted with professional perspectives on health, the layperson is likely to engage in sophisticated information processing in an attempt to establish which behaviours are more 'healthy' than others; this evaluation will then determine their subsequent choice of action (see also Beattie *et al.*, 1993; Davey *et al.*, 1995). Clearly, these findings must be acknowledged by all health professionals and their practice modified accordingly. One of the dangers – particularly with reference to physiotherapy – seems to be that the practitioner's attention is often diverted by the wealth of other research and advice concerning effective methods of communication (see for example Glossop *et al.*, 1982; Wagstaff, 1982; Hasler, 1985; Slack, 1985; Cull, 1986; Holland, 1986; Robinson, 1986; Skinner 1986; Griffiths, 1987; Hargreaves, 1987; Hough, 1987; Jobling, 1987; Ley, 1988, Lask, 1989; Payne, 1989; Bernard, 1992; Webb, 1994; Hough, 1995). This is not to deny the value of such work to practitioners; rather, it is to suggest that much of it focuses on the efficacy of specific communication techniques and – with the exception of Hough's contributions – rarely questions the professional's (predominantly biomedical) attitudes and assumptions concerning the nature and abilities of those persons designated as 'patients'.

In connection with the above comments, it seems pertinent to examine further the role of the health worker. In this connection Sim (1990) notes the biomedical model's failure to acknowledge the 'social, cultural and institutional context in which health care occurs'. He contends that this dimension is crucial for physiotherapists who 'require an "action-oriented" theory that will make sense not only of health, but also of health *care* as an activity' (original emphasis). Significantly, physiotherapists – together with many other professional groups – often identify themselves as 'health care workers' and as members of 'the caring professions' and Sim's request for the development of a theoretical basis for health care practice is surely legitimate. We might further supplement Sim's analysis by suggesting that therapists additionally require a theory of 'care' and 'caring' upon which to base practice. It is relevant to observe that the concepts of 'care' and 'caring', whilst they have been hijacked by members of the biomedical fraternity to serve political ends, seem to be associated with a model of health which conceives of the patient as an integrated and unique human being whose overall concerns and needs form the basis of practice. Although these ideas are apparently of little interest to some members of the physiotherapy profession, they have captured the imagination of other professional groups. The positive view of health associated with notions of 'care' and 'caring' has, for example, been well developed within the context of nursing where these ideas seem to have contributed significantly to the practitioner's understanding of the concepts of 'persons', 'health' and 'health education' (see for example Griffin, 1983; Warren, 1988; Watson, 1988; Watson and Ray, 1988; Barker, 1989; MacPherson, 1989; Morrison, 1989; Ray, 1989; Orem, 1991; Jolly and Brykczynska, 1992; Johns, 1994; Andrews and Boyle, 1995).

Turning to wider issues, the biomedical influence on government ideology and policy is clear and is reflected in the way in which health issues are addressed in the UK (see for example Jacobson *et al.*, 1991; Vallance Owen, 1992; Harrison and Pollitt, 1994). The NHS is increasingly run according to commercial principles: health is a purchasable commodity. Indeed, the gradual shift towards this commercial ethos could be taken as evidence of central government's public sanction of the continued and unrivalled dominance of the biomedical model within healthcare practice.

Whitty and Jones (in Davey *et al.*, 1995) argue that because public health physicians – the primary exponents of this model – 'enthusiastically embraced' the 'purchaser-provider split introduced by the NHS reforms', their reaction 'was exploited by the former Secretary of State for Health as support for changes'. The concepts of 'health' and 'health education' are now inextricably linked with such notions as cost-effectiveness, cost-efficiency, customer satisfaction and value for money, principles which increasingly dominate the thinking and dictate the practice of executives within purchasing health authorities and managers of provider units. As Webb (1994) reminds us: 'The Health Education Authority (HEA) is the government-funded body in the UK responsible for health education of the public' and observes that 'it is expected to work fully with the Department of Health on government policies such as the major projects "Look after your Heart", vaccination campaigns and AIDS education'.

The biomedical model's negative view of health colours its interpretation of the related notions of 'protection' and 'education', considered by Tannahill (1985) to fall under the umbrella concept of 'health promotion'. Since concentration is on the elimination of disease within the individual, 'health promotion' becomes a restricted activity, directed solely towards the ' "maintenance" or "restoration" ' of individuals' health (Sim, 1990). Leathley, (1988) makes a similar point, although her notion of 'prevention' seems to carry biomedical overtones. She suggests that 'the general orientation of the National Health Service towards sickness rather than health' presents 'obstacles to increasing the preventive and educational aspects of' physiotherapists' work. Not surprisingly, this negative orientation is reflected in central government's general approach to health matters as revealed in Whitehead's (1989) investigation into health trends in Britain. Whilst she is encouraged by 'the evidence of growing interest in education for health ... during the 1980s', Whitehead concludes that 'the total amount of effort and resources put into education for health is still significant in relation to the size of the task and in relation to the resources allocated to other policies of arguably lower priority'. She continues:

> 'There is much rhetoric about how important health education is ... But there is very little substance behind the rhetoric. The issue has been and still is of low status and low priority in many organisations, with consequent underfunding, under-resourcing and haphazard implementation. The fact that the national health education bodies have only been allocated approximately £1 in every £1000 of NHS expenditure is one indicator of the continuing low status according to health education in the country'.

Whitty and Jones (1995) echo Whitehead's sentiments. They note the 'tripartite' ... components of the public health function as laid down in the Acheson report: to survey the health of the population; to promote and maintain health; and to ensure that the means are available to evaluate existing health services'. Whitty and Jones are concerned, however, about the 'growing misconception that "purchasing for health gain" ' is the process by which ... ' "promoting and maintaining health"... will be achieved'. They contend that 'this confusion has been fed' by the government's paper *The Health of the Nation*, which, because it equates health promotion with 'changes in individual life-style as the means of preventing disease', demonstrates a 'misunderstanding of effective health promotion strategies'. That the government requires evidence of 'health service utilization' testifies to its wish to perpetuate the 'myth that purchasing health services will improve the health of the population', a myth with which members of the medical profession seem all to eager to comply in order to retain their 'clinical autonomy' (see below). Additionally, it is particularly worrying to witness the 'strong political direction' to which the health service is becoming increasingly subjected and to observe the relentless process whereby its financial and human resources are, under the tight control of administrators, being continually pruned.

Within the reactive approach characteristic of the biomedical model, there is little room to embrace the positive idea of health as going beyond the mere absence of disease in collections of isolated, freely choosing individuals. Because it cannot accommodate the concept of 'social health' the model fails to reflect crucial areas of human experience. It rejects the Aristotelian conception of society as comprising interdependent human beings. It ignores the painful truth of social inequality: that peoples' life-chances, and therefore their opportunities to make choices, are necessarily unequal (Hart, 1985; Rodmell and Watt, 1986; Morgan et al., 1988; Townsend et al., 1992; Beattie et al., 1993; Jones, 1994; Benzeval et al., 1995; Davey et al., 1995). Furthermore, as noted above, the model conceives of health as a commodity rather than as a basic human right. Policy based on this philosophy shows no genuine desire to create a society in which the current disparities in peoples' health would be minimized. Acknowledgement of the validity of subjective human experience would prompt central government to adopt more positive health strategies since its principal concern would be the restoration and maintenance of social health. Burkitt (1986), Coutts and Hardy (1989), and Ewles and Simnett (1995) describe sociological models of health education which appear to be based on a recognition of the need to encompass 'lay perspectives and experiences' concerning health and illness (Sim, 1990). Acknowledging the socio-economic determinants of health, the practitioner 'stresses the need for social planning, e.g. housing estates that allow family generations and social networks to be maintained, challenging the power relationship between the professional and the client' (Burkitt, 1986). As Sim (1990) suggests, this model provides an additional – and distinct, conceptual framework within which a professional may work; its importance lies in its ability to 'show that strictly medical concepts and definitions are insufficient if we are to understand the way in which individuals conceive of health and illness and how this understanding shapes their behaviour'. Certainly, the biomedical model is unable to accommodate the important social aspects of 'disability' and 'handicap' (for example Brechin and Liddiard, 1981; Brechin et al., 1981; Oliver, 1983; Brechin et al., 1988; Oliver, 1990; Swain et al., 1993; French, 1994; Morris in Davey et al., 1995).

Perhaps, however, there is a more sinister reason behind central government's apparent preference for the biomedical above other models of health upon which to base policy. It has already been suggested that the NHS reforms have endorsed this above other models and it would be naive to assume that this was accidental. Sim (1990) alerts us to what he perceives as the 'most serious objection' to the biomedical approach: 'it makes those who are experts on disease the sole arbiters of health. The layperson's views and experiences related to health are thereby disqualified'. As many sociologists observe, this has led to the 'medicalization' of health, in which the characteristic inequalities within the clinician/patient relationship are systematically preserved by the 'expert' in the interests of medical hegemony (Hart, 1985; Morgan et al., 1988;

Collier, 1989; Scambler, 1991; Jones, 1994) observe 'the autonomy enjoyed by professional groups' who utilize 'knowledge as a powerful asset to use to attain and maintain power'. Citing Freidson (1970), these authors suggest that 'the medical profession's power to control what constitutes health and illness has been used to extend the medical monopoly over areas of life and behaviour which were not traditionally the concern of the medical profession'. Thus, the medical profession effectively 'creates' illness in order to 'extend its professional dominance, with authority deriving from its professional status and claims of competence'. Morgan et al. (1988) cite childbirth as an area which has become increasingly 'medicalized' by professional intervention (see also Hannay, 1988; Coutts and Hardy, 1989; Armstrong, 1994; Jones, 1994). Farrant and Russell (1986) offer further evidence of this 'vested interest' in relation to the former HEC's literature on CHD:

> 'Furthermore, the "population" versus "high risk" preventive strategy debate, within the medical literature, has, in part, to be seen in the context of the medical profession's own interests in keeping coronary prevention within medical control and within a conventional paradigm of medical intervention. One of the arguments that has been advanced in favour of a high-risk strategy of CHD prevention is that it offers for physicians (and patients) a more familiar and comfortable model of medical practice. The WHO notes that "Doctors often lack the training and hence also the motivation to enlarge their responsibilities beyond the care of the sick". However, Rose points out that much harder to overcome than this ... "is the enormous difficulty for medical personnel to see health as a population issue and not merely as a problem for individuals". Thus, whilst epidemiological theory points towards a population approach to CHD prevention, reviews of current practice and initiatives in the medical literature ... suggests an emphasis by the medical profession on the role of high-risk screening strategies within a medical setting'.

The above issues are linked to the social questions previously considered. For how long can the professionals continue to ignore the socioeconomic and environmental determinants of disease and disability as identified by so many writers? (for example Hart, 1985; Burkitt 1986; Currer and Stacey, 1986; Morgan et al., 1988; Hannay, 1988; Armstrong, 1994; Jones, 1994). The unwillingness to acknowledge this aspect of health together with the discreditation of people's knowledge and subjective experiences by professionals (Farrant and Russell, 1986) seems to be a practice in which central government covertly, but actively, colludes.

Other models: some further problems

The 'illness' model of health which validates the subjective experience of being unwell has limitations, however, not dissimilar to some of those identified in the biomedical 'disease' model. Firstly, 'health' is a negative concept, derived from the notion of 'illness': its presence implies a corresponding absence of illness. This perspective therefore fails to reflect the potentially complex relationship between 'health' and 'illness', either at an individual or social level. It cannot, for example, accommodate the possibility of the co-existence of both in a permanently disabled person. This individual may not feel 'ill' but it would not be meaningless or inappropriate for a physiotherapist to discuss strategies directed towards enhancing that individual's 'health'. Conversely, a person who is considered to be in good 'health' might nevertheless testify to 'feeling unwell' and may be unable to identify the reasons for these feelings. Second, the 'illness' model focuses on the importance of restoring and maintaining a person's 'health' rather than on its positive improvement. Thus the sociological and environmental health education strategies described by Burkitt (1986) and by Ewles and Simnett (1995) could be viewed in this light and not necessarily as examples of proactive policy.

This positive aspect is captured in the WHO's (1946) definition, cited by Burkitt (1986) and Sim (1990), which presents health as a multi-dimensional, all-embracing concept that could apply to almost any aspect of a person's life. The WHO defines health as 'The complete physical, mental and social well-being and not simply the absence of disease or infirmity' (see also Webb, 1994b). The definition, however, raises many problems, not the least of which is related to its terminology. For example, how are we to understand the notion of 'well-being'? Is it identical with that of 'health'? On an Aristotelian analysis, the association between 'well-being' and human flourishing suggests that 'health' is a necessary, but not a sufficient condition for eudaimonia – happiness (see Aristotle, EN bk. I, Trans. Ross, 1986). The attainment of a happy life is to some extent dependent upon good fortune; thus it would seem possible for a person to be 'healthy' but not to experience 'happiness' or 'well-being'.

Together with these theoretical difficulties, adopting the WHO's (1946) concept of 'health' poses potential practical problems. Insofar as it purports to reflect a generally shared ideal, the WHO's notion of 'health' does not fully acknowledge the view expressed by Ewles and Simnett (1995) that ' "Being healthy" means different things to different people'. A similar allegiance to (liberal) individualism is embodied in exhortations to 'be open-minded in approach to people and to be aware that health is a matter of opinion rather than of fact' (Coutts and Hardy, 1989). In any case, as implied earlier, the WHO's notion of 'health' is utopian and therefore probably unattainable by the majority of individuals. With reference to health education, it proves difficult to implement. Because 'health' is equated with all the positive aspects of life experience, the clear identification and, indeed, achievement, of a person's health goals becomes extremely problematic. (For further discussion of definitions of 'health' see Webb, 1994).

From theory to practice

In an attempt to crystallize the arguments adduced above concerning the disadvantages of the biomedical model, it now seems appropriate to examine one health educator's account of practice. The account highlights further difficulties associated with this particular health educator's (unsuccessful) struggle to extricate himself from a fundamental conviction in the efficacy of a biomedical approach. To focus on these kinds of ideological problems seems to be particularly relevant to a discussion whose chief aim is to encourage a more analytical and critical approach to physiotherapy practice.

David Muir, Promotions Officer at the *Look After Yourself* Project Centre, Christchurch College, Canterbury, outlines a training course which comprised part of the popular *Look After Yourself* programme in which many UK health authorities have been involved. That Muir's fundamental allegiance is to the biomedical model of health is evident from the authoritative and censorious tone of his opening claim: 'Good health is considered by most people to be the single most important thing that they want in their lives, and yet many do little about it'. (Muir, 1989). In a characteristically Cartesian manner, he then compares bodily health with inanimate objects such as 'cars and household appliances' and condemns people because 'they prefer to wait until something goes wrong' rather than taking preventive action. Although Muir's intention seems to be to discredit the biomedical model, his language betrays an allegiance to its tenets. He asserts that: 'Health is sometimes mistaken for fitness' but rejects this limited perspective because it neglects 'other important aspects of a healthy life-style' such as making 'sound' dietary choices, maintaining 'correct' physical weight and the ability to 'cope adequately' with life stress, all of which he sees as playing 'an integral part in helping to achieve the sort of health which makes you feel good'.

For Muir, then, 'health' is detectable in individuals by the application of prescribed objective criteria (including those of aesthetics, rational ability and emotional resilience). That 'health' is also identified with 'lifestyle' and 'well-being', however, seems to indicate Muir's recognition of the shortcomings of a biomedical model and, it appears, his wish to convey an indebtedness to other models. For example, the model that incorporates the subjective notion of 'illness' (Sim, 1990) against which 'wellness' is judged (see also Hannay, 1988; Williams, 1989; Scambler, 1991; Armstrong, 1994). In this context, we may now enquire as to whether Muir believes that the notions of 'health' and 'well-being' refer to synonymous states? Does his concept of 'health' incorporate the Aristotelian idea of 'eudaimonia'? (Harré, 1990). If Muir equates 'health' with 'flourishing', perhaps he also has in mind a positive conception of 'health' based on the somewhat utopian definitions of the World Health Organization (cited in Hart, 1985; Burkitt, 1986; Whitehead, 1989; Sim, 1990; Webb, 1994; Ewles and Simnett, 1995).

However eclectic Muir's conception of 'health' may appear to be, he takes it to be a self-evident truth that 'health' comprises an appropriate subject for education. The premise is characteristic of the biomedical model of 'health education' (Burkitt, 1986; Hyland, 1988). This premise, which carries the status of an *a priori* truth, is that if teachers 'equip individuals' with 'skills and knowledge that are appropriate to their health needs', those 'individuals' will be able to 'take positive steps' towards achieving what Muir considers to be this desirable state. Indeed, such tuition will enable class participants to 'make gradual changes' to 'their life-style'. Muir is keen to demonstrate a commitment to a 'progressive' educational philosophy: his 'integral' group training scheme is participative. Significantly, however, its objectives are couched in familiar terminology: 'gaining an understanding of relevant health topics', instructing individuals how to exercise 'safely and regularly' and teaching 'understanding and coping with stress and knowing how to practise simple relaxation techniques'.

Finally, Muir manages to introduce another concept: 'holism' (as described by Flew, 1983; Burkitt, 1986; Newbeck, 1986, Newbeck and Rowe, 1986; Pietroni, 1987; Seedhouse and Cribb, 1989; Davey *et al.*, 1995; Barnitt and Pomeroy, 1995; Ewles and Simnett, 1995). He seeks to link his concepts to 'health' and 'health education' by advertising his training programme as an example of an 'holistic' approach to management. Muir is confident that, 'The importance of this "holistic" or "total" approach to health and well-being is recognized by an increasing majority of those involved in promoting good health, and many see it as essential to their work …' In common with some physiotherapists (see for example Williams, 1986; Jackson, 1987), Muir perceives it to be a legitimate (and professionally advantageous) strategy to synthesize 'science' and 'art' and 'orthodoxy' and 'alternativism' within practice. Since 'holism' represents a philosophy whose principles stand in direct opposition to those of scientific reductionism, however, further questions arise. Is it empirically likely, and indeed, theoretically consistent, for a health educator to subscribe, seriously, to both these philosophical perspectives? To indicate an indebtedness to both within the scope of one paper, therefore, would seem to reflect either a genuine, or a contrived metaphysical inconsistency, neither of which can pass unobserved. Certainly, to base practice on such a philosophical confusion cannot be countenanced, irrespective of other demonstrable weaknesses associated with the biomedical approach.

Towards a philosophy of health and health education

That our discussion of some of the problems associated with the biomedical approach to health and health education has inevitably exposed other difficulties in some alternative concepts of health should not disconcert us. Disadvantages, as well as advantages, are to be found with any model which can inform practice. There are no simple solutions to this complex problem. Acceptance of these conclusions need not, and indeed, should not, lead us to abandon our search for an attractive theoretical foundation upon which to base physiotherapy. Our response to such intellectual challenges should be positive and constructive if qualitative improvements in physiotherapy practice are to be effected.

Sim (1990) believes that physiotherapists require a primary, proactive model of health on which to base practice. He contends that , 'a more ambitious and wide-ranging definition is necessary' if management is to incorporate 'activities concerned with enhancing health and extending its boundaries'. Sim then cites two theorists, Whitebeck (1981) and Seedhouse (1986), who conceive of health in terms of human aspiration or potential. For Sim, the attractions of such a concept are twofold. First, 'a high degree of health may coexist with illness or disease'; second, 'health as a concept extends beyond the sphere of medical care, and may even be incompatible with certain aspects of medicine'. 'Health', thus 'embraces all spheres of the individual's life in which human aspirations can be realised'. Katherine Mansfield's description of health (cited in Coutts and Hardy, 1989) and the WHO's (1984) definition (cited in Whitehead, 1989) embody this ideal.

Certainly, Seedhouse's philosophy is attractive in many respects, as reflected in his concept of health:

'A person's optimum state of health is equivalent to the state of the set of conditions which fulfil or enable a person to work to fulfil his or her realistic chosen and biological potentials. Some of these conditions are of the highest importance for all people. Others are variably dependent upon individual abilities and circumstances'. (Seedhouse, 1986).

Because they comprise the foundations of Seedhouse's general philosophy, it is worth expanding on some of the ideas contained within the above definition. The fundamental, ethical premise is that 'health' is 'an undefined "good" about which discussion is barely necessary' (Seedhouse, 1994). Seedhouse's concept of a person (Seedhouse, 1988) seems to owe much to the Aristotelian ideology discussed earlier, which conceives of persons as interdependent social human beings whose individual potential for achievement is inextricably linked with that of the flourishing of society in general (see MacIntyre, 1985). For Seedhouse, each person possesses certain basic rights, among which is the right to 'health'. Since the attainment of a person's health is necessarily linked with the realization of 'his or her realistic chosen and biological potentials' it is evident that Seedhouse is committed to a fundamental belief that each person has the right to claim personal autonomy, central to which is the notion of 'choice' (Seedhouse and Cribb, 1989; Seedhouse and Lovitt, 1992; Seedhouse, 1994; see also Raz, 1986 for a full discussion of personal autonomy). Seedhouse's concept of persons is also informed by his stated commitment to other ethical principles: equality; fairness; and justice (Seedhouse and Cribb, 1989; Seedhouse and Lovitt, 1992; Seedhouse, 1994). Persons are, for Seedhouse, intrinsically valuable: they have the right to be treated according to specific moral precepts.

Given that he adopts this particular concept of a person, it is consistent for Seedhouse to conceive of the health worker as having a duty to guarantee these basic rights. He thus characterizes 'Work for health' as 'essentially *enabling*' (Seedhouse, 1986, original emphasis) and associates it with 'providing the appropriate foundations' to facilitate the achievement of personal potentials. The health worker is encouraged to remove obstacles to the attainment of a person's 'biological and chosen goals' and to provide 'the basic means by which (such) goals can be achieved'. Seedhouse openly acknowledges the 'fuzzy' boundaries of the concept of health: 'The world is an interconnected whole: nothing is finally clear-cut'. Using a time-honoured metaphor, Seedhouse makes a crucial point, pertinent to all those engaged in health work:

'Work for health is work on building a solid stage, and keeping that stage in good condition. The roles that people perform, and how they choose to perform these roles upon that stage is up to the individuals provided that the platform is sound' (Seedhouse, 1986, original emphasis.)

Turning to the concept of 'education', Seedhouse (1986) contrasts it with 'training' which he equates with 'indoctrination' and 'which involves imparting a single set of ideas'. He proposes a theory of education which contrasts with that espoused by the biomedical model. Seedhouse regards education as having two principal aims: first 'To provide the learner, either directly or indirectly, with all relevant information about a subject area'; second, 'To instil a childlike curiosity ... to encourage a questioning attitude, a confidence to select and to criticise; to promote the sense that the information that is being presented is what we have now – it is not the final word; and to encourage the idea that each of us is part of a continuing inquiry'. To suggest that all our knowledge is tentative, provisional and changing and that everyone (professional and layperson alike) is engaged in an on-going inquiry is to challenge the fundamental premises upon which the biomedical model is based. This challenge, in itself, is liberating and therefore empowering.

Seedhouse's concept of health education is derived from the synthesis of his ideas on health and education. He contends that health education 'should not indoctrinate' or be 'a propaganda exercise' (Seedhouse, 1986). Its aim should be: first, 'To ensure that all people have a good standard of general education' and second, 'To develop people's powers of conceiving, and so to enable them to make the most of the information they have'. Seedhouse identifies what he believes to be the benefits – to professionals and to lay people – of a health education programme which embodies these aims and exhorts the health professionals to strive towards them (Seedhouse, 1986).

Some implications for physiotherapy practice

Some of the implications of adopting Seedhouse's philosophy need to be identified. These seem to fall into two broad categories: those associated with personal attitude change and those related to the practical aspects of health care and the manner of its delivery. With reference to the former category, it behoves all of us to undertake a regular re-examination of our metaphysical and ethical beliefs in relation to our role as health care workers. How we conceive of 'health', 'health education' and 'persons' will determine the quality of our services. For example, many of us regard the patient/therapist relationship as central to clinical practice without ever questioning either the underlying assumptions associated with these concepts or, more fundamentally, our own frame of linguistic reference. That language reflects ideological beliefs and attitudes is confirmed by the periodic need to revise dictionaries. The language we use to describe the world, however, also defines the parameters within which we perceive that world. Thus the very use of the terms 'therapist' (agent) and 'patient' (passive recipient) dictates how we conceive of this relationship, and may, indeed, contribute to the perpetuation of that attitude. The fact that these terms continue to be used supports the contention that many professionals wish to preserve the inherent inequalities which characterize their relationships with members of the general public. Had there been a genuine wish to eliminate this inequality and establish a relationship founded on egalitarian principles, the traditional nomenclature would have been replaced by terms deemed to reflect these ideals. It therefore seems to be necessary to introduce a new linguistic frame of reference in order to precipitate an attitude change which has hitherto been slow to evolve. Interestingly, it has been suggested by a music therapy colleague that the terms 'researcher' and 'co-researcher' deserve serious consideration as contenders. Within this frame of reference, 'education' for 'health' would be a socially shared goal, a collective enterprise, with each participant demonstrating mutual respect for personal autonomy reflected in a willingness to engage in the processes of both teaching and learning.

To focus briefly on the second category concerning the various aspects of health care delivery, many physiotherapists currently seem to encounter numerous extrinsic as well as intrinsic barriers to good practice. Lyne and Phillipson (1986) catalogue a number of these barriers and identify 'the pressure of acute referrals' as being 'the most significant barrier to health education'. They cite other problems associated with 'workload and work organization' and lack of resources (see also Leathley, 1988; Tonkin, 1995) and report that 'problems of professionalism' and 'communication between professions' further mitigate against educational activities. Whitehead (1989) echoes these problems and identifies additional obstacles to good practice. The first of these 'is almost certainly inadequacies in pre-service and in-service training' which is often 'treatment orientated'.

Whitehead (1989) alludes to the unsatisfactory practice of ' "crisis" treatment' and the fact that some professionals do not consider 'educational work' as 'their role', some report 'lack of confidence in educational skills, and lack of support from managers who may give the impression that it is not a legitimate activity for their staff'. The results of a survey undertaken by Sluijs *et al.* (1993) reveals that 'Those therapists with high expectations about the effects of educational compliance paid more attention to the education of their patients' and that those 'who spent more time with their patients had a better relationship with them'.

Conclusion

How, then, are we to effect attitudinal and organizational change? How are we to overcome these various obstacles to the establishment of good practice? As Whitehead (1989) laments, 'the over-riding impression … is one of health educators attempting to swim upstream, against the current of forces which have operated to damage health or undermine educational efforts …'. Her report of lay participation in community health projects, however, provides an encouraging example of what is surely good practice of the kind in which more physiotherapists could become increasingly involved, given opportunities and encouragement to do so by their managers. Furthermore, Whitehead's account of community-based health education illustrates that change, although a difficult process to manage, is possible, given the initial commitment amongst professional health workers. And this is the crucial point. In order to establish and maintain good practice, we, as physiotherapists, must be genuinely committed to this ideal; we must find the energy to examine and evaluate our knowledge, skills and attitudes on a regular basis and be receptive to new perspectives. Where possible, we must initiate and manage change within both the educational and clinical context and, perhaps most importantly, we must work to dismantle inter-professional barriers. It is, however, encouraging to observe that, in some countries (for example, South Africa), physiotherapists are becoming increasingly involved in community-based rehabilitation projects.

If these exhortations are summarily dismissed as the incoherent ravings of an inveterate idealist, it is difficult to find a rational argument which might serve to combat such a reaction. The only hope, perhaps, lies in directing the reader to Mary Warnock's writings on educational practice and, in particular, to her valuable observation that, 'It is the function of an ideal to be unattainable. It is no argument against adopting an ideal, therefore, to show that it is impossible to attain it' (Warnock, 1977). To aim for the establishment of physiotherapy practice based on Aristotelian principles does not, therefore, imply a naive belief that this aim will be fully realized; rather, it demonstrates a genuine commitment to those principles and a serious intention to strive towards their realization.

References

Adamson B. J. and Nordholm L. A. (1994) A comparison of Australian and Swedish physiotherapists' view of professional practice. *Physiotherapy Theory and Practice*, **10**(3) 161–169.

Andrews M. M. and Boyle J. S. (1995) *Transcultural Concepts in Nursing Care* (2nd edn). Philadelphia: J. B. Lippincott.

Aristotle (1986) *The Nicomachean Ethics*, Transl. Ross, D. Oxford: Oxford University Press.

Armstrong D. (1994) *An Outline of Sociology as Applied to Medicine* (4th edn). Oxford: Butterworth–Heinemann.

Balfour C. (1993) Physiotherapists and smoking cessation. *Physiotherapy*, **79**(4) 247–250.

Barker P. (1989) Reflections on the philosophy of caring in mental health. *International Journal of Nursing Standards*, **26**(2), 131–141.

Barnitt R. and Pomeroy V. (1995) An holistic approach to rehabilitation. *British Journal of Therapy and Rehabilitation*, **2**(2), 87–92.

Beattie A. (1993) The changing boundaries of health. In *Health and Wellbeing: A Reader* (Beattie A., Gott M., Jones L., Sidell M. (eds) Hampshire and London: McMillan Press, 260–271.

Beattie A., Gott M., Jones L., Sidell M. (eds) (1993) *Health and Wellbeing: A Reader*. Hampshire and London: Macmillan Press.

Benzeval M., Judge K., Whitehead M. (eds) (1995) *Tackling inequalities in Health: An Agenda for Action*. London: King's Fund.

Bond J., Bond S. (1994) *Sociology and Health Care: An Introduction for Nurses and Other Health Care Professionals* (2nd edn). Edinburgh, London: Churchill Livingstone.

Brechin A., Liddiard P. (1981) *Look at it This Way: New Perspectives in Rehabilitation*. Sevenoaks: Hodder and Stoughton in association with The Open University Press.

Brechin A., Liddiard P., Swain J. (eds) (1988) *Handicap in a Social World*. Sevenoaks: Hodder and Stoughton.

Burkitt A. (1986) Health, health education and the physiotherapist. *Physiotherapy*, **72**(1), 2–4.

Burnard P. (1992) *Effective Communication Skills for Health Professionals*. London: Chapman and Hall.

Campbell, K. (1970) *Body and Mind*. London: MacMillian.

Chartered Society of Physiotherapy and Health Education Authority (1987) *Health Education and Physiotherapy: A Venture in Collaboration*. London: CSP and HEA.

Chartered Society of Physiotherapy (1988) Health education workshop: a venture in collaboration. *Physiotherapy*, **74**(12) 602–606.

Collier J. (1989) *The Health Conspiracy*. London: Century Hutchinson.

Condie E. (1991) A Therapeutic approach to physical disability. *Physiotherapy*, **77**(2), 72–77.

Coutts L. C., Hardy L. K. (1989) *Teaching for Health: The Nurse as Health Educator*. Edinburgh: Churchill Livinstone.

Creswell J. (1995) Occupationally challenged. *Physiotherapy Frontline*, **1**(22), 13–14.

Cull P. (1986) Using audio and visual aids. *Physiotherapy*, **72**(11), 539–542.

Currer C., Stacey M. (eds) (1986) *Concepts of Health, Illness and Disease: A Comparative Perspective*. Leamington Spa: Berg Publishers Ltd.

Davey B., Gray A., Seale C. (eds) (1995) *Health and Disease: A Reader* (2nd edn). Buckingham, Philadelphia: Open University Press.

Descartes R. (1989) *Selected Philosophical Writings*, Transl. Cottingham, J. Stoothoff R., Murdoch P. Cambridge: Cambridge University Press.

Downie R. S. (1988) Health promotion and health education. *Journal of Philosophy of Education*, **22**(1), 3–11.

Doyal L. with Pennel, I. (1991) *The Political Economy of Health*. London: Pluto Press.

Edmonds B. (1988) The certificate of health education: a personal perspective. *Physiotherapy Practice*, **4**(1), 26–29.

Ewles L., Simnett I. (1995) *Promoting Health: A Practical Guide* (3rd edn). Middlesex: Scutari Press.

Farrant W., Russell J. (1986) *The Politics of Health Information: 'Beating Heart Disease' as a Case Study of Health Education Council Publications*, Bedford Way Papers, No. 28, London: Institute of Education, University of London.

Fatchett A. (1994) *Politics, Policy and Nursing*. London: Baillière Tindall.

Flew A. (ed.) (1983) *A Dictionary of Philosophy* (2nd edn). London: Pan Books.

Frank A. O., Maguire G. P. (eds) (1988) *Disabling Diseases: Physical, Environmental and Psychosocial Management*. Oxford: Butterworth-Heinemann.

French S. (ed.) (1994) *On Equal Terms: Working with Disabled People*. Oxford: Butterworth-Heinemann.

Friedson E. (1970) *The Profession of Medicine*. New York: Aldine Publishing.

Friend B. (1995) Promoting health in schoolchildren. *Physiotherapy Frontline*, **1**(15), 14.

Galler R. (1993) The myth of the perfect body. In *Health and Wellbeing: A Reader* (Beattie A., *et al.*, eds). Hampshire and London: MacMillian Press, pp. 152–157.

Glazer-Waldman, H. R., Hart J. P., LeVeau B. F. (1989) Health beliefs and health behaviors of physical therapists. *Physical Therapy*, **69**(3), 204–210.

Glossop E. S., Goldenberg E., Smith D. S., Williams I. M. (1982) Patient compliance in back and neck pain. *Physiotherapy*, **68**(7), 225–226.

Griffin A. P. (1983) A philosophical analysis of caring in nursing. *Journal of Advanced Nursing*, **8**, 289–295.

Griffiths P. (1987) Creating a learning environment. *Physiotherapy*, **73**(7), 328–331.

Hannay D. R. (1988) *Lecture Notes on Medical Sociology*. Oxford: Blackwell Scientific Publications.

Hargreaves S. (1987) The relevance of non-verbal skills in physiotherapy. *Physiotherapy*, **73**(12), 685–688.

Harré R. (1990) Health as an aesthetic concept. *Cogito*. 4(1), 35–40.

Harrison S., Pollitt C. (1994) *Controlling Health Professionals: The Future of Work and Organisation within the NHS*. Buckingham: Open University Press.

Hart N. (1985) *The Sociology of Health and Medicine*. Ormskirk: Causway Books.

Hassler J. C. (1985) Communication and relationships in general medical practice. *Physiotherapy*, **71**(10), 435–436.

Hayne C. R. (1988) The preventive role of physiotherapy in the National Health Service and Industry. *Physiotherapy*, **74**(1), 2–3.

Higgs J., Titchen A. (1995) The Nature, generation and verification of knowledge. *Physiotherapy*, **81**(9), 521–530.

Hills R. (1995) The Role of the physiotherapist in health education. Abstract of Higher Degree Thesis, *Physiotherapy*, **81**(5), 270.

Holland S. (1986) *Teaching Patients and Clients.* Managing Care Pack 6, London: The Distance Learning Centre, South Bank Polytechnic.

Hough A. (1987) Communication in health care. *Physiotherapy,* **73**(2), 56–59.

Hough A. (1995) *Physiotherapy in Respiratory Care: A Problem-solving Approach.* London, New York: Chapman and Hall.

Hyland T. (1987) Value-Free? *Education and Health,* **5**(4), 89.

Hyland T. (1988) Values and health education: a critique of individualism. *Educational Studies,* **14**(1), 23–31.

Jackson D. A. (1987) Where is the physiotherapy profession going? *Physiotherapy,* **73**(11), 590–591.

Jacobson R., Smith A., Whitehead M. (eds) (1991) *The National Health: A Strategy for the 1990s.* London: King's Fund Centre.

Jaggi A., Bithell C. (1995) Relationships between physiotherapists' level of contact, cultural awareness and communication with Bangladeshi patients in two health authorities. *Physiotherapy,* **81**(6), 330–337.

Jewson N. D. (1993) The disappearance of the sick man from medical cosmology. 1770–1870. In *Health and Wellbeing: A Reader* (Beattie A. *et al.* eds). Hampshire and London: MacMillian Press, 44–54.

Jobling M. H. (1987) Cognitive styles: some implications for teaching and learning. *Physiotherapy,* **73**(7), 335–338.

Johns C. (ed) (1994) *The Burford NDU Model: Caring in Practice.* Oxford: Blackwell Science.

Jolly M., Brykczynska G. (eds) (1992) *Nursing Care: The Challenge to Change.* London, Melbourne, Auckland: Edward Arnold.

Jones L. J. (1994) *The Social Context of Health and Health Work.* Hampshire and London: MacMillian Press.

Keith L. (1994) *Mustn't Grumble: Writings by Disabled Women.* London: The Women's Press.

Lask S. (1989) Teaching health education. *Nursing Times,* **85**(50), 43–44.

Leathley M. (1988) Physiotherapists and health education: report of a survey. *Physiotherapy,* **74**(5), 218–220.

Leathley M., Stone S. (1986) Shared concerns: reflections on some health education issues which are common to four of the professions allied to medicine. *Physiotherapy,* **72**(1), 12–13.

Ley P. (1988) *Communicating with Patients: Improving Communication. Satisfaction and Compliance.* London: Croom Helm.

Lilley M. (1993) Preventive medicine and the benefit of exercise programmes for the sedentary worker. *Physiotherapy,* **69**(1), 8–10.

List M. (1986) Physiotherapy: a mobile profession in health care. *Physiotherapy,* **72**(3), 122–124.

Lyne P. A. (1985) Health education and the professions allied to medicine. *Physiotherapy Practice,* **1**(1), 46–47.

Lyne P. A. (1986) The professions allied to medicine – their potential contribution to health education. *Physiotherapy,* **72**(1), 8–10.

Lyne P. A., Phillipson C. (1986) The barriers to health education. *Physiotherapy,* **72**(1), 10–12.

MacClarity J. (1986) The fitness programme for Marks and Spencer Head Office. *Physiotherapy,* **72**(1), 54–56.

McGinn C. (1982) *The Character of Mind.* Oxford, New York: Oxford University Press.

McIntosh J. M. (1989) Women – the captive audience. *Physiotherapy,* **75**(1), 10–13.

MacIntyre A. (1985) *After Virtue: A Study in Moral Theory* (2nd edn). London: Gerald Duckworth & Co. Ltd.

MacPherson K. I. (1989) A new perspective on nursing and caring in a corporate context. *Advances in Nursing Science,* **11**(4), 32–39.

Marshall K. and Walsh D. M. (1994) Health of mother and child: striking the balance. *Physiotherapy,* **80**(11), 767–771.

Morgan M., Calnan M., Manning N. (1988) *Sociological Approaches to Health and Medicine.* London, New York: Routledge.

Morris, J. (1995) Pride against prejudice: 'lives not worth living'. In *Health and Disease: A Reader* (2nd edn) (Davey B., Gray A., Seale, C., eds). Buckingham, Philadelphia: Open University Press, 107–110.

Morrison P. (1989) Nursing and caring: a personal construct theory study of some nurses' self-perceptions. *Journal of Advanced Nursing*, **14**(5), 421–426.

Muir D. (1989) Look after yourself. *Nursing Times*, **85**(36), 59–61.

Newbeck I. (1986) The whole works. *Nursing Times*, **82**, 48–49.

Newbeck I., Rowe D. (1986) Going the whole way. *Nursing Times*, **82**, 24–25.

Oliver M. (1983) *Social Work With Disabled People*. London: MacMillian Press.

Oliver M. (1990) *The Politics of Disablement*. Hampshire and London: MacMillian Press.

Orem D. E. (1991) *Nursing: Concepts of Practice* (4th edn). USA, London: Mosby Year Book Inc.

Parry A. W. (1991) Physiotherapy and methods of enquiry: conflict and reconciliation. *Physiotherapy*, **77**(7), 435–438.

Patrick D. L., Scambler G. (eds) (1991) *Sociology as Applied to Medicine*. London: Baillière Tindall, Cassell Ltd.

Payne R. (1989) Glad to be yourself: a course of practical relaxation and health education talks. *Physiotherapy*, **75**(1), 8–9.

Pietroni P. (1987) Holistic medicine: new lessons to be learned. *The Practitioner*, **231**, 1386–1390.

Popper K. (1972) *Conjectures and Reflections: The Growth of Scientific Knowledge*. London: Routledge and Kegan Paul.

Pratt J. W. (1989) Towards a philosophy of physiotherapy. *Physiotherapy*, **75**(2), 114–120.

Ray M. A. (1989) The theory of bureaucratic caring for nursing practice in the organizational culture. *Nursing Administration Quarterly*, **13**(2), 31–42.

Raz J. (1986) *The Morality of Freedom*. Oxford, New York, Toronto: Oxford University Press.

Ritchie J. E. (1989) Keeping Australians healthy: The challenge to physiotherapy practice posed by the concept of the new public health. *Australian Journal of Physiotherapy*, **35**(2), 101–107.

Roberts H., Smith S., Bryce C. (1995) Prevention is better … In *Health and Disease: A Reader* (2nd edn) (Davey B., Gray A., Seale C., eds). Buckingham, Philadelphia: Open University Press, 170–177.

Roberts P. (1994) Theoretical models of physiotherapy. *Physiotherapy*, **80**(6), 361–366.

Robinson Y. K. (1986) Teaching adults: some issues in adult education for health education. *Physiotherapy*, **72**(1), 49–52.

Rodmell S. and Watt A. (eds) (1986) *The Politics of Health Education: Raising the Issues*. London: Routledge and Kegan Paul.

Ryle G. (1973) *The Concept of Mind*. Harmondsworth: Penguin Books.

Scambler G. (ed.) (1991) *Sociology as Applied to Medicine* (3rd edn). London: Baillière Tindall.

Seedhouse D. (1986) *Health: The Foundations for Achievement*. Chichester: John Wiley and Sons.

Seedhouse D. (1988) *Ethics: The Heart of Health Care*. Chichester: John Wiley and Sons.

Seedhouse D. (1994) *Fortress NHS: A Philosophical Review of the National Health Service*. Chichester, New York, Brisbane, Toronto. Singapore: John Wiley and Sons.

Seedhouse D., Cribb A. (eds) (1989) *Changing Ideas in Health Care*. Chichester: John Wiley and Sons.

Seedhouse D., Lovet L. (1992) *Practical Medical Ethics*. Chichester: John Wiley and Sons.

Shore M. (1986) The Health Education Council 'look after yourself programme'. *Physiotherapy*, **71**(1), 14–16.

Sim J. (1990) The concept of health. *Physiotherapy*, **76**(7), 423–428.

Skinner C. M. (1986) Talking to small groups: a specialised skill. *Physiotherapy*, **72**(11), 535–538.

Slack P. (1985) Projecting the facts. *Nursing Times*, April 3, 24–27.

Sluijs E. M. (1991) Patient education in physiotherapy: towards a planned approach. *Physiotherapy*, **77**(7), 503–508.

Sluijs E. M., van der Zee J., Kok G. J. (1993) Differences between physical therapists in attention paid to patient education. *Physiotherapy Theory and Practice*, **9**(2), 103–117.

Smith, P., Jones, O. R. (1987) *The Philosophy of Mind: An Introduction*. Cambridge: Cambridge University Press.

Stachura K. (1994) Professional dilemmas facing physiotherapists. *Physiotherapy*, **80**(6), 357–360.

Strawson P. F. (1984) *Individuals: an essay in descriptive metaphysics*. London and New York: Methuen.

Swain J., Finkelstein V., French S., Oliver M. (1993) *Disabling Barriers – Enabling Environments*. London: Sage Publications.

Tannahill A. (1985) What is health promotion? *Health Education Journal*, **44**(4), 167–168.

Teichman J. (1974) *The Mind and the Soul: An Introduction to the Philosophy of the Mind*. London: Routledge and Kegan Paul.

Tonkin J. (1995) At the heart of the community. *Physiotherapy Frontline*, **1**(21), 14.

Townsend P., Whitehead M., Davidson N. (eds.) (1992) *Inequalities in Health: The Black Report and The Health Divide*. London: Penguin Books.

Turner B. S. (1988) *Medical Power and Social Knowledge*. London: Sage Publications.

Twomey L. (1986) Physiotherapy and health promotion. *Physiotherapy Practice*, **2**(4), 153–154.

Vallance Owen A. (1992) *The Health Debate Live*. London: British Medical Journal.

Wagstaff G. F. (1982) A small dose of common sense: communication, persuasion and physiotherapy. *Physiotherapy*, **68**(10), 327–329.

Warnock M. (1977) *Schools of Thought*. London: Faber and Faber.

Warren C. D. (1988) Review and synthesis of nine nursing studies on care and caring. *Journal of the New York State Nurses Association*, **19**(4), 10–16.

Warren M. D. (1985) Promoting health and preventing disease and disability – an introduction to concepts, opportunities and practice: a review: Part I. *Physiotherapy Practice*, **1**(2), 57–63.

Warren M. D. (1986) Promoting health and preventing disease and disability – an introduction to concepts, opportunities and practice. Part II. *Physiotherapy Practice*, **2**(1), 3–10.

Watson M. J. (1988) New dimensions of human caring theory. *Nursing Science Quarterly*, **1**(4), 175–181.

Watson J. and Ray M. A. (eds) (1988) *The Ethics of Care and the Ethics of Cure: synthesis in chronicity*. National League for Nursing, University of Colorado Publication Center for Human Caring.

Webb P. (ed.) (1994a) *Health Promotion and Patient Education: A Professional's Guide*. London: Chapman and Hall.

Webb P. (ed.) (1994b) The sociology of health and illness. In *Health Promotion and Patient Education: A Professional's Guide* (Webb P., ed.). London: Chapman and Hall, 3–20.

Whitebeck C. (1981) A theory of health. In *Concepts of Health and Disease: Interdisciplinary Perspective*. (Caplan A. L., Englehardt H. T., McCartney J. J., eds). Reading, Massachusetts: Addison-Wesley.

Whitehead M. (1989) *Swimming Upstream: Trends and Prospects in Education for Health*. Research Report No. 5, London: King's Fund Institute.

Whitty P., Jones I. (1995) Public health heresy: a challenge to the purchasing orthodoxy. In *Health and Disease: A Reader* (2nd edn) (Davey B., Gray A., Seale C., eds). Buckingham, Philadelphia: Open University Press, 384–387.

Wilkinson, S., Kitzinger C. (eds) (1994) *Women and Health: Feminist Perspectives*. Bristol, London: Taylor and Francis.

Williams B. (1985) Are persons bodies. In *Problems of the Self*. Cambridge: Cambridge University Press.

Williams J. I. (1986) Physiotherapy *is* Handling. *Physiotherapy*, **72**(2), 66–70.

Williams J. I. (1989) Illness behaviour to wellness behaviour: the 'school for bravery' approach. *Physiotherapy*, **75**(1), 2–7.

28 Psychological treatment in physiotherapy practice

Tina Everett

It is a common human experience that minor physical illnesses increase when one is 'run down', perhaps before an overdue holiday or when family relationships are strained. In a similar way pain is increased by fear of its possible causes and outcomes, but reduced by reassurance and empathy. The medical and nursing professions now recognize that any treatment outcome may be influenced by psychological factors (Pearce, 1987). Within the physiotherapy profession increased attention is being paid to psychological processes and their influence on health and illness. Physiotherapists are involved with inter-disciplinary work with groups and individuals, including stress management groups, pain clinics, cardiac rehabilitation and preparation for childbirth, where this influence is of paramount importance.

There has also been an increased focus in psychological treatments in physiotherapy over the last decade, both within the specialist area of mental health (Everett *et al.*, 1995) and within general physiotherapy practice. A recent report by the Chartered Society of Physiotherapy (CSP, 1991) states that, 'the analysis by chartered physiotherapists of their patient's physical problems takes account of the patient's current psychological, cultural and social factors and is based on an assessment of movement and function' it goes on to say 'physiotherapists must be skilled … in the related educational and self-care approaches to prevent, cure or alleviate physical manifestations of somatic and psychological disease'.

The increased attention being paid to psychological processes and their influence on both health and illness in physiotherapy has been driven by several forces including the move towards a holistic approach in medicine and a graduate profession. it is apparent from a recent study, where questionnaires were sent to 26 physiotherapy educational establishments (of which 20 replies were received), that psychology has gained some ground as a subject area in the physiotherapy under-graduate curriculum (Everett, 1995). The study showed that psychology was given between 19 and 40 hours of teaching time and up to 40 hours of private study (with the exception of one establishment with 100 hours of each). Almost all physiotherapy students are assessed in psychology through either compulsory examination questions, continuous assessment, or both. Psychology is generally taught by a psychology lecturer and/or a physiotherapy lecturer who may have a degree in psychology.

The field of mental health and mental disorder is given much less priority and is non-existent in some physiotherapy curricula. Only 11 of those replying to the questionnaire were able to offer students a placement in the mental health field and some of these placements were only optional. It appears, therefore, that at least 50% of physiotherapy graduates will have no experience of working in the mental health field and a significant number will have received no teaching in this area. It is likely, however, that all physiotherapists will treat some patients suffering from major symptoms of anxiety and depression within their first year of practice.

It is my belief that some clinical understanding of mental health and the problems of mental disorder, will increase the student's awareness of the psychological factors influencing the health of their future clients. In this chapter psychological influences, particularly communication and stress, that impinge on all treatments will be discussed, as well as specific treatment approaches relating to pain, chronic fatigue and mental disorder. Case studies will be included in the discussion.

It could be argued that psychological treatment takes place all the time in physiotherapy practice. The paradigm of the 'lived-body' (Thornquist, 1994), emphasizing its basic function as the source of experience, is consistent with how we function in daily life. Yet this is not the paradigm on which western medicine has been based. Thornquist argues that in professional practice health care workers separate mind and body. He states: 'The dualistic perspective permits the body to be treated as an object extrinsic to the self, as a collection of parts and one's attention to be focussed on a single body organ or region only. It allows treating the body deprived of life as a passive impersonal object for professional scrutiny'. In her research, Thornquist found that physiotherapists related well to their patients at first on an interpersonal level but when they started their assessments and treatments the mind/body split occurred. The physiotherapists in her study formed their own impressions of the patient but were unable to link this with their physical findings. This led to a power-based relationship. Some of the important information given by patients was ignored as it did not fit into the therapists' pattern of assumptions. One patient commented after her treatment that the therapist was concerned only with her joints and muscles and did not make connections between her life and her health problems.

Klaber Moffet (1994) states: 'Many attempts have been made to label patients as 'organic' or 'functional' depending on whether or not a physical foundation for the problem can be found. However this dichotomy appears to be neither conceptually valid or of practical value (Rosen et al., 1980; Murray, 1982; Weinman, 1987) and it has been suggested that this distinction should be discarded in favour of an approach which also assesses current emotional stressors and available coping mechanisms'. It is interesting to note that in a recent revision of the International Classification of Diseases of Mental and Behavioural Disorders (WHO, 1992) the term 'psychosomatic' as a category has been omitted because it would imply that 'psychological factors play no role in the occurrence, course and outcome of other diseases not so described'.

Research reported in the psychological literature has demonstrated that the development of pain and the individual's perception of it may be influenced by many different, though often interrelated, psychological variables (Klaber Moffet, 1994). (For further information on the psychology and sociology of pain, the reader is referred to Chapter 10.)

Communication

Communication is one important psychological variable in the therapeutic relationship. In the busy NHS purchaser/provider out-patient department of the nineties it is not easy to pay attention to good communication and the rights of the individual. Yet physiotherapists believe in the whole person approach and recognize the need to question some of their accepted practices. I will now pose some questions to which each individual or individual department must work out its answers. These questions have arisen from my experience of working with patients with mental health problems and adaptations I have had to make to traditional treatment approaches. Perhaps these questions could form the basis of a staff meeting or an in-service training session. Would a student dare to ask these questions on placement?

1. Do you have at least one treatment or consultation room in your department which is private and sound proof or are all patients treated behind curtains?
2. If a patient is late for treatment do you:
   a) see them briefly as soon as you have a moment?
   b) give them another appointment as soon as possible?
   c) put them back on the waiting list? (I have known this to happen when both the cultural differences in the concepts of time and the unreliability of the local bus service were ignored. The woman concerned had acute neck pain).
3. Is it always necessary to ask patients to undress fully before assessment? What is your approach if they are not happy to do this?
4. If a patient misses an appointment and has not let you know do you
   a) send another?
   b) inform the GP?
   c) cross him or her off the list?

The next set of questions come from John Swain's book *The Use of Counselling Skills: A Guide for Therapists* (Swain, 1995). If you wish to take these questions seriously it would be wise to refer to this book and at least to read Chapter 7 and 8.

1. How do you use questions? The most common mistake is to ask closed questions, which can be answered in a word or two, rather than open questions which allow some expression of feeling.
2. Do you leave silences or do you jump in as soon as the client hesitates?
3. Do you ever reflect back to the person the ideas or feelings being communicated to you?
4. Do you help the person talk about what he or she wants to talk about or only what you want to hear?

Responses to stress   It is well recognized that stressful life events correlate with episodes of physical illness and that the social environment can affect health (Goldberg and Huxley, 1992). In order to maintain homeostasis, three independent yet related systems must remain in balance; the central nervous system, the neuroendocrine system and the immune system (Perez, 1988). If the immune system is not functioning well due to increased stress, lymphocytes may fail to recognize changes in cellular identity and thus ignore cancer cells. In the same way, failing to communicate about emotional concerns may lead the individual to deny stress and to internalize emotions which may lead to further stress.

There are two important components to the stress response; the stressors (relationships, work, families, financial problems, poverty, illness) and the stress mediators (social support, financial security and personal characteristics such as high self-esteem). The stress mediators moderate the stress or, if they are lacking, the effect of the stressors increases. It should be noted that many factors, for example relationships, families and work, can serve both as stressors and stress mediators.

Goldberg and Huxley (1992) assert that humans respond to stress with symptoms of anxiety or depression or, more commonly, both sets of symptoms. The evidence from the research points, as one might expect, to an increased vulnerability to stress in those who have suffered some form of parental neglect or a chronic lack of social support. Goldberg and Huxley describe three ways in which individuals try to recover from mental distress; psychological, chemical and neurotic. They maintain that the psychological strategies depend on the availability of social support, confiding relationships and opportunities for a fresh start. The chemical attempts at recovery include alcohol and recreational drugs, self-medication and prescribed psychotropic medication. Neurotic strategies lead to mental illnesses such as phobias and hysterical paralysis which will be discussed later in the chapter.

There is a growing body of evidence that shows that exercise can play an important role in both psychological and chemical restitution (Smeaton, 1995). Mutrie (1988) demonstrates a strong positive correlation between exercise intensity and an anti-depressant effect. She showed in her research that it is exercise itself and not just the participants' expectations or the attention they get which provides the benefit. The recently proposed 'organic unity theory' views the distinction between the mental and physical as a semantic one (Goodman, 1991) and would see no contradiction in exercise being described as a psychological treatment. Recent studies have found non-aerobic exercise to be as an effective anti-depressant as aerobic exercise (Doyne, 1987; Martinsen et al., 1989). In his chapter on exercise and mental health where he looks at these studies, Smeaton (1995) concludes: 'As the effects of exercise on depression are comparable with those of psychological therapy and given the undesirable side-effects of anti-depressant medication and ECT, the emergence of exercise, cheap and relatively side-effect free as a potential treatment for depression is an exciting prospect'.

Exercise as a psychological treatment can take many forms and individual preferences, as well as local availability, will influence choice.

Physiotherapy departments are often able to provide a multi-gym and circuit training facilities both in the mental health and cardiac rehabilitation settings. Tai chi, yoga and dance movement therapy all provide a gentle form of exercise where individuals develop an awareness of themselves and their relationships to the people and world around them. Exercise assists relaxation and may improve both posture and self-esteem. One of the pioneers of movement therapy in the USA puts it like this:

> 'If psychoanalysis brings about a change in mental attitude, there should be a corresponding physical change. If dance therapy brings about a change in the body's behaviour, there should be a corresponding change in the mind. Both methods aim to change the total human, mind and body'. (Schoop, 1974).

This chapter will now focus on the three areas where psychological treatment approaches are essential: pain, chronic fatigue and mental disorder. Treatment will be discussed and illustrated with case studies. The importance of touch and the psychotherapeutic concept of holding will be examined.

Pain

Physiotherapists are rightly concerned with their patients' posture and know that a change in posture can lead to pain relief and a reduction in future mechanical problems. How often, however, do we stop and consider the psychological effect of criticism? When in pain how does it feel to be told 'all you need to do is to stand up straight'? Would it not be better to ask the person how he or she is feeling or what changes he or she would like to make? As Skelly (1995) points out 'self-esteem is largely bound up with how we feel about ourselves, whether we feel clumsy, ugly, ungainly, unapproachable, etc., whether we feel fit and physically capable, at home being a body, or whether we feel that we "have" a body which is somehow not "us", which is both alien and a kind of trap'.

One only has to look at the work of the Alexander Technique practitioners to know that posture correction is not just a matter of pointing out the faults. It is a sharing of oneself with the client and working on one's own body energy and release of tension thereby enabling the client to do likewise.

Lessons using the Alexander technique consist of two parts:

1. Helping the pupil detect and let go of excessive tension that has been held unconsciously in the body.
2. Helping the pupil find different ways of moving that are easier and more efficient, thus reducing 'wear and tear' on body structures and internal organs (Brennan, 1991).

According to many researchers (Turk, *et al.*, 1993; Reesor, 1988) problems of life and an individual's interpretation of them are all important in chronic pain and relevant to the development, perception and maintenance of pain.

In her research into chronic back pain, Klaber (1986) found that 'in the early stages (of low back pain) of diagnosis and assessment, anxiety levels can be greatly reduced by clear simple explanation to the patient of the problem as far as this is possible. In the chronic stages (6 months to a year) anxiety cannot now be reduced by reassurance alone. The patient has to be taught methods by which he or she feels able to control the pain his or herself. This may be achieved by a number of different approaches or a combination of them including cognitive-behavioural therapy (Beck, 1976; Hawton, 1989), biofeedback (Birk, 1980) and relaxation training (Mitchell, 1977) as well as progressive exercise programmes. One the anxiety levels are reduced the patient generally feels more able to cope with the pain although the pain reported may not have altered greatly in intensity.

It is believed that some people are more prone to develop recurrent back pain and other psychosomatic disorders due to parenting deficiencies in their early development (Crown, 1980). Early childhood socialisation and learning determines how an individual in adult life perceives painful stimuli and responds to physical symptoms (Fordyce, 1976; Pennebaker, 1982; Craig, 1986). The physiotherapist working with these clients needs to have some knowledge of the psychodynamic counselling (Jacobs, 1995) and cognitive-behavioural approaches to pain management (Beck, 1976), but more especially to work closely with other members of the inter-disciplinary team (e.g. psychologist, psychotherapist, community psychiatric nurse, etc.). An inter-disciplinary approach appears to be the most effective method of treating patients with chronic intractable low back pain. The case study used to illustrate the treatment of chronic pain is found in the section on mental disorder as it relates more specifically to that area. (For further information on the psychology and sociology of pain, the reader is referred to Chapter 10.).

Chronic fatigue

Clear objectives of helping the individual gain control over his or her pain seems to be key to the relative success of teatment of chronic pain. The same appears to be true for the treatment of chronic fatigue (ME) sufferers. An incomplete study in Leeds (Pemberton et al., 1994) is expected to show that significant life style changes occur when the focus is on coping rather than on the cause, and when psychological approaches, such as stress management, are combined with treatment where graded activity is used.

Case study

Carol, a dental receptionist, suffered chronic fatigue for 4 years following an influenza virus. She was able to work part-time but was unable to have any social life. She felt under-valued and exploited in her job. At home her teenage children made the tea every day and her husband did the shopping and house work while Carol lay exhausted on the settee. Carol joined a group for chronic fatigue patients, run by a physiotherapist and a specialist nurse trained in cognitive therapy. For the first time Carol met people with similar problems. She found it a relief to talk about her symptoms. The aims of the chronic fatigue group were:

1. To enable members to benefit from shared experience.
2. To promote an understanding of the causes of muscle fatigue and the importance of graded activity.

3. To help members consider and develop desired life style changes.
4. To increase skills in relaxation and assertiveness.

Over the weeks the group discussed coping strategies to improve sleep and the quality of rest, and the gradual increase of activity (Hatcher, 1993). They worked on assertiveness skills (Holland and Ward, 1990) and practised relaxation (Mitchell, 1977; Everett, 1990). By the end of the ten sessions Carol had changed her job – still a part-time receptionist but with people who respected rather than exploited her. She had bought herself a bicycle and was cycling slowly on non-work days for 30–40 minutes, enjoying the fresh air and discovering countryside of which she was previously unaware.

Mental disorder

The psychological and chemical forms of restitution from mental disorder are the most common. The neurotic response is generally a maladaptive response to relieve anxiety and reduce responsibility, often totally interfering with the person's life as in phobic avoidance, somatic pains and hysterical paralysis. Phobias are usually the easiest to treat and are generally seen by clinical psychologists. The physiotherapist is more likely to meet the person with somatic pains and dysfunction or with the less common hysterical paralysis. A team approach is essential and there are no easy solutions. The patient must be an informed member of the team and be aware that playing one member against another is not acceptable. The therapist should be aware of the patient who says 'you are the only one who can help me, none of the others can'. This is not to deny the importance of individual therapeutic relationships, or that people relate more easily to some individuals than others, but rather to guard against the splitting of the team. Patients who see total perfection in their therapists usually have a very poor self-image and see themselves as bad and worthless. They do not necessarily admit to this but it can be apparent in their behaviour. People who consistently somatise their distress and permanently occupy the sick role have probably suppressed their lack of self-worth into the subconscious. The pain and disability is very real and not something people can 'snap out of' or come to terms with easily.

Case study

June was referred to the psychiatric hospital for physiotherapy for her persistent back pain. She arrived in a lie-back wheelchair carrying elbow crutches. She was wearing a soft collar and wrist splints and using a TENS machine. Her case notes revealed a long history of back pain, repeated hospital referrals (many of which were due to drug overdoses) and many investigations. The diagnosis was Munchausen's syndrome (chronic factitious illness). The family history was one of a disturbed and disrupted childhood with possible abuse causing her many problems in adolescence. Further abuse followed in her first marriage as she struggled to bring up her two children. Her second marriage is much more successful. Her husband supports her financially and socially but often encourages her belief that she has a chronic disabling illness. Two years prior to this referral June had been working as a part-time cashier in a supermarket – she had given up the job because of back pain. In planning a treatment programme it was important to help June give up her chronic illness behaviour while attending to her very real pain and distress. At times there were clinical signs of sciatica but repeated assessments showed marked changes in symptoms and no evidence of relevant organic disease. The aims and goals of treatment were:

1. To take the pain seriously but to help June acknowledge that no further tests or procedures were going to take place.
2. To attempt to ration drug analgesia.
3. To increase muscle strength, flexibility and stamina as an important part of her general rehabilitation.
4. To increase social activity outside hospital.

Regular case reviews were held with June and her husband which included the physiotherapist, occupational therapist, consultant and GP. As frequent visits were made to the Accident and Emergency department (including repeated overdoses of paracetamol) the consultant devised a care plan with June's consent which was attached to her notes. June attended the physiotherapy multi-gym for general exercise three times a week and gradually built up her exercise tolerance. She also started swimming classes for disabled people and became quite competitive with other swimmers and with herself. She enjoyed socialising at the hospital and with the ambulance personnel. It took over 2 years for June to decrease her attendance at the hospital and to build a social life with her husband away from health care provision. At present her only contact with the hospital is a 3 monthly review in accordance with the care programme approach which operates at the hospital.

Holding

Holding is an important psychological treatment and one the physiotherapist, in some circumstances, is able to provide. The psychotherapist is able to 'hold' a patient in his or her mind to help the patient re-experience being held as a baby when the context prohibits physical contact (Winnicott, 1960). It is possible that some patients cannot experience being held in the mind without the physical containment (Richer and Zapella, 1989). In the case study below the physical containment is provided in the guise of physiotherapy which was also essential for physiological reasons. Regular meetings of the care team enabled changes in physiotherapy (mainly requested by the patient herself) to be seen in terms of her need to be held (in a way acceptable to a very independent teenager) and her need to face the fear of falling (Winnicott, 1957). It is essential that the patient is seen by the same physiotherapist each time, and that the team works together with support from a psychotherapist.

Case study

Rachel is a bright, intelligent 15-year-old girl, fiercely argumentative but easy to engage in conversation. She lost the use of her legs 1 year prior to her first psychiatric admission. At first the paralysis was temporary, a few minutes at a time, but within a few months it became more permanent requiring the use of a wheelchair.

Initially Rachel's legs were flaccid and physiotherapy involved passive movements, trunk exercises and transfers between wheelchair and floor – a manoeuvre she managed with remarkable ease. Physical investigations proved negative but the symptoms did not change and were not within conscious control. Rachel's first visit to the hospital was interrupted by the death of her mother for whom she seemed unable to mourn.

At the start of the next term she returned to boarding school in her wheelchair. Within 2 months her legs and trunk became rigid, necessitating a 'lie-back' wheelchair with leg extensions and her return to hospital. She then started psychotherapy twice a week and daily physiotherapy. Her school work continued with the hospital teachers but her motivation and concentration were impaired. She was now able to stand in a large padded walking frame and to take some steps with gentle assistance to her legs. During sleep her legs moved freely. When Rachel was informed of this she said it was 'no big deal' as her legs often moved of their own accord but would never do what she wanted them to do. She had gradually become doubly incontinent and had no sensation in her legs. Horse riding was started weekly and through this Rachel was gradually able to sit up and to bend her knees. Eventually she was able to return to a standard wheelchair but only with her legs tied to the footrests – otherwise they would spring forward into extension.

At the same time as making enormous progress in her psychotherapy Rachel lost the use of and sensation in her left arm. She was beginning to admit cautiously to staff that she felt some sadness at the loss of her mother. Her father visited regularly but communication was limited.

One goal of physiotherapy treatment was to ensure that function and mobility were not impeded when conscious control of her limbs returned. Therefore the aims of treatment were:

1. To maintain full range of movement in all joints.
2. To maintain or improve muscle strength.
3. To increase independence in all activities of daily living.
4. To maintain or improve proprioception and balance.

Another goal was to allow Rachel to experience both a physical holding (as a baby is held by its mother) and a letting go as experienced in her request to fall onto a soft surface.

Physiotherapy now involved holding Rachel from behind with hands on the front of her hips, sometimes just to balance her, sometimes with an assistant gently moving her legs to walk forwards. Progress was being made, some active steps had been taken but there was still a long way to go. One treatment a week now takes place in a playroom with a foam mattress flooring where Rachel is able to experience falling and rolling.

Rachel now attends as an out-patient for physiotherapy and psychotherapy. Good liaison with her boarding school is a priority.

Touch

The growing demand from the public for complimentary therapy may indicate a psychological need for therapeutic touch. Krieger (1975) states that 'touch is a transference of energies from one person to another – an act of healing or helping that is akin to the ancient practice of laying on of hands'. Christine Jones (1995), writing about reflex therapy, states that the 'general overall effect may have far reaching implications in alleviating emotional and mental imbalances and may assist patients with anxiety, panic attacks, hyperventilation, phobias and fears and many other imbalances and disorders of the mind. Treatment may provide deeper relaxation or the release of some stored emotion held within the linked tissues or in the conscious or sub-conscious mind'. (Linked tissues refer to tissues linked to a site of past trauma). This unconscious release may be manifested in tears, in sleep or in a feeling of greater connectedness of mind and body – a feeling that the body is part of oneself rather than an uncomfortable appendage. Preston (1973) stated that 'some elderly people's need for touch may supersede their need to talk', and that 'touching confused and demented patients may be more useful than verbal communications'. It has been found that some people in psychiatric care will behave in such a way as to necessitate some form of restraint as it is their only opportunity for physical contact. These clients may benefit from therapeutic massage provided it is part of an agreed care plan. The individual differences in the need for and the acceptance of touch must be recognized.

Case study

Susan is a mother of three in her early thirties who developed anorexia nervosa soon after the birth of her first child. During her first long hospital admission she had, for many months, shrunk from physical contact with staff. In time Susan built up a trusting relationship with her key worker and was gradually able to accept and enjoy hand massage, later she enjoyed foot massage and eventually massage to the back and face. During her second hospital admission Susan felt very tense and anxious and was referred for physiotherapy treatment. The aims of treatment were:

1. To relieve tension and assist relaxation.
2. To improve her self-esteem.
3. To help her to be kind to her body rather than to punish it.

Susan was unable to benefit from a relaxation group, or from individual relaxation using standard techniques. Time was spent developing a trusting therapeutic relationship and eventually Susan began to enjoy gentle exercise and hydrotherapy. As she progressed in her psychotherapy she found that massage prior to lunch enabled her to relax sufficiently to eat a cooked meal. Susan was also able to encourage other anorexic patients to try some gentle hand massage.

Conclusion

This chapter has illustrated the importance of physiotherapists meeting people 'where they are', that is focusing on the 'whole person'. This is not only important in the treatment of patients suffering mental distress but in all areas of physiotherapy practice. From the case studies it has been shown that patients with long-term, adverse illness behaviour or functional paralysis need long-term goals and consistency in treatment delivered by an inter-disciplinary team. The stress involved in this work should not be under-estimated; skilled support and supervision must always be available to physiotherapists working in the mental health field.

References

Birk L. (1980) *Biofeedback: Behavioural Medicine*. New York: Grune and Stratton.
Beck A. T. (1976) *Cognitive Therapy and the Emotional Disorders*. New York: International Universities Press.
Brennan R. (1991) *The Alexander Technique*. Shaftsbury: Element Books.
Crown S. (1980) Psychosocial factors in low back pain. *Clinics Rheumatic Diseases*, 6(1), 77–92.
Craig K. (1985) Social modelling influences: pain in context. In *Psychology of Pain* (2nd edn) (Skernbach R., ed.). New York: Raven Press.
Chartered Society of Physiotherapy (1991) *Curriculum of Study*. London.
Doyne E. J., Chambliss D. L., Beutler L. E. (1993) Aerobic exercise as a treatment for depression in women. *Behaviour Therapy*, 14, 434–440.
Everett T., Dennis M., Ricketts E. (1995) *Physiotherapy in Mental Health*. Oxford: Butterworth-Heinemann.
Everett T. (1990) *Relax and Release, Speak Easy Audio Cassettes*. Sounds Good Ltd. Available from Winslow Bicester.
Fordyce W. (1976) *Behavioural Methods for Chronic Pain and Illness*. St. Louis: C. V. Mosby.
Goldberg D., Huxley P. (1992) *Common Mental Disorders: A Bio-social Model*. London: Routledge.
Goodman A. (1991) Organic unity theory: the mind body problem revisited. *American Journal of Psychiatry*, 148(5), 553–563.
Hatcher S. (1993) Unpublished series of booklets from the Leeds Fatigue Clinic at Seacroft Hospital.
Holland S., Ward C. (1990) *Assertiveness: A Practical Approach*. Bicester: Winslow Press.
Jacobs M. (1985) *The Presenting Past – An Introduction to Practical Psychodynamic Counselling*. Oxford: Oxford University Press.
Jones C. (1995) *Physiotherapy in Mental Health*. (Everett T., Dennis M. and Ricketts E., eds). Oxford: Butterworth-Heinemann.
Klaber J. (1983) Chronic back pain: a study of pain response and its correlation with psychological variables. *M.Sc. Dissertation*. Birmingham: University of Aston.
Klaber Moffet J. A. (1994) The Role of psychological variables in the assessment and physiotherapeutic management of musculoskeletal disorders. *PhD thesis*. London: University of London.
Klaber Moffet J. A., Richardson P. H. (1995) The influence of psychological variables on the development and perception of musculoskeletal pain. *Physiotherapy Theory and Practice*, 11, 3–11.
Kreiger D. (1975) Therapeutic touch, the imprimaturs of nursing. Searching for evidence of psychological change. *American Journal of Nursing*, 75(5) 784–787.
Martinsen E. W., Hoffart A., Solberg O. (1989) Comparing aerobic and non-aerobic exercise in the treatment of clinical depression: a randomised trial. *Comprehensive Psychiatry*, 30(4), 324–331.
Mitchell L. (1977) *Simple Relaxation*. London: John Murray.
Murray J. (1982) Psychological aspects of low back pain. *Psychological Reports*, 50, 50.
Mutrie N. (1989) Exercise as a treatment for moderate depression in the UK Health Service. In *Sport, Health, Psychology and Exercise Symposium*. London: Sports Council.
Pearce S., Richardson P. (1987) *Chronic Pain: Investigations. A Handbook of Clinical Adult Psychology* (Lindsay S., Powell G., eds). Aldershot: Gower.
Pemberton S., Hatcher S., House A., Stanley P. (1994) Chronic fatigue syndrome: a way forward. *British Journal of Occupational Therapists*, 57(10), 381–383.

Pennebaker J. (1982) *The Psychology of Physical Symptoms*. New York: Springer-Verlag.

Perez M., Farrant J. (1989) Immune reactions and mental disorders. *Psychological Medicine*, **18**, 11–13.

Preston T. (1973) When words fail. *Ann J Nurs*, **73**(12), 2064–2066.

Reesor K., Craig K. (1989) Medically incongruent chronic back pain. physical limitations, suffering, and ineffective coping. *Pain*, **32**, 35–45.

Richer J. M., Zapella M. (1989) Changing autistic children's social behaviour – the place of holding communication. *Communication*, **23**, 35–41.

Rosen J., Frymoyer J., Clements J. (1980) A further look at the validity of the MMPI of low back patients. *Journal of Clinical Psychology*, **36**(4), 994–1001.

Schoop T. (1974) *Won't you Join the Dance? A Dancer's Essay into Treatment of Psychosis*. California: Mayfield Publishing.

Skelly M. (1995) Community care and working with carers. In *Physiotherapy in Mental Health* (Everett E. D., *et al.*, eds). Oxford: Butterworth-Heinemann.

Smeaton J. (1995) Exercise and mental health. In *Physiotherapy in Mental Health* (Everett E. D. *et al.*, eds). Oxford: Butterworth-Heinemann.

Swain J. (1985) *The Use of Counselling skills – A Guide for Therapists*. Oxford: Butterworth-Heinemann.

Thornquist E. (1994) Profession and life separate worlds. *Social Science and Medicine*, **39**(5), 701–713.

Turk D. C., Meichenbaum D. H., Genest M. (1983) *Pain and Behavioural Medicine – A Cognitive-Behavioural Perspective*. New York: Guildford Press.

Weinman J. (1987) *An Outline of Psychology as Applied to Medicine* (2nd edn). Bristol: Wright.

Winnicott D. W. (1960) The contribution of direct child observation to psychoanalysis. Cited in *Maturational Processes and the Facilitating Environment* (1982). London: The Hogarth Press.

Winnicott D. W. (1960) The theory of the parent/infant relationship. Cited in *Maturational Processes and the Facilitating Environment* (1982). London: The Hogarth Press.

World Health Organization (1992) *ICD-10 – Classification of Mental and Behavioural Disorders. Clinical Descriptions and Diagnostic Guidelines*. Geneva: World Health Organization.

Index